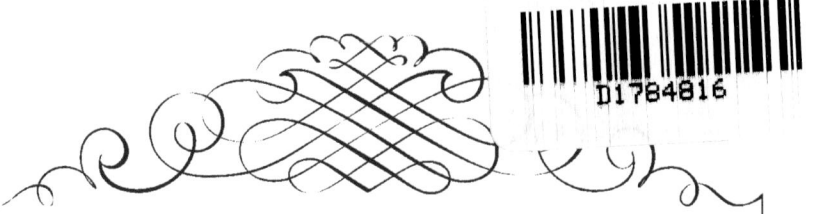

1,000,000 Books

are available to read at

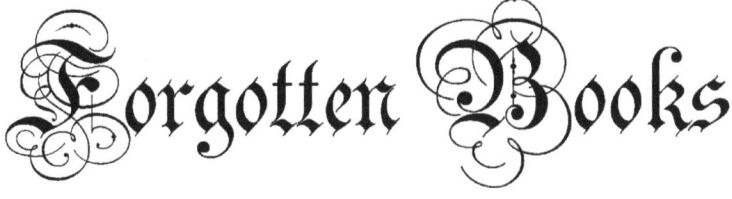

www.ForgottenBooks.com

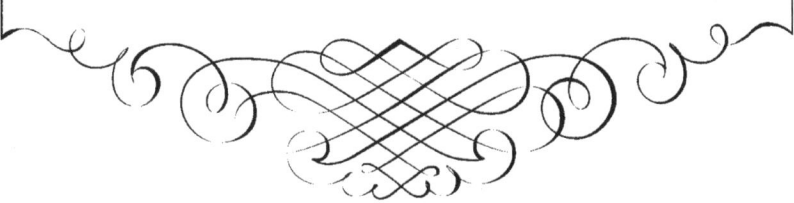

Read online
Download PDF
Purchase in print

ISBN 978-1-5280-0239-4
PIBN 10156917

This book is a reproduction of an important historical work. Forgotten Books uses
state-of-the-art technology to digitally reconstruct the work, preserving the original format
whilst repairing imperfections present in the aged copy. In rare cases, an imperfection in
the original, such as a blemish or missing page, may be replicated in our edition. We do,
however, repair the vast majority of imperfections successfully; any imperfections that
remain are intentionally left to preserve the state of such historical works.

Forgotten Books is a registered trademark of FB &c Ltd.
Copyright © 2018 FB &c Ltd.
FB &c Ltd, Dalton House, 60 Windsor Avenue, London, SW19 2RR.
Company number 08720141. Registered in England and Wales.

For support please visit www.forgottenbooks.com

1 MONTH OF FREE READING

at

www.ForgottenBooks.com

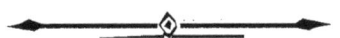

By purchasing this book you are eligible for one month membership to ForgottenBooks.com, giving you unlimited access to our entire collection of over 1,000,000 titles via our web site and mobile apps.

To claim your free month visit: www.forgottenbooks.com/free156917

* Offer is valid for 45 days from date of purchase. Terms and conditions apply.

English
Français
Deutsche
Italiano
Español
Português

www.forgottenbooks.com

Mythology Photography **Fiction**
Fishing Christianity **Art** Cooking
Essays Buddhism Freemasonry
Medicine **Biology** Music **Ancient**
Egypt Evolution Carpentry Physics
Dance Geology **Mathematics** Fitness
Shakespeare **Folklore** Yoga Marketing
Confidence Immortality Biographies
Poetry **Psychology** Witchcraft
Electronics Chemistry History **Law**
Accounting **Philosophy** Anthropology
Alchemy Drama Quantum Mechanics
Atheism Sexual Health **Ancient History**
Entrepreneurship Languages Sport
Paleontology Needlework Islam
Metaphysics Investment Archaeology
Parenting Statistics Criminology
Motivational

897 MARLBOROUGH ST.
BOSTON, MA 5.

INJURIES AND DISEASES

OF THE

ENITAL AND URINARY ORGAN

BY

HENRY MORRIS

M.A., M.B. LOND., F.R.C.S.

SURGEON TO, AND LECTURER ON SURGERY AT, THE MIDDLESEX HOSPITAL;
MEMBER OF THE COUNCIL AND OF THE COURT OF EXAMINERS OF
THE ROYAL COLLEGE OF SURGEONS, ENGLAND;
EXAMINER IN SURGERY IN THE UNIVERSITY OF LONDON

WITH NINETY-SEVEN ILLUSTRATIONS

NEW YORK

WILLIAM WOOD & COMPANY

1895

17 A 90

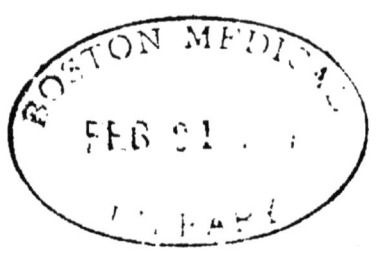
BOSTON MEDICAL
FEB 21
LIBRARY

PREFACE.

THE MS. of this work was completed in September, 1894, and was then put aside during the busy months of the winter session. It has since been carefully revised, and somewhat added to, with the wish that it might be fairly representative of surgical opinion and practice at the moment of its publication. It is in a way a continuation of my book on the "Surgical Diseases of the Kidney," a second edition of which is now in course of preparation for the Press.

For many years it has been my intention to publish a treatise on the Surgery of the Genital and Lower Urinary Organs. In 1885 I undertook a series of articles on these subjects, but the pressure of other work made it difficult for me to write them in the allotted time, and I was graciously allowed to withdraw from my engagement. It is only too probable that my intention would still have remained unrealised, had I not made a promise to contribute the articles on these subjects to the "System of Surgery" edited by Mr. Frederick Treves. This promise has influenced me not only to write this book without further procrastination, but to write it on the lines adopted in that work.

To the practising surgeon who has also to lecture, two methods suggest themselves. He can either adopt the method of the clinical lecturer, who takes a case as his text and builds his teaching upon and around it. Or he can adopt the form of the lectures given in a systematic course; and, whilst making only occasional reference to individual cases, describe in a methodical manner all that is requisite to be known about his subject, basing his teaching not on his own experience only, but also on that of others.

The former plan is perhaps the more attractive, and it certainly is the less laborious to the author; but I have chosen the latter because it is the method adopted in the "Surgical Diseases of the Kidney," and also because it is the one most likely to be useful to the busy practitioner who has but little time to read, as well as to the student who, it is to be feared, has more to read than he has time to read it in.

I have endeavoured to make my descriptions as clear and complete, but, at the same time, as brief as possible; and with this object I have, in reference to "operative treatment," generally confined myself to "principles," referring my readers to works on operative surgery for details as to the technique of the various operations.

I may be criticised for omitting to give a separate chapter on "Urinary Fever" in a work which includes the affections of the urethra. But the phenomena of urinary fever I consider to be more closely connected with the affections of the kidney than with those of the lower urinary organs.

In every variety of this fever we know there is always a morbid condition of the kidneys: either a simple temporary congestion of healthy organs, or an acute inflammation of those which are the seat of chronic organic disease. These renal changes are reflex effects, and are generally caused by some urethral nerve disturbance. We have no proof that any urethral lesion by itself, or that the poisonous effects of absorbed urine can cause it; whilst the rapidly transient character of the acute paroxysmal attacks tends to disprove, at any rate so far as this group of cases is concerned, the theory that the fever is due to microbic infection of the blood from the urine. In describing the treatment of urethral affections I have repeatedly mentioned the precautions which should be taken against urinary fever, and this is all I have thought it necessary to do in this work, as I have very fully described all forms of the fever in the "Surgical Diseases of the Kidney."

In compiling the several parts of the present treatise I have drawn largely upon the notes of cases in my own practice, extending now over a period of twenty-five years; and I have not hesitated to state my own conclusions, and to give my own preferences as to treatment, even though they do not in every respect coincide with the generally accepted teaching.

I have, however, in all instances also given the views of acknowledged authorities, and have made very free use of the writings of well-known authors. I am especially indebted to the works of Curling and Jacobson; of Sir Henry Thompson and Guyon; of Reginald Harrison and the contributors to the admirable "Traité de Chirurgie," edited by Simon Duplay and Paul Reclus; as well as to many others whose names are quoted in the text.

Many of the illustrations have been specially executed for this work; others were done under my direction several years ago from specimens in the Middlesex Hospital Museum, and were used subsequently by Mr. Mansell Moullin for his article in the "Manual of Surgery," edited by Mr. Treves, and published by Messrs. Cassell and C^{o}. Others are from works published by the firm just named, and by Messrs. J. & A. Churchill, or have been copied from French or German works; but in all cases their source has been, I hope, duly acknowledged.

To my friends Mr. Frank Steele and Mr. Arnold Lawson I am indebted for their care in reading the proof-sheets, and to my colleague Dr. Wynter for help in the matter of references.

To the Publishers, to Mr. Berjeau the artist, and to Mr. Butterworth the engraver, I desire to express my sincere thanks for their courteous assistance and advice, and for the able way in which they have done their respective parts in this work.

HENRY MORRIS.

8, *Cavendish Square, London,*
   September, 1895.

CONTENTS.

Part I.

GENITAL ORGANS.

Part II.

GENITO-URINARY ORGANS.

Part III.

URINARY BLADDER.

LIST OF ILLUSTRATIONS.

Injuries and Diseases

OF THE

Genital and Urinary Organs.

Part I.

GENITAL ORGANS.

CHAPTER I.

INJURIES AND DISEASES OF THE SCROTUM.

INJURIES OF THE SCROTUM.

WOUNDS of the scrotum may be incised, contused, lacerated, punctured, or gunshot; they may extend through the tunica vaginalis, and may be followed by the protrusion of the testicle.

Contusions of the Scrotum are often followed by the escape of a very large amount of blood into the loose connective tissue beneath the skin and dartos. In this way a considerable purple-coloured swelling (scrotal hæmatocele or hæmatoma) is formed, which from its uniform outline may be mistaken for a hæmatocele of the tunica vaginalis (ordinary vaginal hæmatocele). Indeed, the one may be produced by the same violence which causes the other: and in some instances the vaginal hæmatocele communicates through a rent in the tunica vaginalis with the scrotal hæmatoma.

In some cases of scrotal hæmatoma there is only a trifling discoloration of the skin at the bottom of the scrotum. In other cases the extravasation and discoloration extend very wide of the scrotum, reaching up along the abdomen and down the thighs. Sloughing or abscess of the scrotum is apt to follow contusions.

Scrotal hæmatocele may occur as the result of tapping for hydrocele, as in the following case :—A gentleman aged sixty-seven had had double hydrocele for many years. The right

B

had been radically cured, the left had frequently been tapped at intervals of several months.   In April, 1894, it was tapped

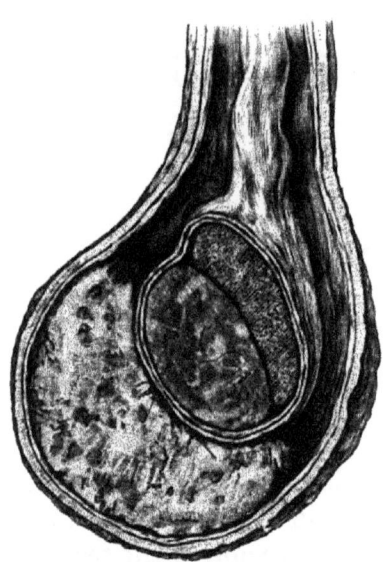

Fig. 1.—Hæmatoma in Scrotal Space.
(*After Paul Reclus.*)

as usual, and without, at the time, any appearance of injury to any vessel; but within half an hour afterwards the patient felt his scrotum "refilling" and blood trickling down his leg, but no pain.   In two hours the left side of his scrotum was so large he could not sit down.   The swelling increased, and bleeding from the puncture continued till the next morning.   By the middle of the day after the tapping, the groins, hypogastrium, and the front and sides of the upper half of both thighs were darkly ecchy-mosed.   In a few days the blood began to be absorbed, and at the end of three weeks the case presented the appearance of an ordinary hæmatocele, and was painful, tender, and cômmencing to be inflamed.   The testicle was not made out.   In front and near the raphe of the scrotum was a soft fluctuating prominence, red and not specially tender.   An incision was made over the front and outer part of the swelling, the contents were turned out, and then a definite false membrane was seen limiting the space everywhere but on the inner side where the untorn sac of the

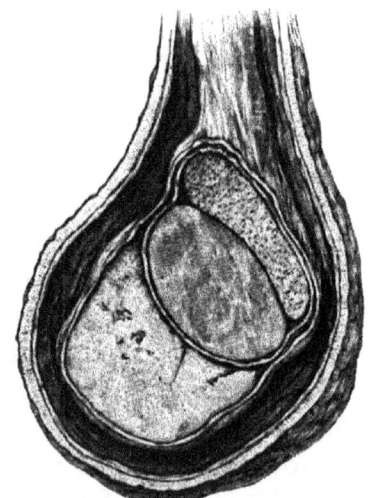

Fig. 2.—Intravaginal Hæmatocele.
(*After Paul Reclus.*)

tunica vaginalis was situated.   The vaginal sac contained two or three ounces of straw-coloured fluid, and had formed the fluctuating prominence above mentioned. The testicle was of normal size and appearance, having a small fibrous pedunculated body attached at its upper part close to the globus major. In detaching the false membrane the scrotal tissues, which were soft and rotten, tore easily; and as in places they were inflamed and threatening to slough, I performed castration, and at the same time removed a considerable part of the left side of the scrotum. Iodoform was sprinkled over the raw surfaces, and the cut edges of the skin were united by sutures. During the first six hours after the operation a large quantity of blood-stained serum escaped. The patient rapidly recovered.

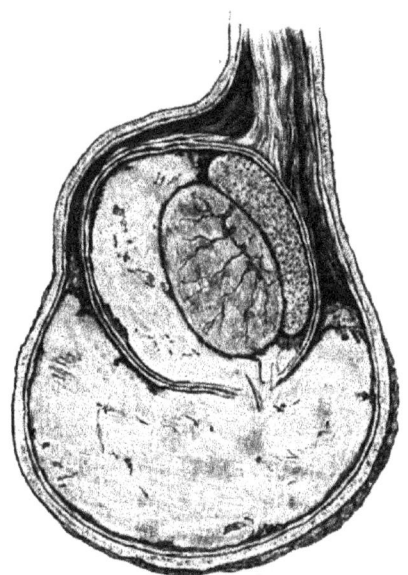

The *treatment* of wounds, contusions, sloughing, and abscess of the scrotum is the same as that required for the corresponding conditions in other parts of the body. Incised and lacerated wounds heal very rapidly, the contraction of the dartos tissue favouring the apposition of

Fig. 3.—Intravaginal Hæmatocele communicating with Scrotal Hæmatoma. (*After Paul Reclus.*)

the divided edges. Sutures, however, are advantageous, though primary union is often obtained without them.

GENERAL DISEASES OF THE SCROTUM.

Prurigo and Eczema of the Scrotum arise in children from the dribbling of urine due to phymosis, stone in the bladder, atony, and incontinence from other causes. Eczema occurs also in adults from the constant wetting with urine in some cases of stricture and enlarged prostate; and it is frequently caused by diabetes and disturbances of the digestive organs. These affections are apt to spread to the thighs, perinæum, and hypogastrium. They are attended with much itching, and, as a result of scratching, they are often associated with excoriations and cracks, and the skin becomes thickened and hypertrophied, and discharges a fluid having a very unpleasant odour derived largely from the perverted secretion of the sebaceous glands.

The *treatment* must be directed to the cause. The itching, which is often almost unbearable and paroxysmal, will be much relieved by frequent washings with weak eau-de-cologne water, the application of boracic powder, or linen wrung out of boracic, or lead lotion made up with elder-flower water.

Parasites.—The pediculi pubis often invade the scrotum. They are to be seen by the naked eye, and their eggs are found as minute whitish masses on the hairs of the part. A solution of corrosive sublimate (2 grs. to ℨj of water) or mercurial ointment are effective remedies for these loathsome lice.

Varicose veins.—The veins of the scrotum sometimes become greatly enlarged, especially in persons whose dartos tissue has been weakened by age, debility, hernia, varicocele, or hydrocele. Cold bathing and a suspensory bandage are the remedies.

Emphysema of the scrotum is present in gangrene of the scrotum when putrefactive changes occur in the dead and dying tissues. Simple emphysema has been sometimes produced by malingerers and showmen artificially. This condition can be easily and painlessly produced by inserting the point of a small tube or syringe through a small hole in the skin and blowing in air. The air is very readily absorbed, and the parts restored to their normal size.

Œdema of the Scrotum occurs either as a primary affection, or as secondary to disease of some other organ, such as the heart, kidneys, or liver—in cardiac, renal, or hepatic dropsy. It occurs too as a secondary condition in epididymo-orchitis and from obstruction to the circulation by inguinal and pelvic swellings and tumours. Kocher refers to peritonitis, inflammation of the seminal vesicles and ejaculatory ducts, and of the cellular tissue around the base of the bladder as causing secondary œdema of the scrotum. Primary œdema is seen in erythema and erysipelas, in cases where there is any local irritation, and in cases of inflammation from injury or the bites of insects. The primary cases are always inflammatory.

The *symptoms* are a uniform and general swelling of the

scrotum of a doughy, inelastic consistence, and of a pale and often shiny and glossy or translucent appearance, pitting readily and deeply on pressure; or, in other cases, the scrotum may have a reddish opaque appearance, and a tough and brawny feeling. The swelling commences at the lowest part of the scrotum, and increases in an upward direction until at length it involves the penis; and the prepuce, especially, may become enormously enlarged and distorted. All the rugæ and the raphe of the scrotum are obliterated as a rule; but, in rare instances, the swelling has been limited to one-half the scrotum. On one occasion Pott punctured a localised œdema and let out two ounces of limpid serum, under the impression he had to deal with a hydrocele, but subsequently convinced himself that it was an anasarca of the scrotum on one side only, having much of the fluid in one distended space and the rest diffused through the cellular tissue in the usual manner.

Œdema of the scrotum is distinguished from inflammation by the absence of tenderness and of constitutional symptoms, although when the œdema results from epididymo-orchitis, there are the tenderness and feverishness of the inflamed testicle.

The *treatment* consists in remedying the disease or condition on which the œdema depends, if possible. When the cause is removed the effusion rapidly vanishes by rest or elevation of the scrotum. Southey's tubes, or a few minute punctures with a tenotomy knife, will allow of the fluid draining away. It is seldom necessary or desirable to make large incisions.

Inflammation of the Scrotum is always the cause of primary œdema. It is generally erysipelatous in character, occurs in the intemperate and debilitated, and is usually excited by the irritation due to dribbling of urine, or from some puncture, abrasion, eruption, boil, or sore on the surface of the scrotum. Inflammation of the scrotum may be started by an acute phymosis due to gonorrhœa, or to chancre. The skin becomes dusky red, œdematous, and shining, the swelling and redness spread to the penis and to the inner sides of the thighs, and these local symptoms are accompanied by thirst, shivering, high temperature, foul tongue, constipation, and the other signs of fever. Liston, who published several such cases, named the condition "acute anasarca of the scrotum," because of the rapid and excessive transudation of serum into the loose and abundant connective tissue.

The inflammation usually terminates by resolution, but suppuration is not uncommon. Occasionally, owing to the rapidity and excess of the exudation, extensive sloughing of the subcutaneous tissue occurs, leaving the testicles more or less exposed, and sometimes even gangrenous. Agnew states that he has twice seen almost the entire scrotum destroyed, and retention of urine and general typhoid symptoms caused, by rapid and intense exudation.

Extravasation of urine into the scrotum rapidly excites inflammation and sloughing; it will be diagnosed by the previous history of stricture or injury, the commencement of the swelling in the perinæum, and very probably by the difficulty in introducing a catheter into the bladder, and the discharge of blood from the urethra.

The *treatment* is, as a rule, simple and successful, and consists in keeping the patient in bed, elevating the scrotum, applying some warm, soothing lotion, such as Goulard water; and administering, at first, a brisk purge, and subsequently an effervescing saline mixture. Under this treatment the symptoms usually subside in three or four days, and the patient is quite recovered by the eighth or tenth day.

When, however, the symptoms do not yield, and suppuration is threatened, a few incisions should be made to relieve tension and prevent sloughing, and then fomentations of weakly carbolised Goulard water should be applied. If sloughs occur, their separation should be hastened by charcoal or carrot poultices, and the removal with forceps and scissors of all parts as they become loose. As soon as the dead tissues have come away, even though the testicles are left in great part bare, cicatrisation rapidly ensues under a dressing of an antiseptic oil or ointment and a general tonic and stimulating treatment.

Sloughing of the Scrotum may follow accidental injury, frostbite, scalds, embolism, or may result from the damage due to extravasation of urine, or from inflammation. A considerable portion of the scrotum may thus be lost, and the testicles become exposed to a corresponding degree. It is remarkable, however, with what rapidity and completeness these losses are repaired and how soon the testicles become covered over again. When sloughing follows erysipelas, or occurs in the course of one of the continued fevers, the prognosis is very grave; and in these cases tonics, stimulants, and nutritious food, as well as antiseptic local treatment, will be very requisite.

EPITHELIOMA OF THE SCROTUM.

This is commonly named "chimney-sweep's cancer." Sometimes it is spoken of as "soot cancer," and this name directly denotes the cause of this disease. Soot when applied constantly to other parts of the body, has been known to excite epithelioma. Sir J. Earle met with it on the hands of a gardener who had used soot for the destruction of insects on leaves. Epithelioma scroti occurs in others than sweeps. Dr. Paris saw it in smelters; Dr. Schaffner in muleteers in Mexico; and of ten cases at Guy's Hospital, mentioned by Jacobson, three occurred in labourers in gasworks, three in workers at tarworks, one in a chemical labourer, one in a lampblack maker, one in a shoemaker, and one in a labourer. Paraffin, tar, and the distillation of crude carbolic acid from tar, are each of them excitants of scrotal epithelioma. Volkmann, Joseph Bell, and Ball of Dublin, have published such cases. Scrotal epithelioma is rare in comparison with epithelioma in other situations. The proportion of sweeps affected was always comparatively small, so that, doubtless, a predisposition on the part of those affected is required, as well as the action of the special irritant. Nor was the disease ever very common, and there is good reason for believing that it is becoming appreciably less so than formerly, owing to the great precautions in regard to baths and clothes which of late years have been taken by the workers in these materials.

There are no statistics of the disease from fifty to one hundred years ago to compare with those of the present time; and the impressions drawn from memory as to the comparative frequency of diseases are notoriously deceptive. Still, there is an uniformity of opinion on the part of surgeons whose memories extend back to hospital practice before the commencement of the second half of this century that chimney-sweep's cancer is much less often met with now than formerly.

The action of soot in causing epithelioma is very slow, and consequently the disease has been very rarely indeed met with before middle life, even in men whose childhood and boyhood have been passed in constant contact with soot. From observations made by Mr. Spencer (Med.-Chir. Trans., vol. lxxiv. p. 59), it appears that the cells of the rete Malpighii of the healthy skin beyond the margin of soot cancer are sometimes filled with black granules; and it is probable that soot may thus remain in the skin tissues harmless for years, till the " predisposition " to cancer, which comes with adult life in some persons, favours its actual development. In this way is explained the occurrence of chimney-sweep's cancer in men years after they have ceased to follow their vocation as sweeps.

In the same way is explained the occurrence of soot cancer in the lymphatic glands as a primary affection (Lawson, *Lancet,* 1878, vol. ii. p. 576; Paget, "Surg. Path.," p. 447); as well as the delayed recurrence of secondary disease in the inguinal glands years after removal of scrotal epithelioma, and without any recurrence in the scar (Butlin, *Brit. Med. Journ.,* 1892, p. 1343). The disease is much more rare in other countries than in England. It is said to be unknown in France, rarely seen in Germany, and Agnew states that he had never seen a case in Philadelphia or elsewhere in America.

Scrotal epithelioma is very slow in its progress, seldom. proving fatal in less than six or eight or more years; often. existing a very long time, even several years, before implicating lymphatic glands, and even at the last not extending beyond the nearest group of glands. Secondary affection of the glands may be deferred for several years, and when it occurs it may be not till years after the excision of the primary affection.

Symptoms.—It generally begins as a small single wart or pimple on the most dependent part of the scrotum; but frequently the skin is dry and harsh, or there are several warts or scaly patches of skin around the spot which is advancing, or has advanced, to the epitheliomatous stage. In other instances it begins as a horn-like excrescence or papilloma; or as a small subcutaneous nodule in connection with a sebaceous gland or hair follicle; or as a cauliflower-like outgrowth of a papillomatous nature. At first the disease, in whatever form it begins, appears to be of a simple nature, and may so remain for a long time; but, sooner or later, it softens, becomes more vascular, and excoriates or ulcerates, and then becomes covered with a thin scab at one part, whilst perhaps it sloughs at another, and, maybe, sends out a cauliflower-like excrescence at another. The sore usually yields a thin ichorous discharge; its edges are irregular, hard, and everted, and its base is also much indurated. As the disease advances, it does so in depth as well as in area, and though it has little tendency to invade the testicle, it may destroy the underlying part of the tunica vaginalis and spread beyond the scrotum to the penis, groins, or perinæum.

The inguinal glands are not early affected by chimney-sweep's cancer. They may become inflamed during the warty stage of the disease; but later, when ulceration has set in and epitheliomatous elements reach them, the glands become indurated with malignant disease, and subsequently soften and break down into deep, open, foul, discharging sores. By slow degrees the general health fails, the strength is exhausted by pain and discharges, and perhaps recurrent hæmorrhages, and in this way death is brought about.

It is very rare for the disease to reach the lumbar glands or to give rise to secondary deposits in lungs, liver, or other abdominal viscera.

Treatment.—Excision, wide and free of the disease, at as early a period as possible, is the only proper treatment. When the inguinal glands are invaded, they, too, should be excised. When the disease has advanced beyond the limits of an operation, as when the penis and perinæum are deeply affected, or the whole groin from pubis to spine of ilium is infiltrated and deeply ulcerated, then the only rational treatment consists in anodynes locally and internally; frequent irrigation with some antiseptic lotion; and the application of eucalyptus or iodoform ointment to counteract the offensive discharges. The prophylactic treatment comprises strict cleanliness both as to clothes and skin, and the removal of any wart or papilloma before it becomes cancerous. Mr. Butlin's lectures in the *Brit. Med. Journ.* of 1892 may be consulted for much interesting information respecting this disease.

OTHER FORMS OF MALIGNANT DISEASE OF THE SCROTUM.

These are very rare. Medullary cancer, scirrhus, and melanotic sarcoma, and a mixed adeno-chondro-sarcoma, have all been described (Jackson, pp. 552 and 563); and Dr. Crocker (Path. Soc. Trans., 1888) has put on record a case of so-called Paget's disease, in which a superficial ulceration began on the scrotum and adjoining under-surface of the penis somewhat resembling eczema. It was quite intractable to treatment, and at length two nodules formed, and the whole affected area of the scrotum was excised. The structure of the growth was very like that of rodent ulcer.

With regard to melanotic growths of the scrotum, Mr. Jacobson writes: "They are often extremely insidious, both in their commencement and their course. Yet in spite of this insignificant commencement and apparently unimportant progress, there are no growths which can be more malignant. They do not always infect the glands. Histologically, the growth is usually a melanotic sarcoma, containing round and spindle cells, and presenting a matrix which very often forms definite alveoli. Finally, it is a growth which is especially liable to commence in and to be hastened by any irritation. Thus removal by the knife at the earliest possible moment is imperatively needed."

NON-MALIGNANT TUMOURS OF THE SCROTUM.

There are several varieties, but all are rare.

Angeiomata or Vascular Growths.—Scrotal nævi are not very uncommon in infants. They should be treated as are nævi in other parts. If left alone, they may undergo cystic, fibroid, or fatty change, and in these forms are occasionally met with in later life.

I have had two cases in young adults of congenital venous tumours amongst varicose veins, lying along the course of the cord and the upper part of the scrotum. In some similar cases on record the angeioma has involved the penis, and there has been hæmaturia due to the rupture of an enlarged vein into the penile part of the urethra.

In all cases it is best to remove these nodules and, with them, some of the dilated veins with which they are connected. If left, it is probable they may inflame, ulcerate, and bleed, or pass into some sarcomatous condition later in life.

Cystic Tumours.— These are of different nature, but they are all very rare. There are two kinds both probably of sebaceous origin. One is a simple dilatation of a sebaceous follicle containing cheesy sebaceous matter; the other is a dense sac of connective tissue containing clear serous or yellow viscid fluid, and probably also originating in a sebaceous follicle.

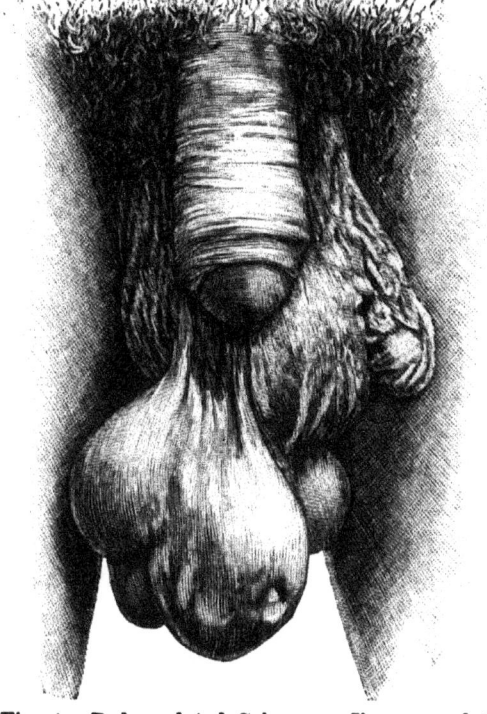

Fig. 4.—Pedunculated Sebaceous Tumours of the Scrotum. (*After Mr. A. Sheen, of Cardiff.*) (*Brit. Med. Journal*, July 6th, 1895.)

They are commonly multiple, and vary in size from a swanshot to a hen's egg.

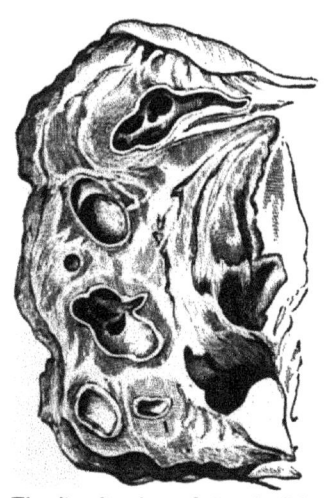

Fig. 5.—Section of Cystic Disease of the Scrotum. (*After Curling.*)

Two other forms of scrotal cyst deserve mention, namely, the hydatid and urinary cysts. Dr. Muskett, of Sydney, has recorded a case of hydatid cyst in the *Medical Press and Circular*, 1889 (vol. i. p. 142), which attained to the size of two closed fists. It was tapped several times and ultimately suppurated, and when the sac was about to be laid open, a hydatid cyst forced its way through the cannula used for drawing off the pus, and the patient was thereupon cured without incision.

Urinary cysts are caused by the gradual escape of a small quantity of normal urine through an abnormal opening in the urethra. In some cases an abscess has preceded the formation of the cyst, urine escaping into the cavity after the evacuation of the pus. In such cases the size of the cyst will depend upon the size of the preceding abscess, but they are larger when occurring in the scrotum than in the perinæum.

Mr. Page (*Med. Chron.*, 1887, vol. vii. p. 194) reported a case of urinary cyst the size of a small apple, in the mid-scrotal region, indistinctly fluctuating and apparently connected with the urethra, about an inch in front of the bulb. It contained offensive fluid composed of urine and pus, and was cured by being laid open and scraped out. It followed a blow received eighteen months previously.

The best treatment for the sebaceous forms of cysts and the hydatid cysts is removal. The urinary cysts should be laid open and scraped, as was done successfully in Mr. H. W. Page's case.

Lipoma.—Adipose tumours having definite capsules and an aggregation of distinct lobules are developed in the sub-cutaneous connective tissue of the scrotum. They are very rare, have a doughy, soft feeling, and give rise to an imperfect sense of fluctuation—symptoms which are apt to cause mistakes in diagnosis when the lobulated outline cannot be distinguished. Sir J. Paget speaks of the shifting of fatty tumours from the groin or region of the spermatic cord into the scrotum. These scrotal lipomata may be continuous, with masses of fat over the abdomen and penis, as in cases recorded by Curling and Sir Henry Thompson.

Mr. Hutchinson (*Arch. Surg.*, vol. iii. No. 60, pl. lxiii.) has described and illustrated a case of **diffuse lipoma** of large size, in a man of middle age, which affected the pubic region and almost buried the penis and scrotum in masses of fat.

The treatment is excision, as practised by Mr. Birkett, Mr. Lane, and Dr. Kimball. When too diffuse for operation, the patients should abstain from malt liquors, sugar, and starchy food, and take frequent doses of sulphide of calcium, with the view of checking the growth of the tumours.

Fibromata.—These are occasional growths of the scrotum occurring as single tumours of varying density, some being hard and others loosely woven and œdematous. They are usually encapsulated, often lobulated, and sometimes attain a large size. Twenty-three and twenty-four pounds, and in one case forty-four pounds, are weights which have been reached by these tumours. These fibrous tumours are sometimes blended with other forms of new growth. Thus cartilage, fatty tissue, myxomatous or sarcomatous elements may be mixed with the fibrous ; or the tissue may undergo calcareous changes, or slough and give rise to troublesome hæmorrhage. They affect men well advanced in age; but in one case mentioned by Curling the patient was only two and a half years of age. Their great density, and the absence of translucency, will distinguish these tumours from encysted hydrocele.

The proper treatment is excision; but the disease may not improbably recur, as in a case operated upon by Sir W. Fergusson.

Enchondromata.—These are the rarest of all scrotal tumours. In one case, that of a Chinaman in Canton, reported by Dr. Kerr, the growth was the size of a child's head, and consisted of cartilage and true bone intermixed.

ELEPHANTIASIS SCROTI

is an affection of India, Arabia, China, West Indies, Syria, the Delta of the Nile, and other hot countries, but is rarely seen in Europe or North America.

It is a chronic inflammatory disease associated with much œdema, set up by repeated attacks of erythema, and resulting in chronic hypertrophy of the skin and cellular tissue. This œdema and subsequent hypertrophy in cases of endemic elephantiasis are due, according to Dr. Manson, to obstruction of the scrotal lymphatics by the filaria sanguinis hominis. The causes of non-filarial elephantiasis, sporadic cases of which are met with in persons who have never been abroad, are less well known. The obstruction in these latter may be due to simple inflammatory matting, or to cicatricial contraction of the lower abdominal lymphatics or of the thoracic duct itself. Mr. Hutchinson records two cases in which, as he believes, the disease was due to œdematous inflammation of syphilitic origin. He is of opinion that there is no real distinction between elephantiasis of the Tropics and that which occurs in Great Britain; and that the filaria sanguinis hominis, whilst probably aggravating the disease, is not the sole cause of it, nor of any peculiar form of it.

Heat and moisture seem to have a powerful influence in

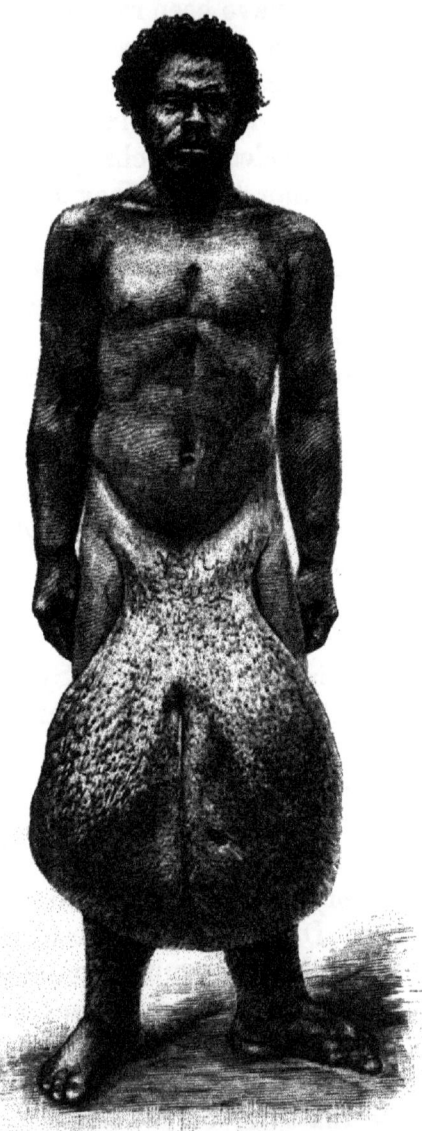

determining the production of the disease. The pathological changes are similar in character to those seen in the Barbadoes leg, and in the hypertrophied external genitals of females which have been the seat of repeated attacks of inflammatory œdema from gonorrhœa, or erysipelas. The chief alteration in the tissues of the scrotum is the enormous hypertrophy of the subcutaneous connective tissue, which becomes so dense as to cut almost like cartilage. Lymphatic vessels, dilated or varicose, and filled with a gelatinous fluid, are found in this œdematous, dense, white, fibrous, and elastic tissue, and the lymph spaces of the cutis are enlarged. Sir Joseph Fayrer found erectile growths in some instances; and in others, masses of fat and earthy concretions have been seen scattered

Fig. 6.--Elephantiasis Scroti. (From a photograph given to me by Mr. Sutton.)

through the hypertrophied connective tissue. The veins are enlarged, tortuous, and patulous when cut. The testicles lie embedded in the posterior part, and the penis is covered with similarly hypertrophied tissue in the anterior part of the swelling. Vaginal hydrocele is commonly associated with the elephantiasis, and hæmatocele occasionally so. The testicles are unchanged, but the spermatic cord is much elongated by traction, and the cremaster much thickened.

Symptoms.—In the early stages elephantiasis is associated with frequent attacks of feverishness, local heat and pain, by erysipelatous œdema, and swelling of the inguinal glands. Each attack leaves the scrotum more enlarged, and, when once thoroughly established, the scrotal enlargement goes on increasing without fresh pyrexial attacks. The shape of the swelling is pyriform or ovoid, having a broad, thickened peduncle extending the whole area of the perinæum from anus to pubes. Owing to the drag upon the skin of the hypogastrium, the hair of the pubes is spread out over the front and upper part of the sides of the tumour ; and the penis is gradually drawn in till it is represented only by an umbilical-like aperture. The surface of the skin may be smooth, though thickened and indurated, but it is more generally rugose, and fissured, and superficially ulcerated between the rugæ. Crusts cover the superficial ulcers, and an offensive sanious discharge oozes from beneath the crusts. Sometimes there is a discharge of lymph from some of the more prominent knots or rugæ, and in some cases sloughing occurs, and the testicles become thereby exposed. Agnew refers to six cases in which this happened. When not inflamed or ulcerated, the skin is very little sensitive. The chief, almost the only, inconvenience is the dragging and great weight. The growth sometimes attained is enormous, amounting to 120 lbs., and even to 200 lbs.

Prophylactic treatment.—For culinary and drinking purposes, only boiled water should be used, and stagnant water should be avoided even for washing. In fact, every prophylactic measure against the filaria sanguinis hominis should be taken. Operation should not be undertaken during an attack of fever or of local inflammation, nor in old age, or in persons with visceral disease. Stricture of the urethra should be inquired for, and treated, if existing, prior to operation, as there is often difficulty in passing urine for a few days after operation. Hernia, abscesses in the scrotum, hydroceles, and hæmatoceles, though they enhance the risks, do not contraindicate operation.

Operative treatment.—The *operation* should be performed under the best hæmostatic and aseptic conditions. Turner's (of Samoa) clamp, consisting of two parallel wooden bars approximated by screws, or Esmarch's bandage, should be applied; then the body of the penis, and subsequently the testicles, should be dissected out, and the whole of the coverings of these organs, as well as the raphe of the perinæum,

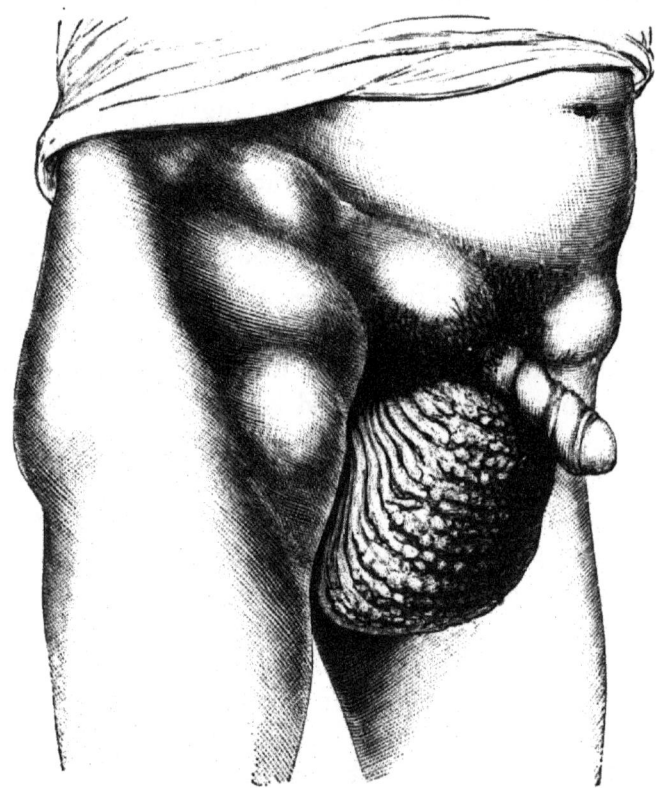

Fig. 7.—Lymph Scrotum with Hypertrophied Lymph Glands in Groins.   (*Carter.*)

should be dissected away. No portion of the diseased tissues should be left behind, otherwise recurrence is certain. All bleeding vessels should be ligatured or twisted. The wound must heal in chief part by granulations, and, whilst doing so, care must be used to keep the penis free. In successful cases the sexual functions, as well as the general health, are restored.

LYMPH SCROTUM.

In men of any age from puberty upwards who reside, or have resided, in the Tropics (China and India), the condition known as lymph scrotum, or varix lymphaticus, may be met with, but in these only. It is allied to elephantiasis of the scrotum, being probably dependent upon the same cause.

The patient, having been the subject of previous malarial attacks, gets his scrotum and inguinal glands, and perhaps, too, his testicles, inflamed during a paroxysm of fever. Then an abscess forms in the scrotum, and vesicles occur upon its surface and burst, discharging straw-coloured, serous-looking fluid. The discharge continues for a few days; the scrotal swelling diminishes; the discharge ceases, reaccumulates, and refills the vesicles, which again burst and go through the same process. In all cases the inguinal glands enlarge.

The fluid discharged is lymph mixed with chyle. Lymph scrotum has hitherto been met with only in persons who are residing, or have resided, in countries in which elephantiasis is endemic. Dr. Manson believes that both diseases are due to filaria sanguinis hominis, which causes obstruction in the thoracic duct or in the lymphatics. The treatment consists in excision as in the case of elephantiasis scroti.

SCROTAL FISTULÆ AND CALCULI.

Fistulæ occasionally open upon and burrow through the scrotum; they arise from urethral stricture, or burrowing suppuration outside the urethra in connection with the epididymis, testis, or inguinal glands.

Scrotal Calculi consist either of uric acid or of phosphate of lime, and are formed by deposition from the urine, either within the urethra or along some fistulous track. They have been met with after many years of existence and growth, and in some cases of large size. Having made their way by ulceration through the urethra, they increase by the deposition of salts from the urine which escapes through the urethra fistula. Sometimes, it is probable, they have been formed by deposition from urine which has escaped into a peri-urethral abscess cavity and without the previous escape through the urethra of a calculus formed within the urinary track. They should be removed and efforts made to get the fistula to heal. They have been known to attain to great sizes. Holmes mentions a case in which the stone weighed eight ounces; Von Graefe one in which the stone, weighing twenty-six ounces was

c

discharged spontaneously from the scrotum.   Lippman reports a case where four phosphatic calculi weighing one ounce and a half were removed from a fistula situated a little behind the junction of the penis and scrotum.   Fifteen years before, a calculus weighing four ounces and a quarter had been removed from the same part after it had given rise to obstructed micturition.   In the *Brit. Med. Journ.* for July 11, 1885, a case is recorded in which seven uric acid calculi were removed by incision from a sac in the connective tissue of the scrotum. They had been forming for many years, and had caused hæmaturia, and pain on micturition and in coitus.   Calculi may begin to form in boyhood, and either continue to increase in size through a long life or give rise to urgent symptoms in young adult life.

CHAPTER II.

CONGENITAL ABNORMALITIES OF THE TESTIS: HYPERTROPHY AND ATROPHY OF THE TESTIS.

ABNORMALITIES of the testicle have relation to either the development or the transit of the organ. The two classes are closely related to each other: any fault in descent interferes with the proper development, and conversely any defect in its development may interfere with the descent of the testicle.

The following is a tabular statement of all the various congenital abnormalities and defects of the testicle grouped under these two heads (Le Dentu, " Des anomalies du testicule," *Thèse d'agr. de Paris*, 1869) :—

Abnormalities in development.	Excess in number	=	Polyorchism.
	Deficiency in number	=	Anorchism. Monorchism.
	Fusion of testis	=	Synorchism.
	Hypertrophy		
	Atrophy		

Abnormalities in descent.	Undescended—retained along the normal track.
	Ectopia, or descent to a point outside normal track.
	Inversion of the descended testicle.

ABNORMALITIES IN DEVELOPMENT.

Polyorchism is undoubtedly rare, and in the majority of the cases in which a third testicle has been supposed to exist it has turned out to be an encysted hydrocele, or a movable fibrous body in the tunica vaginalis, or an omental hernia.

Anorchism is the absence of both testicles. **Monorchism** is the absence of one testicle. These conditions are rare, and are sometimes erroneously thought to exist when, in reality, the testicle is either retained, imperfectly descended, or atrophied. Either the testicle as a whole, including epididymis and more or less of the vas deferens, may be absent; or the testicle proper may be absent, the epididymis and all the rest of the parts being present; or the epididymis and vas may be absent and the testicle proper may be present. These deficiencies of part only of one testicular apparatus can be easily understood if it be remembered that the vasa efferentia, the epididymis, and the vas deferens are derived from the Wolffian body and its duct, whereas the testis is developed separately from the genital mass. When these abnormalities affect one organ only, the scrotum on the same side is usually present, though probably not perfectly developed. In some cases of monorchism malformation or absence of the ureter and kidney on the same side has been observed. In some cases of anorchism the external genitals have usually existed only in a rudimentary state, and abnormalities affecting the urinary apparatus and the rectum and anus have co-existed with those of the testis.

In monorchism, if the single testicle is well formed and in normal position, the sexual function and bodily and mental powers are unaffected. In anorchism (both testicles absent) the individual is impotent, sterile, with impaired energy and feeble mental and physical powers, and the puerile manner and puny voice of the eunuch.

ABNORMALITIES IN TRANSIT OF THE TESTIS.

When one or both testicles are retained within some part of the abdominal track, the word *cryptorchism* is used to describe the condition. When the testicle descends into some abnormal position, it is spoken of as " *ectopia of the testis.*" It is to be regretted that this expression, "ectopia of the testicle," is sometimes used for those cases also in which the testicle has incompletely descended, being retained at some point in its normal course. It is excessively rare for both testes to be undescended. A testis may be retained at any point in its normal course from loin to scrotum. In many cases the position of an undescended testicle varies, the organ being sometimes within the abdomen, at others in the canal ; or as in other cases, sometimes in the canal, at others at the top of the scrotum.

In most cases of undescended testis, the epididymis and vas have their normal relation to the body of the organ, but in some exceptional cases the epididymis and vas have passed beyond the testis proper towards or into the scrotum, thus looking as if the obstacle which had prevented the testis proper from descending had not been able to hold back the epididymis and vas.

Ectopia Testis occurs in three situations: (1) The testis, having traversed the inguinal canal, goes to the perinæum instead of to the scrotum—*perinæal ectopia* (Fig. 8); this is the most common form. (2) The testis leaves through the crural instead of the inguinal canal, and remains near the saphenous opening—the *crural ectopia*; this is a very rare

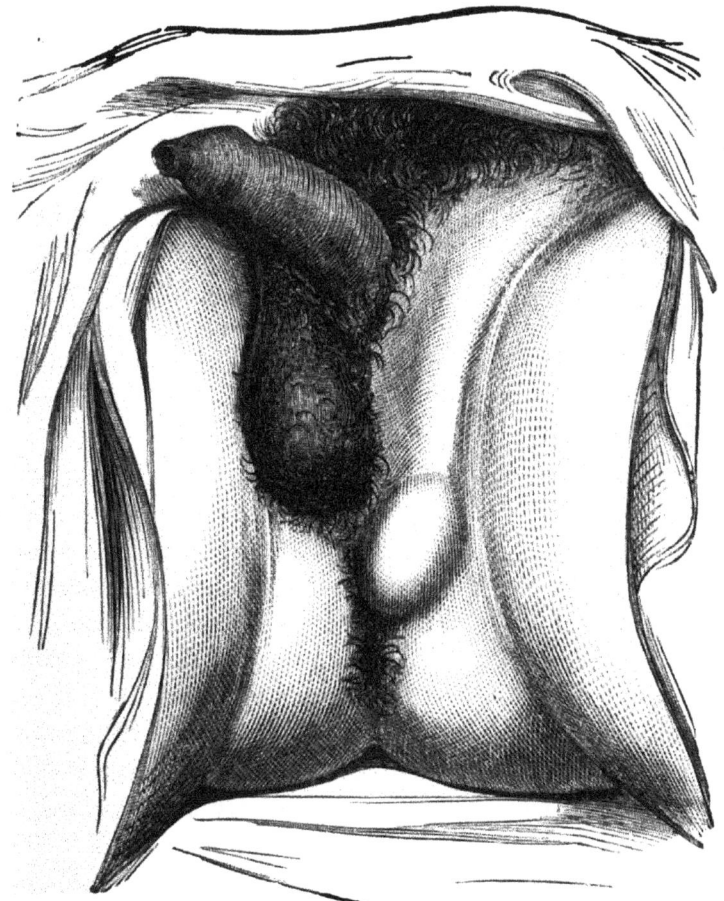

Fig. 8.—Perinæal Ectopia. (*Godard.*)

variety (Fig. 9); and (3) the rarest of all, the *peno-pubic ectopia*, is where the testis is situated in front of the pubes at the root of the penis. In the perinæal ectopia the testis occupies a pouch beneath the deep layer of the superficial fascia, and is surrounded by its tunica vaginalis. The scrotum of the corresponding side is often ill-developed. The cord can be traced down to the testis along the outer side of the scrotum, and in an adult the testis and epididymis can be distinguished. It is usually congenital, but a testicle which for years has been retained in the inguinal canal has been known to migrate subsequently into the perinæum. Perinæal ectopia is almost invariably unilateral, though Mr. Curling has alluded to one case in which it was said to have been bilateral. The probable cause of perinæal ectopia is the inser-

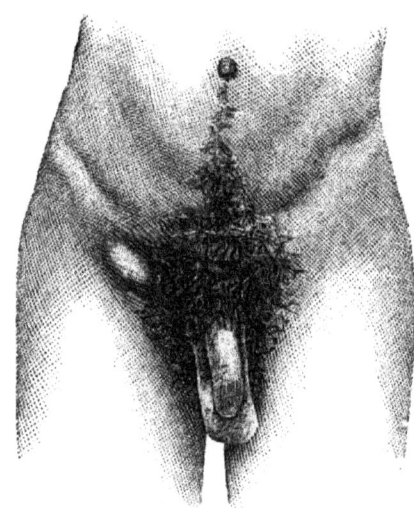

tion of the middle fasciculus of the gubernaculum into the subcutaneous tissues of the perinæum. The testis when so misplaced is liable to injury and inflammation and to inconvenient pressure in sitting and riding.

The other two forms of ectopia testis are very rare and need no special description.

Causes of Ectopia. — *Perinæal ectopia* is attributed to the faulty insertion of the middle fasciculus of the gubernaculum testis; *peno-pubic* to atrophy of the external and scrotal

Fig. 9.—Ectopia of the Testis. Male of 29 years of age. Ruptured in first year. Right testis in Scarpa's triangle the size of a filbert 1½ in. to 2 in. below Poupart's ligament. Scrotum absent on right side. (*After Macready.*)

fasciculi, the internal fasciculus alone exercising its influence.

In the *crural ectopia* the testis passes under Poupart's ligament through the crural ring in exactly the same way as a femoral hernia.

Retention of the Testis. *Causes.*—Many are ascribed, but few are known. Intra-uterine peritonitis, contracted size of external ring, ill-development of inguinal canal, a long mesorchium, absence or malposition of one or more of the attachments of the gubernaculum testis, shortness of the vas deferens, or of the vessels of the cord, the excessive size of the epididymis, and the forcible contraction of the cremaster have all been regarded as causes, and illustrative cases have been published. (*Vide* Jacobson, "Diseases of Male Organs of Generation," pp. 39–44.) Mr. Hulke had under his care in the

Middlesex Hospital a man, aged twenty-seven, with bilateral oblique inguinal hernia, the hernial sacs descending into the scrotum and ascending over the external oblique ; this man's testes were retained in the abdomen, owing probably to long mesorchia, allowing the testicles to float about instead of entering the inguinal canal (Med.-Chir. Trans., vol. xlix. p. 189).

Retained and ectopic testicles, though small, ill-developed, and sometimes the subject of fibrous and fatty degeneration, must not be regarded as being invariably functionless. It is pretty certain that a misplaced testis is healthy and functional, though small, until by pressure and repeated attacks of inflammation it degenerates and becomes sterile. Even then the man need not be sexually incapable. This is a question sometimes of importance in medico-legal cases.

Misplaced Testes. *Complications.*—The complications of misplaced or retained testes are hernia (either congenital or acquired), inflammation, gangrene, peritonitis, atrophy, hydrocele, hæmatocele, and in adult life malignant disease. A testicle, whether retained or ectopic, is liable to attacks of *inflammation* (epididymo-orchitis) from blows, strains, sudden twists of the body, or from muscular contraction, from extension of inflammation, from a local peritonitis, from gonorrhœa, or the passage of instruments. A testicle retained in the upper part of the canal or in the abdomen, if inflamed, may set up a local or general peritonitis, and when retained in the inguinal canal it may simulate strangulated hernia.

Gangrene of a retained or misplaced organ may occur as a result of inflammation, either where there is or where there is not torsion of the cord. Where there is no torsion of the cord, the gangrene follows repeated attacks of inflammation ; where torsion occurs, the gangrene is the direct result of the interference of the blood supply by the twisting of the vessels.

Hydrocele, either the acute or chronic form, and *hæmatocele,* occasionally, affect an undescended or ectopic testicle. It has already been stated that such testicles may undergo either *fibrous* or *fatty degeneration* and *atrophy.* They are also prone to be the seat of *malignant* disease (Fig. 10), and they not unfrequently become *complicated with hernia.* The hernia may be of the congenital order and descend along

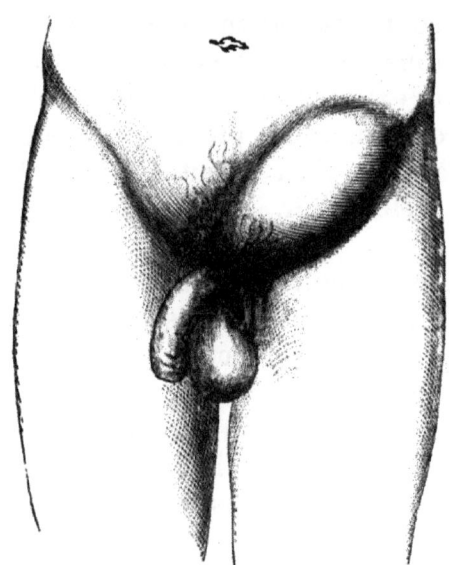

Fig. 10.—Malignant Disease of retained Testis. (*Osborn.*)

the entirely or partially unobliterated funiculovaginal process (Fig. 11). Or it may be of the acquired variety, and the sac may take the course of the inguinal canal and appear (*a*) at the external abdominal ring; or (*b*) it may emerge between some of the fibres of the aponeurosis of the external oblique or (*c*) be bulged into a recess on the deep aspect of the oblique aponeurosis. I have operated upon cases of the last variety (*c*) in which both hydrocele and acquired hernia have co-existed with an undescended testicle situated above the middle of Poupart's ligament. Syphilis is not recorded as having affected an undescended testis, and only a few cases have been published in which such testes have been the seat of tubercle.

Treatment of Ectopic and Misplaced Testicle.—If such a testicle becomes inflamed, as it is very apt to do, the treatment should at first be palliative, as for ordinary epididymo-orchitis. Where, from frequent recurrence

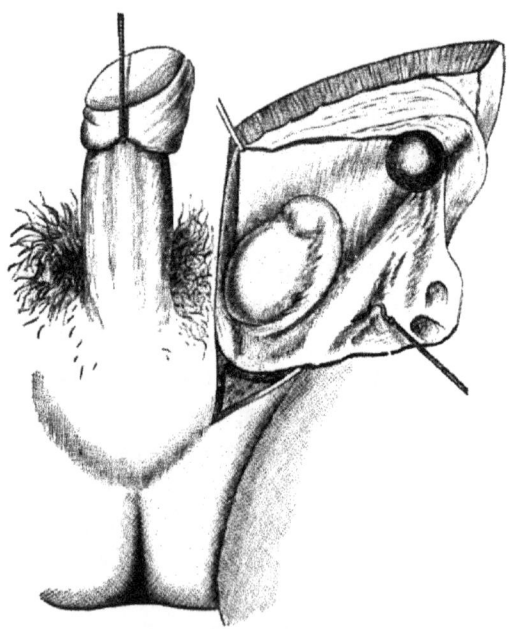

Fig. 11.—Cruro-scrotal retained Testis. Inguinal canal laid open and exposing a knuckle of strangulated bowel projecting at internal ring. (*Jacobson, after Godard.*)

of inflammation, more must be done, the testicle should be transplanted by operation to, and fixed in, the scrotum by one or more sutures if the organ is healthy and the scrotum fairly normal. If otherwise, castration must be performed.

If gangrene has commenced, either from torsion of the cord or otherwise, castration is to be recommended ; for even if the inflammatory and sloughing processes cease, the testis, if allowed to remain, is sure to atrophy. When complicated with malignant disease, castration is the only treatment, the rules for its performance being the same as for malignant disease elsewhere. When the testis is retained in the abdomen, the risks of the operation are increased by adhesions to abdominal viscera, and the operation has to be conducted on the lines of an abdominal section. Secondary deposits and extension to the lumbar and pelvic glands, of course, contraindicate an operation. When complicated with hernia, the treatment varies in different cases. If the rupture can be returned and the testis pulled down, Woods' truss, with a horseshoe-shaped pad, should be worn continuously. When this cannot be accomplished, or when, on account of the rupture becoming strangulated, an operation is required, either transplantation of the testicle or castration should be performed. I have, on several occasions, adopted one or the other plan, and have been well satisfied with the results of transplantation in properly selected cases—*i.e.* where the testicle is well formed and can be drawn down into the scrotum without too much traction, and where the scrotum is fairly well formed. It is not necessary, however, that the testis should be drawn down to, and held in, the very lowest part of the scrotum. Whilst stitching it as low as is compatible with moderate traction, it will be sufficiently out of harm's way if it acquires attachment to the upper end of the scrotal tissues. In some cases, to avoid too much traction on the end, it is best to detach the lower end and body of the epididymis from the testis, leaving the testis suspended only by the globus major, or the testis may be inverted before fixing it in the scrotum. Transplantation may be performed for cases complicated with strangulated hernia, as well as for cases in which the hernia is not strangulated, but as a rule castration is the best treatment.

In some cases of imperfectly descended testicle in children, adhesions are stretched and the cord elongated by the nurse or surgeon daily dragging lightly upon the testicle with the finger-tips, pressing it towards the scrotum and retaining it there for four or five minutes at a time. Transplantation by this means, or by operation, should be tried also in cases of ectopic testis. When an operation is performed, care should be taken to divide any process of the gubernaculum which may be holding the testis to the ischium, to fix the testicle in the scrotum by means of one or two sutures, and to keep the wound in an aseptic state during the whole period of healing.

TORSION OR AXIAL ROTATION OF THE SPERMATIC CORD.

Nicoladoni drew attention to torsion of the spermatic cord as a complication of a testicle retained in the inguinal region of a young man in 1885 (Langenbeck's "Archives of Clinical Surgery," p. 180). At the same time he described a similar condition affecting the spermatic cord of a man aged sixty-two, but in this instance the testicle was in the scrotum. Bramann followed by recording a case in the same "Archives" in the year 1890. But the attention of the profession in this country was first specially directed to the subject by my friend and former house surgeon, Mr. W. Gifford Nash (now of Bedford), in June, 1891. The patient, a lad of sixteen years, was under the care of Mr. Connell Whipple, in the South Devon and East Cornwall Hospital, Plymouth, where Mr. Nash was house surgeon at the time. The case was described as one of "strangulated epididymis of an incompletely descended testis, producing symptoms like those of strangulated hernia," for which castration was successfully performed (*Brit. Med. Journ.*, June 6, 1891).

The specimen removed from this boy was sent to the Hunterian Museum of the College of Surgeons, and was examined by Mr. J. H. Targett. who reported upon it as follows:—"The preparation consists of the body and epididymis of the left testis, and the adjacent portion of the mesorchium. The body of the testis is normal. Between it and the globus major is a deep groove, at the bottom of which lies a loop of omentum, which encircles the attachment of the body of the testis to the epididymis. The mesorchium measures nearly two inches across, and is irregularly swollen on either side from distension of the vessels and extravasation of blood between the layers of the peritoneum. At the junction of the mesorchium and epididymis, in the position of the globus minor, there is a well-marked constriction, which appears to have resulted from a severe twisting of the epididymis upon

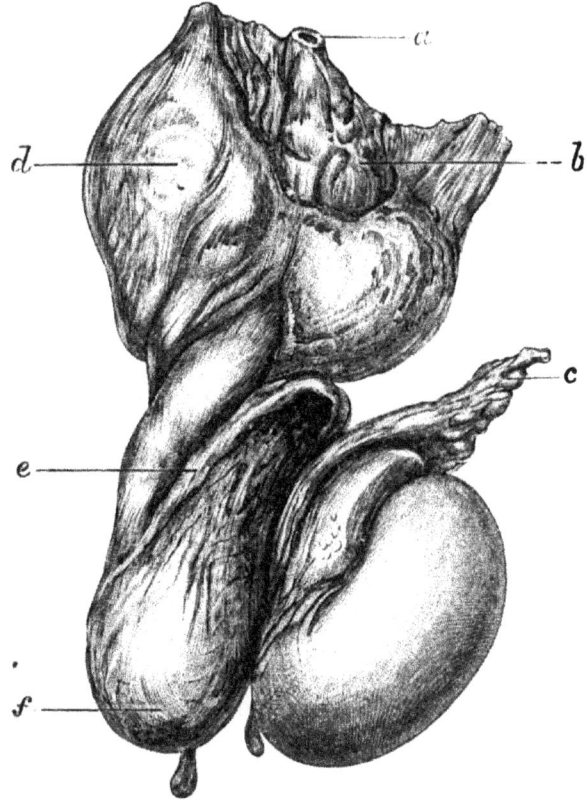

Fig. 12.—Strangulation (from Torsion) of imperfectly-descended Testis. Body of testis is normal. (*Nash.*)

a, Vas deferens ; *b*, mesorchium ; *c*, torn end of loop of omentum : *d*, blood extravasated between layers of peritoneum and mesorchium ; *e*, twist of epididymis on the mesorchium ; *f*, globus major.

the mesorchium. To this torsion the acute strangulation of the epididymis was probably due, as well as the hæmorrhage into the fatty tissue of the mesorchium " (Fig. 12).

Since the publication of Mr. Nash's paper several cases have been recorded, and papers written on the subject. Mr. Edmund Owen has recently given a summary of these in the seventeenth volume of the Medical Society's Transactions (volume for 1894, pp. 61 *et seqq.*). Torsion or axial rotation of the spermatic cord is generally associated with *imperfect descent of the testis*, and Nicoladoni thought that delayed descent rendered a testis liable to torsion of its cord; the absence of a mesorchium, by allowing the testicle freedom of movement, he also thought was an important factor. In some cases a too long mesorchium has facilitated the rotation (Gervais). Whilst it appears that retention of the testis, in the inguinal region particularly, renders the cord liable to torsion, this accident is by no means limited to undescended, imperfectly descended, or misplaced testis. It is stated above that in one of Nicoladoni's cases, the testicle was in the scrotum; and in a second case published by Mr. Nash (St. Bartholomew's Hospital Reports for 1893, vol. xxix. p. 163, and *Brit. Med. Journ.*, April 8, 1893, p. 742), of torsion of the right spermatic cord of a school-boy aged nineteen, " the testicle was in its proper place, and there was no undue patency of the external abdominal ring." In some cases of torsion of the cord of an undescended testis congenital hernia has been associated with it; and most of the recorded cases of strangulation of an undescended testis by torsion of the cord have evinced symptoms resembling more or less closely those of strangulated hernia. The testicle on either side may be affected; but hitherto, out of fourteen cases, the right has been concerned in eight. No satisfactory account of the cause of axial rotation has yet been given which will apply to all the recorded cases. The absence of a mesorchium, or an extreme length or laxity of the mesorchium, has been supposed to account for some cases; twists and other violent efforts for others; but in others, again, no cause seemed forthcoming. This, however, is no more than has to be admitted with regard to the axial rotation of other organs, such as the kidneys, spleen, ovaries, and gravid uterus, and of certain ovarian and hydatid cysts, and uterine myomata. Mr. Owen remarks, "there is one thing quite certain—namely, that a testis in the scrotum which possesses a normal mesorchium cannot be twisted. A scrotal testis with a long mesorchium may, perchance, undergo rotation, but this accident is far more likely to affect an undescended testis which has no mesorchium in the proper sense of the term."

The testis may be twisted either towards, or away from,

the median line. In all cases the epididymis has been more swollen than the testis; the testis itself in some cases has appeared normal to the naked eye. A good deal of blood may be extravasated into the epididymis, and between the layers of the peritoneum forming the mesorchium. The testis may be black and gangrenous, as may be also the epididymis; and the latter may be constricted into lumps or masses by tight bands of tissue.

The *symptoms* have in all cases been pretty much the same, namely, the more or less sudden occurrence of pain and swelling in the groin attended with vomiting. In several instances the true nature of the swelling has only been discovered on performing an exploratory operation.

Most have been diagnosed as strangulated hernia. In Mr. Nash's second case the testicle and epididymis were very tender, especially the epididymis. There was a very tender lump on the spermatic cord, about the size of a cobnut, one inch above the testis; and the cord, whilst not altered in any way, and quite normal above this lump, was much swollen between the lump and the epididymis. The epididymis lay in front of the body of the testis. The external abdominal ring was not unduly patent.

The fact that the epididymis was in front of the body of the testis, that the testis and epididymis were swollen and tender, that there was a distinct lump or knot involving the cord, above which the cord was normal and below which there was swelling, led Mr. Nash to a correct diagnosis, and to the immediate and very successful adoption of the plan of untwisting the cord without operation by rotating the testis in the reverse direction. This was easily accomplished by rotating the testis to the patient's right, when the organ quickly resumed its position with the epididymis behind the body of the testis. All symptoms rapidly disappeared, and by the next day there was no trace of anything unusual about the parts.

Diagnosis.—In many instances the surgeon can only be sure of the nature of the case by cutting down upon the swelling. In other cases—such as that of Mr. Nash's, just related, and in one related by Mr. Owen—the diagnosis can be made by (1) the empty condition of the inguinal canal; (2) the unobscured cord; (3) the imperfectly descending testis; (4) absence of the testis on one side of the scrotum; (5) by the epididymis being in front of the testis; and (6) by the existence of a lump or knot in the cord with swelling between the knot and the testis, and the natural state of the vas deferens above the knot. If, as Mr. Nash so successfully effected, the cord can be untwisted, and the symptoms thereby at once relieved, the diagnosis is complete. If not, the swelling must be exposed and the actual condition inspected. The surgeon will then see the tense plum-coloured gland, mesorchium, or epididymis, and will detect the twist in the cord.

Treatment.—If the cord, either without or after exposure by operation, can be untwisted, and if the testis or epididymis is not in a state of gangrene, it will not be necessary to remove the organ. If the twisted cord cannot be satisfactorily put right, or if gangrene is threatened, or actually exists, it will be best to tie the cord high up and excise the swollen discoloured and hæmorrhagic mass. If the testis has never properly descended and cannot be fixed in the scrotum, it is most likely it will be a permanent inconvenience and trouble even if it is (and it very probably is not) functionally perfect. And even if it has been well developed, it is highly probable that it will suppurate, or atrophy, after a tardy convalescence, in cases where the twist of the cord has been tight and the engorgement of the testicle or epididymis has been great. It is possible that Mr. Bryant may be right in his surmise that unsuspected and overlooked axial rotation may have been the cause of sterility, and atrophy of the testis occurring after what was considered to be simple inflammation of an ectopic testicle. (*See* Medico-Chirurgical Transactions, vol. lxxv. p. 247.)

ABNORMAL POSITION OF THE TESTIS IN THE SCROTUM.

The testicle is occasionally anteverted—*i.e.* the posterior and attached border becomes anterior; so that, if a hydrocele occurs, the testicle is situated in front and the tunica vaginalis behind and below. The testis is also sometimes, though very rarely, inverted (Fig. 13)—*i.e.* its upper end is below, so that the vas deferens starts from an epididymis, the tail of which is above the testis. In these cases the vas is shorter than normal. The relation of the tunica vaginalis to the testis is not affected by this inversion of the organ, as it is in the condition of ante-version. Imitating this condition, I have sometimes fixed the testes thus in transplanting the undescended organs to the scrotum.

HYPERTROPHY AND ATROPHY OF TESTIS.

The average weight of the normal adult testicle is six drachms, according to Mr. Curling, but variations both above and below this average occur.

Hypertrophy may occur when the other testicle has become atrophied, or has failed to be developed, or after removal of the other testicle. In some cases in which one testicle has been retained in the abdomen, or has been absent altogether, the other testicle has been more than double the normal size and weight.

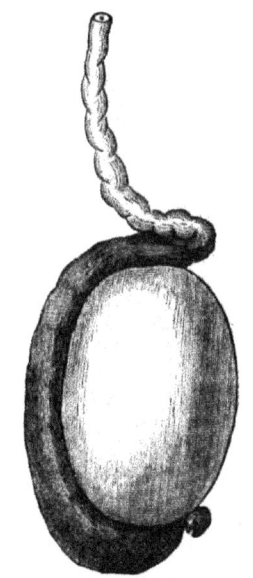

Atrophy occurs in two forms, as the result of different kinds of changes. (1) In those cases which are due to inflammation, whether traumatic, syphilitic, or otherwise, there is a marked shrinking and sclerosis of the testis; all the connective tissue of the gland —perilobular, peritubular, and perivascular—is increased and shrunken, and by its compressive effects the

Fig. 13.—Inversion of Testis, the globus minor being uppermost. (*Jacobson, after Royet.*)

secreting structure is destroyed. The gland shrinks to the size of a horse-bean, or even less, and is hard and nodular; and on section shows nothing but bands of connective tissue, with, perhaps, here and there, a few scattered seminal tubules. (2) The other form of atrophy is much rarer, and results from the cutting-off of the arterial supply, or from nerve lesions, and not from inflammation. It is of the nature of a fatty degeneration of the glandular structure, unaccompanied by any sclerosis of the connective tissue. The testicle in this form of atrophy becomes much reduced in size, but is soft and flabby instead of being hard and nodular. On section, the gland is anæmic; tubules are present, but in different stages of fatty degeneration ; and fatty tissue may also be found beneath the visceral tunica vaginalis between the epididymis and back of the testis.

In both forms the epididymis shares in the atrophy. With the shrinking of the organ the vessels and nerves of the cord diminish in size and the cremaster disappears.

Causes.—Atrophy is brought about (*a*) by local causes, (*b*) by causes acting from a distance. The local causes are the more frequent; they include all the varieties of inflammation of the testis, whether due to injury, gonorrhœa, syphilis, mumps, typhoid, etc. Mr. Jacobson and Mr. Curling each record a case in which atrophy followed an injury to the spermatic cord, caused by a strain in lifting a heavy weight, due to the violent contraction of the abdominal muscles upon the cord as it passes along the inguinal canal.

The causes acting from a distance are those which interfere with the blood or nerve supply, such as an aneurysm or other tumour pressing upon the aorta, and obstructing the circulation in one or both of the spermatic arteries. In Wardrop's edition of Baillie's works (vol. ii. p. 315) is recorded a case in which both testicles were completely absorbed, and nothing but a loose vaginal coat remained, owing to obliteration of the spermatic arteries by an aortic aneurysm. Certain injuries to the head and to the spinal cord, especially in the dorsal and lumbar regions, have been followed by atrophy of the testicles. The prolonged administration of iodine and the iodides depresses the sexual functions temporarily whilst they are being taken; possibly in some cases they do permanent damage to them, but there are no sufficient grounds for believing that they cause wasting of either testes or mammæ. Arrest of development is to be distinguished from atrophy of a once well-formed organ. This arrest is commonly found in undescended and ectopic testes. The common sequelæ of atrophy of the testis are neuralgic pains and sterility; and in some cases the development of certain female characteristics, such as enlargement of the mammæ and a feminine, fat, plump outline of figure.

The *treatment* can only be preventive ; the cause should be removed when possible.

WITH the exception of contusions, traumatic lesions of the testis are rare.

Punctured wounds are almost always of surgical origin, their most frequent cause being puncture with a trocar and cannula in paracentesis for hydrocele. A very acute pain, in some cases inducing syncope, and the escape of a little blood through the cannula as soon as the trocar is withdrawn, and then of blood-stained hydrocele fluid as soon as the cannula, retracted from the tunica albuginea, has entered the vaginal sac, are the indications of this accident. Acute inflammation is likely to follow, especially if the tubular structure of the gland has been at all broken up by the vulnerating body. Suppuration and gangrene have been described as actual consequences of punctured wounds; but they are quite exceptional, for, as a general rule, unless the organ is previously diseased, rapid recovery is the result. In many cases little or no inflammation whatever is excited.

Incised Wounds.—These have been made deliberately by Vidal de Cassis and those who have followed him, for the purpose of relieving tension in acute inflammation of the testicle. A few instances of sabre cuts and of surgical accidents in operations on the scrotum occur from time to time. The symptoms are gaping of the cut edges of the tunica albuginea, free hæmorrhage from the tunica vasculosa, and slight protrusion of tubular structures through the wound in the tunics. Unless the testicle is tuberculous or otherwise partly disorganised prior to the injury, hernia or fungus testis does not occur. In the 400 cases of acute inflammation treated by incision by Vidal de Cassis, not one is said to have been followed by fungus testis. Superficial incised wounds heal as a rule by first intention, even without the introduction of sutures; but if the wound deeply involves any considerable length of the organ, it will subsequently atrophy as the glandular tissue is strangled by the contraction of the

D

cicatricial material. Suppuration is very improbable unless the incision is made with a dirty knife or the wound is allowed to become septic.

Contused wounds of the testis are generally complicated by more serious wounds of neighbouring parts and organs. They are commonly gunshot wounds, and Otis gives 586 cases of contused wounds of the testis as having occurred in the American War of the Rebellion. The mortality of these cases was 18 per cent. In most instances the scrotum was much lacerated, and in many the testicles were torn to shreds. Of the comparatively few recorded cases in the Crimean and Italian wars, the majority resulted in total destruction of the organ, and most of those not at once destroyed by the violence subsequently underwent atrophy.

Contusions.—These are the most frequent of the traumatic lesions of the testis. They are caused by blows, falls astride, kicks, squeezes, and other forms of violent pressure.

Monod and Terrillon describe three degrees. The *first* is very slight, and consists in very minute capillary hæmorrhages amongst the tubules, but without the solution of continuity even of their epithelial lining; the *second* consists in somewhat larger extravasations from rupture of somewhat larger vessels than the smallest capillaries, some of the blood-clots being as large as peas, but never, says Monod, forming one large collection deserving of the name of "intra-testicular hæmatocele." In neither of these degrees is the tunica albuginea damaged. In the third degree the gland is crushed, the tunica albuginea is split open, and little masses of the seminal tubules are disintegrated and transformed into sanguineous pulp. Large areas of the glandular tissue may be broken down by effused blood, and are spoken of as intra-testicular hæmatoceles; these are nearly always in communication, through the torn tunica albuginea, with a hæmatocele in the tunica vaginalis. The epididymis suffers to a less extent than the body of the testicle, but it is frequently also contused, and the globus major especially may be the seat of numerous small extravasations.

Symptoms.—These are acute, insupportable pain, often severe enough to produce syncope. Death from shock, even may be the result—sometimes almost instantaneously, more often perhaps after the lapse of several hours. Curling mentions the case of a man who during a struggle was gripped in the testicles, and was instantly seized with convulsions and died. The pain is not seated only in the testicle injured, but radiates to the thigh and extends along the cord, often reaching as high as the kidney in the loin.

Prognosis.—Though fatal results have occurred, they are very rare. The usual course is for the pain to pass quickly, the swelling to disappear by degrees, and the attack to be of but little immediate importance. The subsequent effects are those which give gravity to these injuries. Atrophy so commonly follows that it is to be expected in any case, and in persons with a tubercular tendency these injuries often induce tuberculosis of the testicle.

Suppuration is very rare, and need not be anticipated if the organ prior to the injury was quite healthy. It is orchitis followed by atrophy, or atrophy even where the inflammation has been too trivial to attract notice, which is the common result of injury in men of all ages. In less than six weeks the body of the testis may be no larger than a haricot bean, may be soft and flabby, with its tunica albuginea wrinkled and clearly too large for its contents, and on section of the testicle proper the gland tissue looks anæmic and opalescent or milky white in colour. The epididymis is frequently but little, if at all, changed.

Diagnosis.—The marked feature which distinguishes traumatic orchitis from inflammation of venereal origin is the remarkable immunity of the epididymis in traumatic cases. The swelling at first is entirely confined to the body of the testicle, and though later the epididymis may also suffer, it is never affected to any marked degree. There may be hydrocele of the tunica vaginalis of either slight or very pronounced dimensions.

Treatment.—The treatment of injuries to the testicle is very simple—namely, rest in bed, cold applications, and the general treatment appropriate for orchitis. Punctured and incised wounds soon heal, and sutures are rarely required even for long incisions. For contused wounds sutures are useless. In very severe cases of the third degree, where the gland is completely crushed or pulped, primary castration is proper.

TRAUMATIC DISPLACEMENT AND TRAUMATIC ECTOPIA OF THE TESTIS.

Though rare, these accidents are recorded by well-recognised authorities. Traumatic displacement or dislocation of the testis results from violence applied to the scrotum. Reclus quotes two cases of the right testis caused by the passage of carriage wheels over the scrotum; in both the right side of the scrotum was empty. In one the testis was displaced into a prominent position at the upper part of the scrotum immediately to the inner side of the left testis, and it was reduced four days later; in the other the right testis was situated immediately beneath the skin covering the pubis, and could not be reduced at all, though the man seemed none the worse for the change of position of the organ.

Traumatic or acquired ectopia is caused either by injury or by sudden and forcible contraction, voluntary or involuntary, of the cremaster muscle, by violent effort during coitus or lifting some heavy weight. When the testicle, having properly descended, returns from accident or violent muscular contraction to some higher position along its natural course of descent, acquired ectopia is said to occur. The testicle may either remain permanently out of the scrotum or redescend after an uncertain time and from some unexpected cause.

If orchitis follows either traumatic displacement or ectopia, adhesions may form and fix the testis permanently in its new place; and if the testis has been pushed or drawn back within the abdomen, severe peritonitis is likely to complicate the orchitis. Castration may be required either because of the pain or of the inconvenience and danger to which the inflamed testis may give rise. Some of these cases have ended fatally either after or when no castration has been performed.

Treatment.—In acquired ectopia and traumatic displacement immediate reduction should be effected by manipulation if possible. If not possible, gentle massage may succeed at a later stage; and if it does not, the gland may perhaps be replaced by operation. Strapping, or a bandage, or one or two sutures, should be used to keep the testicle in place after reduction has been accomplished. If the testicle becomes inflamed, or adherent in its faulty position, castration in many cases should be performed.

CHAPTER IV.

FUNCTIONAL DISORDERS IN RELATION TO THE TESTICLES.

1. Irritable testis.   2. Neuralgia of testicle.
3. Masturbation.   4. Spermatorrhœa.
5. Sexual hypochondriasis.   6. Impotence.
7. Sterility.

IRRITABLE AND NEURALGIC TESTICLE.

SOME men have morbidly sensitive testicles, the slightest touch almost causing pain. Such men, in my experience, are nearly always of neurotic and emotional temperament, and effeminate or pusillanimous ; and in some cases the scrotum, penis, and groins are also hypersensitive. To a slight degree it occurs in many at puberty, or as a result of masturbation, or excessive sexual intercourse, or by ungratified sexual desire. Neuralgia of the testis is like neuralgia of the face, characterised by sudden severe and paroxysmal pain, and may be due to a cause situated in the testicle itself, or in some distant part.

Causes situated in the testicle are contractions of inflammatory deposits, minute abscesses, fibrous bodies in the tunica vaginalis, small encysted hydroceles, progressive atrophy, a small new growth, e.g. fibro-myoma, or injury to the vas deferens.

Causes situated at a distance from the testicle are irritation in the prostatic urethra, stone in the bladder or kidney ; oxaluria, lithiasis, gout, rheumatism, and extreme nervous depression associated with phosphuria and constipation, or some fissure or ulcer of the anus or rectum, are also common causal conditions.

Treatment.—Where possible, the cause should be ascertained and removed ; where this is not possible, the testis should be supported in a suspender, the bowels should be daily evacuated, the diet regulated, rest in the horizontal position enjoined, and ice or hot fomentations, or some anodyne liniment—such as opium, belladonna, or atropine—should be applied locally. Morphia may have to be injected occasionally. Division of the nerves of the spermatic cord and castration have been occasionally practised, but are not to be recommended except in the rare cases of neuralgia from a new growth, or from the contraction of some old inflammatory thickening in the epididymis or testis, which no other remedies have succeeded in improving.

MASTURBATION.

Self-abuse, or the excitement of the sexual organs by the individual himself, is what is understood by masturbation. This is commonly practised by the hands, but may be by friction of the parts against the clothes by shifting or writhing movements of the body. It is a habit only too rife at puberty and early manhood as the result of the natural onset of sexual feelings and desire when not controlled, but it may be formed even in quite early childhood as the effect of some pathological irritation in the penis or rectum of the child—e.g. a long tight foreskin, thread-worms—or of the wanton excitement of the child by the nurse. Those who have had experience more especially of children in charge of ayahs, or Oriental servants, will have seen the evil effects of this practice used to quiet peevishness, or for the gratification of their own lustful inquiries and propensities. The act of masturbation may thus be consummated by seminal emission, or it may not, according to the age at which it is practised; but, whether done before or after the development of the secreting powers of the testis, the same deleterious results to the nervous system follow.

Masturbation is practised by female children and adolescents as well as by males, and is by no means an infrequent cause of nervous ailments, defective development, and ungainly manners; but the consideration of this subject falls under the Diseases of the Female Generative Organs.

The effect of masturbation, or of premature stimulation of the sexual organs is shown on the nervous, muscular, and general systems. The child becomes irritable, restless, excited, or languid, and prematurely old in appearance and ways; his limbs get weak and flabby; his appetite fails or varies; he looks pale, pinched, and pasty. The special senses may become dull or temporarily defective. Epilepsy, tubercular disease, or general physical and nervous prostration may be induced. In the young adult, there are added to the physical changes the effects which spring from the consciousness of wrong doing, or at any rate, of a secret habit. His look is downcast or abashed, he is taciturn, solitary, nervous, hesitating, or timid. His eyes are often strained, the cornea of unnatural brightness, the conjunctiva bloodshot, and his skin is often bedewed by a greasy, clammy sweat.

Yet many who confess to a former considerable practice of masturbation are physically robust, mentally active, and open and courageous in manner. The natural temperament of the individual will greatly modify and influence the effect wrought upon him by this demoralising and mischievous habit.

Treatment.—This resolves itself into moral and medical. To take the last first. Any local cause of irritation must be removed ; circumcision should be performed, and, with the view of breaking the habit, the skin of the penis may be painted with nitrate of silver or brushed with blistering fluid. The bowels should be regulated, the bladder emptied at once on waking from sleep, cold or nearly cold sponging and bathing should be daily employed, and the general health improved by wholesome diet, fresh air, healthy exercise, and proper studies and amusements.

The moral treatment consists in properly guarding and overlooking the lad's habits, his friendships, his occupations ; not in a suspicious, mistrusting, and officious manner, but with the judicious kindliness which should inspire a parent, or a guardian, or master.

It matters not where a boy or youth may be placed— whether alone in an austere puritanical household or amongst the brisk and active companions of a large school—the habit may be formed and kept up.

It should be met and combated by parent or master, not in the spirit of a severe judge toward a criminal offender, but in the manner of the man of the world knowing human nature, aware of its weaknesses, and seeking to minimise them by sagacious sympathy and confidence-winning explicitness.

If such a course were taken, often enough, and in good time, there would be much less of this ruinous habit prevalent in school and college and in private study, and many fewer constitutions and nervous systems injured by a vicious practice commenced often more in ignorance than vice.

SPERMATORRHŒA.

By this term is generally understood the uncontrollable escape, more or less frequently, of seminal fluid, at other times than, and not as the result of, the natural sexual excitement of coitus or the injurious sexual excitement of masturbation. It is very important for the medical man to bear in mind that as the result of continence, especially in young men, semen is pressed out of the vesiculæ seminales during defæcation, especially if the stools are hard and attended with much straining. The position of the vesiculæ seminales between the bladder and the lower part of the rectum, both of which organs are at the same time undergoing expulsive efforts, makes such a discharge from time to time of mechanical necessity and quite natural.

Again, nocturnal seminal emissions in men who observe continence and lead sedentary lives, and especially in young men, are quite natural and consistent with perfect sexual health, provided such emissions do not occur at shorter intervals than ten days to a fortnight. Again, let it be borne in mind that spermatozoa may be found in certain samples of a healthy man's urine as the result of the first flushing of the urethra after a coitus or an emission. And, lastly, the medical adviser should satisfy himself that the fluid which escapes from the urethra is really semen, and not mucus from the prostate, or muco-pus from a stricture or a gleet.

When nocturnal seminal emissions occur weekly, or twice or three times a week, or even oftener, they produce a relaxation of mental and physical tone. This is shown by inability for mental exertion or concentration of attention, flaccidity of will, hysteria, despondency, lassitude, aching back and lower limbs, dull pains in the groins, the feeling of something having given way across the loins, palpitation, cold clammy perspiration, and a whole train of dyspeptic symptoms, with constipation of the bowels.

Such a debilitated state of the sexual apparatus may be induced by long or frequently-practised masturbation till seminal emissions occur on the slightest provocation, sometimes without any or only with the most imperfect erection, and with a minimum of pleasurable sensation.

Treatment.—The most important factor is the proper regulation of the daily life of the patient. A nutritious unstimulating diet, especially avoiding beer, wine, and spirits at night; a due amount of walking or other out-of-doors exercise, so as to produce a degree of physical fatigue by bedtime; going to bed in good time; early rising, and then at once plunging into a cold or nearly cold bath, or if this cannot be borne, sponging the genitals, perinæum, and lower part of the abdomen with cold water; well-directed mental occupation, or travelling, or a sea voyage. These are the best remedies to prescribe.

If any local cause of irritation exists, it should be removed. An itching pile, a loaded rectum, intestinal worms, a long or tight foreskin, an engorged prostate, or an irritable bladder, may need attention.

The engorgement of the prostate is a thing of simple occurrence and easy remedy. It occurs in the early morning by the weight of the night's accumulated urine, and then erections and, with them, emission or temptation to masturbate, occur.

If the man who is the subject of too frequent nocturnal emissions, or who has practised masturbation, would empty his bladder immediately on waking, and at once get up and take his bath he would go far towards curing his weakness.

The drugs which are of any use are strychnine, quinine, the mineral acids and bitter infusions, and arsenic. The preparations of iron are sometimes recommended, but they are apt, I think, to excite the sexual organs, and, though admirable as tonics, are not so beneficial in debility of the sexual organs as the other medicines I have named. Sedatives are not often needed, but, when required, hyoscyamus with camphor, or small doses of opium or morphia with camphor, had best be prescribed. The bowels should be kept in regular action, and any errors of digestion corrected by exercise and the proper selection and regulation of diet.

SEXUAL HYPOCHONDRIASIS.

Sir James Paget has directed attention to *sexual hypo-chondriasis*, by which he means the hypochondriasis of men who attach undue importance to a varicocele, or to some slight affection of, or some imaginary evil in their sexual organs. It may be applied also to those who, having some graver form of seminal weakness, or one of the forms of impotence or sterility, allow their minds to dwell upon their sexual organs and functions with unreasonable pertinacity or desponding apprehension. Some of the patients are easily cured by a few words of comfort and the confidence which follows the removal of their ignorant fears. Some, as Sir J. Paget has written, "fall in love and marry, and are cured; some, getting into the weighty responsibilities of life, have things to think about more important than their sexual organs; and in all, as they grow older, the spinal marrow becomes less irritable, so that the emissions become less frequent and are attended with less feeling of exhaustion."

On the other hand, some drift under the influence of quacks and charlatans, and become hopelessly incurable, help-lessly epileptic, or piteously insane. I have had three or four cases of great sexual excitement, associated with frequent emissions, or with feeble erections and hasty ejaculations, in men who have begged of me to castrate them. One man of fine physique and great athletic powers, who, however, as he advanced towards middle age, became stout and bloated in appearance, has appealed to me on two or three occasions, at lengthened intervals, to castrate him, believing that to be the only way to relieve him of his "distressing sexual fire and passion, which could not be gratified because of his imperfect erections and rapid emissions." I declined in each case to adopt this treatment. Castration, ligature of the spermatic arteries, and excision of a portion of each vas deferens has been employed in cases of onanism and of epilepsy and insanity connected with spermatorrhœa; but these operations have, with very few exceptions, been of mere temporary benefit when not absolutely without any effect whatever.

IMPOTENCE.

The *causes* of impotence have been classified by the younger Gross as atonic, psychical, symptomatic, and organic.

The *organic* causes include absence, defects, and deformities of the penis or testes of either congenital or acquired origin; and large scrotal herniæ or hydrocele, by bringing the body of the penis far behind the protruded skin of the organ. Elephantiasis of the scrotum and penis may produce the same result as herniæ or hydrocele.

The *symptomatic* causes are either (a) certain acute or chronic diseases, such as diabetes, albuminuria, and organic and functional affections of the brain or spinal cord; or (b) injuries to the brain or spinal cord, such as concussion or compression of the brain, or fracture of the spinal column; or (c) the prolonged use of certain drugs, such as the bromides, iodides, opium, conium, camphor, arsenic, lead-poisoning, the fumes of antimony, excessive use of tobacco, and the abuse of alcoholic liquors.

The *psychical* causes are generally compound, due in part to some physical weakness or imperfection, and in larger part to the anxiety or sensitiveness of the individual on account thereof. As Mr. Jacobson expresses it, " sexual intercourse requires for its satisfactory performance the co-ordinated and harmonious action of mind and body." Some slight physical imperfection or want of general tone may give rise to a feeling of fear of impotence, or of mistrust of self, or an exaggerated idea of the effects of past masturbation, or the memory of an unsatisfactory coitus may take possession of the mind, and an imaginary or false impotence will be the result. The mere thought that a sexual intercourse will be impossible or unsatisfactory is quite sufficient cause to make it so. Many writers refer to personal repugnance, to suspicion of infidelity, to disgust, and to the dread of some ill consequence following the intercourse as temporary causes of impotence.

The *atonic* causes are attributed to a diseased state of the reflex lumbar centre, whereby a defective condition of the erectile organism is induced, erection being either feeble or impossible, and ejaculation precipitate. Gross recognises three forms of atonic impotence—(1) erection is imperfect, ejaculation quick, but sexual desire is present ; (2) erection very feeble or absent, but the sexual desire is present; (3) entire loss of erection and of desire also.   Professor Gross considered this form of impotence the result of masturbation or excessive sexual intercourse.   Such patients are prone to vesical irritation or to spermatic, gleety, or prostatic discharges, and are the subjects of hypochondriasis.

The *treatment* of impotence must vary with the cause. Some of the physical or organic causes are beyond treatment of any kind; the same must be said of some of the symptomatic causes, though impotence due to others of this class is benefited or removed by remedies which improve or cure the disease.   When caused by the prolonged use of drugs, tobacco, or stimulants, the peccant habit must be discontinued.

The psychical and atonic causes are many of them only temporary, and some are quite imaginary.   When stricture, phymosis, vesical or prostatic irritation, gleet, or prostatorrhœa exist, they must be treated by appropriate means.   Seminal emissions must be met by regulation of diet, stimulants, and habits of life.   When fear, over-anxiety, despondency, or mistrust is the cause, it must be combated by common-sense advice, by the employment of tonics, especially iron, sanmetto, strychnine, and quinine, and by encouraging the patient to allow sexual matters to take their own course, and to avoid any forced efforts at intercourse.

STERILITY.

Impotence is the incapacity for coitus ; sterility is the inability to procreate.   The two conditions may, but do not necessarily, coexist.   A man may be sterile, yet sexually vigorous; he may be partially impotent, with feeble erection and rapid ejaculation, yet his semen may be fertile and be thus capable of impregnating the female; but if completely impotent, then is the man sterile also.

Sterility is caused (1) by the absence of spermatozoa in the seminal fluid—**azoospermia** ; (2) by the absence of any seminal fluid—**aspermia** ; (3) by failure of the ejected semen in reaching the vagina, owing to some malformation of the male organ.

(1) In the first form of male sterility there may be good natural power of erection and ejaculation, but the emitted fluid lacks that which alone can impregnate—namely, spermatozoa. This may proceed from deficient, defective, injured, or diseased *testes,* and may be either permanent or temporary. When the testes are present and form spermatozoa, sterility may be due to obstruction in the *epididymis* or *vas deferens,* the result of a mass of unabsorbed inflammatory deposit, or of new growth in the globus major or minor, or of injury or rupture of the vas deferens. Syphilitic or tubercular affections of the testis may check the formation of spermatozoa; the same affections of the epididymis or vas may obstruct the passage of the semen. Pus derived from any part of the generative tract, when present in the semen, may destroy the vitality of the spermatozoa, as shown in three cases recorded by Terrillon and Jacobson. Past venereal excesses and certain chronic constitutional diseases lead to azoospermia.

It is in the cases of male sterility from absence of spermatozoa in the ejected fluid that the defect in procreating is often attributed wrongly to the wife. The husband's power of copulation and emission being satisfactory, and both husband and wife being anxious for offspring, the wife is often subjected to a variety of useless treatment which a microscopical examination of the husband's fluid would spare her.

(2) In the second form—aspermia—the power of copulation is present, but there is no emission. The causes as given by Professor Gross are—

(*a*) Obstruction in the ejaculatory ducts or urethra from congenital or acquired causes; the formation of concretions composed of mucus, detached epithelium, or of spermatozoa blocking the ejaculatory ducts; possibly stricture of the urethra.

(*b*) Paralysis of the reflex nerve centre presiding over the sexual act which will lead to want of contractility of the muscular structures of the seminal vesicles, ducts, or urethra, such contractility being necessary for emission.

(*c*) Loss of sensibility of the cutaneous nerves of the penis, and of those of the glans penis. This has been known to follow spinal injury, and also to result from ulceration and subsequent formation of indurated scar tissue over the penis.

(*d*) Cerebral inhibition of the ejaculatory centre. This, though given as a distinct group by Professor Gross, is not, however, a form of sterility. The man is not potentially sterile, but through an act of his will prevents an emission by discontinuing coitus before its consummation, or retards the emission till after withdrawal from the vagina.

(3) In certain rare instances of epispadias and hypospadias the semen cannot be injected into the vagina, though the power of copulation may exist.

Treatment.—Many of the above-named causes being permanent and irremediable, nothing can be done in the way of treatment. When the cause is temporary or removable, as in stricture of the urethra, phimosis, concretions in the prostatic portion of the ejaculatory ducts, the proper treatment for these conditions will remedy the cause of sterility.

CHAPTER V.

HYDROCELE.

WHAT is generally understood by the term hydrocele is a chronic affection, the most common form being "Vaginal Hydrocele," that is, a chronic accumulation of serum in the tunica vaginalis of the testicle.

ACUTE HYDROCELE.

When, as the result of contusion, punctured wound, epididymitis, or orchitis, an effusion rapidly takes place into the tunica vaginalis ; and when the same thing occurs during the course of erysipelas, rheumatism, or one of the continued fevers, *Acute Hydrocele*, or what the French call *Acute Vaginalitis*, is said to exist. All such acute effusions are of an inflammatory character, the fluid being rich in cells of various kinds, and much more readily and spontaneously coagulable than ordinary hydrocele fluid. Such effusions may, if very plastic, become organised into permanent adhesions, such as frequently result from the radical cure of common hydrocele by injection ; or if the inflammation is very intense, or the patient in bad general health, suppuration may follow ; but ordinarily, the fluid is rapidly and completely removed by absorption, under the same treatment which is employed for the promotion of absorption of inflammatory exudations in other parts of the body. It is not common, though it happens sometimes that an acute hydrocele passes into the chronic form.

The acute hydrocele is always secondary to some injury, or disease of the testicle or epididymis. The symptoms are at first merged with those of the disease of the testicle upon which the inflammation of the vaginal membrane depends ; and hence the fact that acute vaginalitis is so frequently overlooked. When pus is formed there are the usual local and general signs of suppuration, and if the matter is not let out the skin ulcerates, an offensive fistula results, and a true hernia of the tubules of the testicle may follow. To avoid this untoward termination the serous fluid should be drawn off early by the aspirator if the vaginal sac becomes markedly distended ; and as soon as signs of suppuration appear, a free incision should be made and the cavity of the tunica vaginalis well irrigated with some antiseptic solution.

The following classification of chronic hydrocele is based on that given by Mr. Jacobson in his admirable work on Diseases of the Male Organs of Generation :—

HYDROCELE.

I.—Hydrocele of the testis.

(a) **Hydrocele of the tunica vaginalis—i.e. vaginal hydrocele.**

1. *Ordinary hydrocele.*—The fluid distends the closed sac of the tunica vaginalis.
2. *Congenital hydrocele.*—A communication exists between the cavity of the tunica vaginalis and the cavity of the peritoneum.
3. *Infantile hydrocele.*—The tunica vaginalis and the funiculo-vaginal process are distended with fluid, but are shut off from the peritoneal cavity.
4. *Inguinal hydrocele.*—Hydrocele in relation with a retained testis.

(b) **Encysted hydrocele.**—The fluid is in a sac distinct from the sac of the tunica vaginalis.

1. *Encysted hydrocele of the epididymis.*—The fluid is in a cyst in the neighbourhood of the epididymis.
2. *Encysted hydrocele of the testis.*—The fluid is encysted between the tunica albuginea and the inner surface of the tunica vaginalis.

II.—Hydrocele of the cord.

(a) **Diffused.**—The fluid forms a serous collection of the nature of œdema in the cellular tissue of the cord, and it ought not to be called hydrocele.

(b) **Encysted.**—The fluid is contained in a distinct sac, originating usually in (1) some unobliterated part of the funiculo-vaginal process; (2) in a cyst formed independently of this process.

(c) **Congenital hydrocele of the cord.**—The fluid is contained in the funiculo-vaginal process, which is shut off from the cavity of the tunica vaginalis testis, but not from that of the peritoneum.

III.—Complications of hydrocele.

(a) **With other co-existing hydroceles.**—E.g. (1) Hydrocele of the tunica vaginalis with encysted hydrocele of the testis; (2) hydrocele of the tunica vaginalis with encysted hydrocele of the cord; (3) hydrocele of the tunica vaginalis with diffused hydrocele of the cord.

(b) **With hernia.**—E.g. (1) Hydrocele of the tunica vaginalis with inguinal hernia; (2) hydrocele of the cord with inguinal hernia; (3) hydrocele of the tunica vaginalis of an imperfectly descended testis with a hernia.

IV.—Hydrocele of the sac of a hernia.

HYDROCELE OF THE TUNICA VAGINALIS.

Pathology. Characters of the Fluid.—The fluid, which in this form of hydrocele is contained in the sac of the serous covering of the testicle, is closely allied to ordinary serum. Its specific gravity is a fraction higher than that of healthy urine, 1022 to 1025 ; its reaction is neutral, and it contains about six per cent. of albumen, and a small amount of fibrinogen ;

thus it coagulates readily with any of the ordinary tests for albumen, but the fluid does not, as a rule, spontaneously coagulate. It is odourless and limpid and transparent, but varies in colour from a pale straw to a turbid green, unless mixed with blood, when it acquires a dull red or brownish colour.

Occasionally it is charged with cholesterin crystals, derived probably from the shedding and fatty degeneration of the cells lining the sac; the fluid is then glistening and less limpid. Alkaline carbonates and sodium chloride are contained in hydrocele fluid in marked amount. Under the microscope only a few epithelial and blood cells are to be seen.

The amount of the fluid contained in the sac varies greatly. From four to twelve ounces is common; but it may exceed a pint, and Cline withdrew six quarts from the hydrocele of the historian Gibbon.

Changes in the Tunica Vaginalis and the other Structures involved in Hydrocele.— In large hydroceles and those of long standing the scrotal tissues are thinned, the cul-de-sac between the testis and epididymis

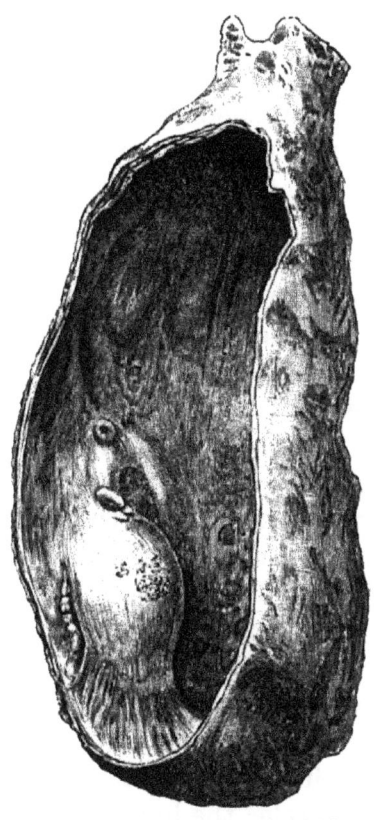

Fig. 14.—Large Hydrocele with a Pouch between the Testicle and Epididymis, the orifice of which is seen in the Figure. (From a specimen in the Hunterian Museum.) (*Jacobson.*)

is distended, and the epididymis is pushed away from the testis, and thus the vasa efferentia are elongated by stretching. If the hydrocele has been unirritated, the tunica vaginalis remains unchanged, except for more or less stretching; but in old, neglected, or injured hydroceles the tunica becomes opaque and thick, or cartilaginous, or calcified throughout or in patches, or it may acquire warty outgrowths on its surface.

E

When the tunica has undergone these changes, the subserous connective tissue and the fibrous tissue of the testicle are thickened and condensed, the testicle sclerosed, flattened, and atrophied, and the epididymis indurated. In some cases the sac of the tunica vaginalis is more or less obliterated; or it assumes an hour-glass shape called by the French the hydrocele *en bissac.* This shape may be due either (*a*) to a localised thickening of the tunica vaginalis, which renders a portion of it less yielding than the rest; or (*b*) to a pouching of the tunica vaginalis, as in a case reported by Mr. Gould (*Lancet*, 1890, p. 894). Glove-like diverticula of the tunica vaginalis may form, and Béraud long ago (1856, " Arch. Gén. de Méd.") suggested that these may give rise to bilocular hydrocele. Mr. Curling drew attention to the occasional formation of a sac or pouch by the depression of the tunica vaginalis between the epididymis and testis. In this manner a pouch distended with the hydrocele fluid is formed on the back and inner side of the testis, the opening into it being seen only on the outer side of the organ (Fig. 14). A typical specimen of this sort exists in the Hunterian Museum, and is often shown to candidates at the examinations at the College of Surgeons.

In some rare cases the vaginal cavity, after the injection treatment, is converted into a number of distinct and separate compartments, having little or no communication with one another. I have met with this condition well marked, following the iodine treatment, in an elderly man with a very large hydrocele; the hydrocele refilled, and, on again tapping, only a part of the reaccumulated fluid was removed until the cannula was pushed in several different directions, by which means one compartment after another was tapped and emptied; the hydrocele was thus eventually cured without further injection. It is rare for a hydrocele to become spontaneously cured, or to rupture, or to suppurate, but each of these terminations has occurred.

The Position of the Testicle is usually below and behind, but in very large hydroceles the sac may reach much lower than the testicle, which is then behind and about half-way down the enla   testicle is anteverted, it will be situated in   ront part of the hydrocele, as it may be, too, if, from inflammatory adhesions, the testicle is adherent to the parietal part of the tunica.

Causes of Hydrocele.—It is a matter of dispute whether common hydrocele is of inflammatory origin and always *secondary* to some other pathological condition—such as disease of the testicle or epididymis,—to urethral stricture, affections of the prostate or suchlike, or whether it is a *primary*, idiopathic, and non-inflammatory affection.

It is quite certain that in the great majority of cases the patients are unaware of having suffered from any of the diseases above named, that their hydroceles have come insidiously and without any apparent cause, and that if secondary to something else the primary affection is unknown and quiescent.

As a rule, I believe the effusion of fluid is quite independent of any inflammation, and is a mere passive process

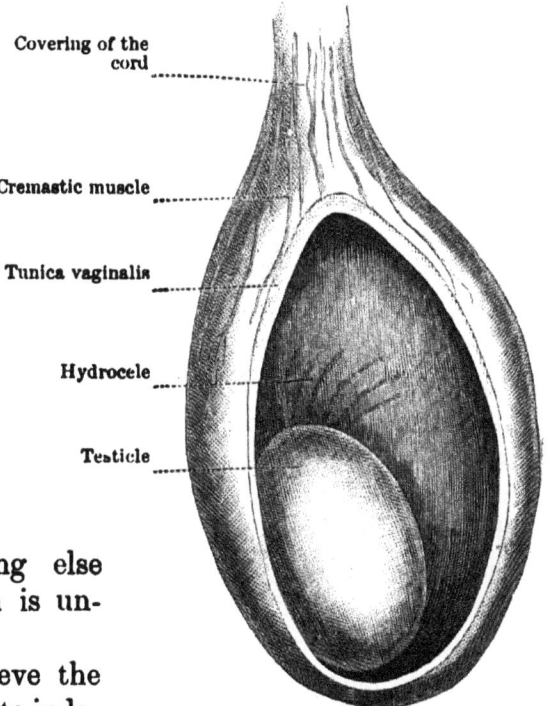

Covering of the cord

Cremastic muscle

Tunica vaginalis

Hydrocele

Testicle

Fig. 15.—Hydrocele of Tunica Vaginalis. (*Sutton.*)

due to the anatomical and mechanical conditions of the vessels and circulation of the cord and testicle. But it must be recognised that there are two classes of hydroceles: (*a*) those *secondary* to some other disease, such as syphilis, tubercle, or chronic inflammation of the testicle, in which cases the hydrocele is generally very small and often acute, and (*b*) *primary idiopathic* hydroceles, which are frequently of large size.

Amongst the exciting causes of vaginal hydrocele, and a very pregnant one in exciting the early reaccumulation of the fluid after tapping, are the *fibrous bodies* which are met with either attached or free in the tunica vaginalis, but much more frequently attached. They are generally solid, but are sometimes cystic. They are very rarely cartilaginous, but occasionally become calcified.

When attached, they may be (1) irregularly scattered over the visceral portion of the tunica vaginalis, and are then of inflammatory origin; or (2) situated between the globus major and the testis proper. The latter form are the result of inflammatory changes in the vesicle or hydatid described by Morgagni, now known to be a relic of the duct of Müller. This vesicle may be quite converted into a small, fibrous, solid body, or, retaining its cystic character, may be converted into one of the forms of encysted hydrocele. These bodies are only met with in adult life, and chiefly in advanced age. They are an exciting cause of vaginal hydrocele, and have been known to excite very severe suffering immediately after the fluid of a hydrocele has been withdrawn. When they are felt through the scrotum, and are a cause of hydrocele or of pain, they should be excised after laying open the tunica vaginalis.

Symptoms.—A pyriform swelling on one side of, and limited to the scrotum, with a smooth and uniform outline, elastic to the touch, translucent, giving no impulse on coughing, dull on percussion, and often giving a thrill on percussion, are symptoms which, when associated, are characteristic of common vaginal hydrocele. But these characteristics may vary or be absent. Both *sides* of the scrotum are about equally often affected alone, and in about one case in every four or five both sides are affected together. The *shape*, instead of being pear-shaped, with the long axis obliquely upwards, may be round or oblong, and may have its longer axis transverse. *Translucency* may be wanting either because of the opacity of the fluid from admixture of blood, or from the milky or syrupy or turbid nature of the fluid in some old hydroceles; or from the opacity and thickening of the tunica vaginalis and other tissues of the scrotum; or owing to adhesions within the vaginal sac, and to the multilocular character of the hydrocele.

Translucency may be present in a scrotal swelling other than hydrocele, though extremely rarely, as in some herniæ of infants (Beck, *Brit. Med. Journ.*, Dec. 2, 1892), and in hydatid of the scrotum. *Fluctuation or thrill* may be marked or absent altogether. When the sac is very tense or its walls thickened, or its contents not limpid, the thrill will not be obtainable at all.

The increase in size is slow and painless, but a dragging effect is experienced in the groin and loin. If the swelling increases along the cord, especially if it reaches upwards to the abdominal ring, an elongated process like the finger of a glove is produced (Fig. 16). When there is a hydrocele on each side, and they are· large, the skin of the penis may be so dragged forwards that the glans penis is quite lost behind it. In a case of an old man with prostatic obstruction and double hydrocele with double scrotal hernia, the glans penis was so far behind the surface that it could not b'e felt; and a catheter to relieve retention could not be introduced until by aid of a tri-valved female urethra dilator the external meatus was found. After tapping the hydroceles the prepuce was still somewhat pressed forwards, but the glans penis could be distinguished.

In some cases this condition leads to eczema or excoriation of

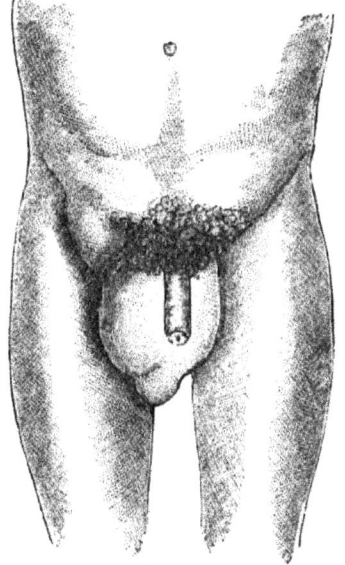

Fig. 16.—Hydrocele of Tunica Vaginalis with Distension of Tubular Prolongation upwards and unusually prominent position of Testis below. (*Morris, American Journ. Med. Sciences.*)

the scrotum from the urine not being projected clear of the patient's body.

Diagnosis.—Hydrocele is to be diagnosed from scrotal hernia, from hæmatocele, from solid tumours, and from other forms of hydrocele.

From Hernia.—Hydrocele increases from below upwards, hernia from above downwards. Hydrocele does not diminish or disappear of itself, hernia often diminishes or recedes entirely in the recumbent position. Hydrocele is always dull, and may give a thrill on percussion; hernia never gives a thrill, unless the sac contains a large quantity of fluid, and is frequently in part or in whole resonant on percussion. When the hernia

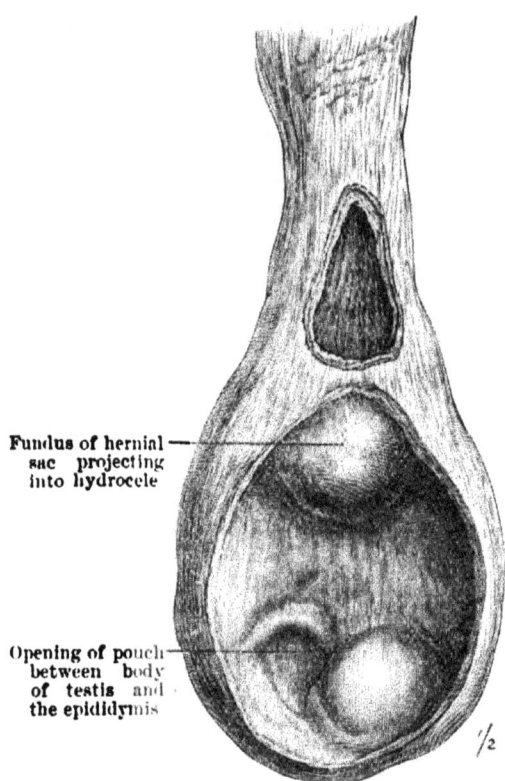

Fundus of hernial
sac projecting
into hydrocele

Opening of pouch
between body
of testis and
the epididymis

/2

Fig. 17.—Sac of Hydrocele of the Tunica
Vaginalis, associated with Inguino-scrotal
Hernia. (Middlesex Hospital Museum.)

contains omentum and is entirely dull on percussion, it feels uneven and nodular —not uniform, like hydrocele. Hydrocele gives no impulse on coughing, hernia does. Hydrocele has a look of standing-off from the body and is tense, hernia has a more pendulous look and the skin over it is not tense. Hydrocele can be pressed bodily towards the perinæum and springs up again when released, hernia cannot be made to do this. Hydrocele is translucent, hernia not (except very rarely in children). In hydrocele the upper part of the cord can be felt, but the testicle is obscure. In hernia the upper part of the cord is obscure, but the testicle is readily made out. Hydrocele, it must be remembered, is often complicated with hernia. (See Figs. 17 and 18.)

From Hæmatocele.—Hydrocele is not usually preceded by violence, hæmatocele is caused by straining or an injury. Hydrocele is elastic, hæmatocele solid and heavy. Hydrocele is translucent, hæmatocele opaque. The skin covering hydrocele is not discoloured, in hæmatocele it is generally ecchymosed, and if the extravasated blood be external to

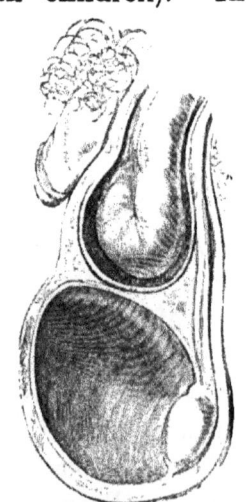

Fig. 18.—The Ordinary
Relation of a Vaginal
Hydrocele and Scrotal
Hernia. (*Curling.*)

the tunica vaginalis the ecchymosis is intense and widespread, reaching sometimes into the inguinal and hypogastric regions.

From solid Tumours.—The want of elasticity, uniformity, and translucency; the rapid enlargement; pain; and, at any rate in the earlier stages of enlargement, the outline of the testicle and epididymis more or less changed, all point to a solid tumour of the testicle. In cancer the affection of the lymph-glands, the solid infiltration along the cord; in tubercle and cancer the ulceration of the skin and formation of a fungus, and the impaired general health are present in the more advanced stages.

From encysted Hydrocele of the Testis. —In the early stages encysted hydrocele is small and round; if the cysts are multiple, they may present a botryoidal outline. They may have existed for years before enlarging sufficiently to simulate vaginal hydrocele. In encysted hydrocele the testicle is commonly below and in front, or to the inner side of the cyst; it may be on the outer side, but is scarcely ever behind.

I have once or twice seen a form of vaginal hydrocele which closely simulated a large cyst between the globus major and body of testis. In these cases the globus major and body

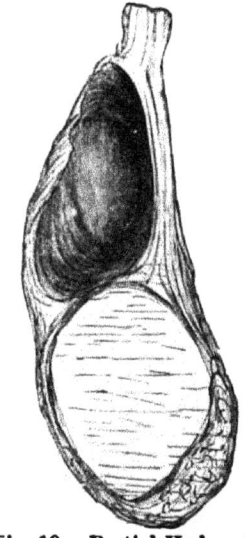

Fig. 19.—**Partial Hydrocele of the Tunica Vaginalis.** The parietal and visceral surfaces of the tunica are everywhere adherent, except above. (*Osborn.*)

of the epididymis were enlarged by tubercular disease and the lower part of the testis was adherent to the parietal tunica vaginalis. Thus the vaginal hydrocele was limited, and formed a circumscribed collection between the globus major and the upper end of the body of the testis, which were widely dragged apart by the fluid. Mr. Osborn has illustrated a hydrocele of a part only of the tunica vaginalis (Fig. 19).

From encysted or diffuse Hydrocele of the Cord.—These forms of hydrocele start in the cord and increase downwards. They are confined to the region of the cord often for months or years before they encroach upon the tunica vaginalis, though they may at length invaginate the vaginal sac from above, and, increasing, occupy a large share of the scrotum (Fig. 20).

From Hydrocele of a Hernial Sac, by the history of the case; but if this is unsatisfactory and the hernia is scrotal, it cannot be distinguished from an infantile hydrocele or a vaginal hydrocele with an inguinal process. Le Dran mentions a case of a man with three forms of hydrocele on the same side—viz. a hydrocele of a hernial sac, a hydrocele of the cord, and a vaginal hydrocele of the scrotum. I have operated in a case where a vaginal hydrocele was associated with an encysted hydrocele of the cord and a bubonocele.

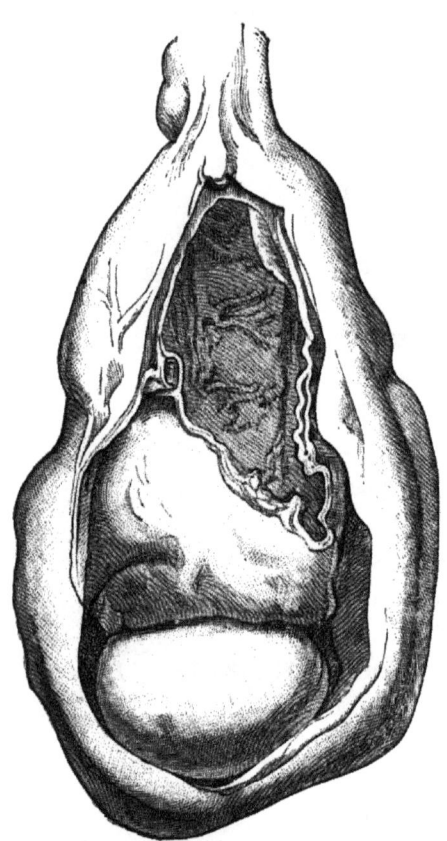

Fig. 20.—Hydrocele of the Tunica Vaginalis and an Encysted Hydrocele of the Epididymis of the same Testis. (Middlesex Hospital.) (*Sutton.*)

Treatment. — Spontaneous cures occur not rarely in children, but are not to be looked for in adults. In young children the fluid may be absorbed by stimulating or discutient lotions; in adults, hydrocele may disappear after an attack of inflammation of the testicle. Acupuncture has also succeeded in boys, but is not to be recommended. It is on account of the bulk, weight, or unsightliness—not because of pain or danger to life—that treatment is required. In children and boys and quite young adults damage may be done, however, to the testicle, owing to the dragging effects on the vasa efferentia and epididymis, and to the atrophy of the testicle by thickening of its tunica albuginea and fibrous sclerosis of the gland tissue. (*See* Atrophy, page 31.)

The *palliative* treatment consists in drawing off the fluid by tapping with a fine trocar and cannula. The patient may either stand against a table, or sit over the front of a chair, or be lying on his back. The surgeon should then make the swelling tense by pressing it forwards between his thumb on one side and his fingers on the other. With a wax match or the flame of a candle he should test the translucency of the swelling, and make out the position of the testicle so as to avoid wounding it with the trocar; he should also avoid puncturing a cutaneous vein. To prevent thrusting the instrument too deeply, he should place the tip of his index-finger at a proper distance from the sharp point. He then pushes the trocar into the front of the sac somewhat below its centre, and in a direction upwards and inwards. The trocar is removed from the cannula, the whole of the contents of the sac evacuated, and the cannula withdrawn whilst nipping the integuments tightly between the left finger and thumb. A flake of cotton-wool is all the dressing which need be applied to the little wound. If, before withdrawing the cannula, the interior of the sac is scratched with its end, and the patient walks a mile or so afterwards, it is possible that sufficient inflammatory action may be excited in the sac radically to cure a recent and medium-sized hydrocele. This cannot be relied upon, but I have known it to succeed. A curious accident has been known to follow the tapping of a large and old hydrocele with a large trocar—the puncture not contracting, the tunica vaginalis became filled with air.

The radical or curative Treatment.—The methods employed for the radical cure of hydrocele are (1) injections, (2) setons, (3) incision, (4) partial excision of the sac.

Injections.—This is a time-honoured treatment, and, on the whole, is very successful when properly performed, and when done for small and moderate-sized hydroceles in which the sac is not cartilaginous, calcified, or greatly thickened, and where no loose or pedunculated bodies are present within the sac.

Many different fluids have been used: alcohol (Munro), port wine (Sir B. Brodie), port wine diluted one-third with a decoction of rose-leaves (Earle), mercury perchloride, zinc sulphate, ergotine, muriated tincture of iron, tincture of iodine (Sir R. Martin and Velpeau), and carbolic acid (Levis) have all had their trial. On the whole, I prefer either the carbolic acid treatment or the linimentum iodi diluted with twice its quantity of water. The hydrocele must be tapped with the precaution against wounding the testicle given on page 57. From half an ounce to an ounce of the iodine solution, according to the size of the hydrocele, should be injected, after the complete evacuation of the sac, by means of a syringe well fitting the cannula. The whole of the iodine fluid should be allowed to remain in the sac for

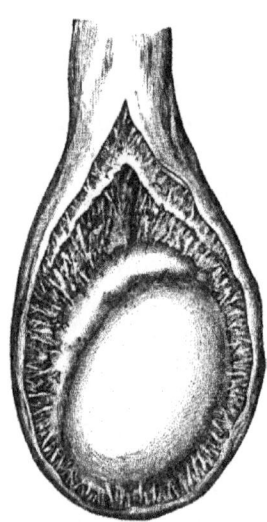

Fig. 21.—Sac of Vaginal Hydrocele obliterated by Adhesions after Injection of Iodine. (London Hospital Museum.) (*J. Cantlie.*)

a minute or two, and be pressed from one part to the other within it; then half of it may be withdrawn by the syringe and the other half left. Care should be taken, when drawing out the cannula, to grip the scrotal tissues firmly round the instrument, so as to avoid the escape of any of the iodine into the cellular tissue. The patient should be lying down during the operation, else he may faint, as a very sharp, burning pain reaching along the groin to the loin, and accompanied with a sensation of sickness, is generally experienced. After the operation the recumbent position should be maintained for three or four days if much inflammatory swelling ensues. The bowels should be well opened before operation, and the diet moderately restricted afterwards. Swelling begins within an hour or two, and is most variable in degree. Sometimes a cure will result without enough to inconvenience the patient; in other cases, the size reached in three or four days is as great as the hydrocele, and seven or eight days will elapse before the patient can move about. In three or four weeks the swelling will have entirely disappeared, and the cure will be complete.

The mode of cure is either by universal or partial adhesion of the parietal to the visceral portion of the tunica vaginalis (Fig. 21), or by converting the serous membrane to a dull, dry, fibrous condition without power of secreting.

When carbolic acid is used, it should be injected by means

of a syringe, with a nozzle sufficiently long and slender to pass through the cannula into the hydrocele sac (Levis) : or by means of a large exploring hypodermic syringe, the needle of which, when charged, should be passed into the sac before withdrawing the fluid ; then the sac should be emptied by a small trocar and cannula in the ordinary way, and when the sac has been quite emptied and the cannula withdrawn the carbolic solution should be discharged from the syringe into the sac. (Jacobson.) By manipulation, the carbolic should be brought into contact with the whole of the interior surface of the sac. Levis advised the injection of a drachm of the crystals of carbolic acid, dissolved in five per cent. of glycerine. Others have used much less (ten to twenty minims), repeating the injection twice, or oftener if required. Others, again, have used much more of the concentrated fluid, but, on the whole, it is best used as Levis advised. The injection gives rise to a sense of warmth, followed by numbness ; it causes no pain, and is said to be more certain, attended with less inflammation, and to require less time for the cure—twenty-four to thirty-six hours being the usual time for confinement to the house.

The untoward effects and accidents which may follow the injection of either iodine or carbolic acid are too much inflammation, cellulitis, sloughing, and suppuration in the sac or abscess in the scrotum. Recurrence takes place occasionally after each method ; indeed, hydrocele recurs after every known method of treatment. As a rare occurrence, carbolic acid poisoning has followed the use of this drug. (Dr. J. Murray, *New York Med. Record*, June 20th, 1891.)

Some of the French surgeons have used with success solid nitrate of silver, fused on to the end of a probe or director. After emptying the hydrocele sac, the instrument carrying the fused silver nitrate is introduced through the cannula, and moved about so as to bring the salt in contact with much of the surface of the sac.

Antiseptic incision, or, better still, *excision* of the whole of that part of the tunica vaginalis which lines the scrotum, but without attempting to interfere with that covering the testis and epididymis, should be employed in preference to injection in the following cases :—(1) where the sac is very thick and opaque, cartilaginous, or calcified ; (2) when there is doubt as to whether the hydrocele is of congenital nature, or is a hydrocele of a hernial sac, with a small opening into the peritoneum; (3) when hernia complicates hydrocele, and a radical cure of both is desired; (4) when a loose or pedunculated, fibrous body is present in the tunica vaginalis; (5) when there is a doubt as to whether there is or is not serious organic disease of the testis; (6) when a vaginal hydrocele is associated with a hydrocele of the cord and an inguinal hernia. (Morris, "Radical Cure of Hydrocele," *The International Journal of Medical Sciences*, August, 1888.) Many of the ancients practised excision of the parietal portion of the sac. In the eighteenth century Saviard, Garengeot, and Le Dran in France, and Douglas, Percival Pott, and Joseph Bell in this country, and Mr. S. Sharp (of Guy's), the great advocate of incision later, adopted partial excision. Formerly, with the incision treatment, the sac was stuffed with lint, and left to suppurate and granulate; Volkmann, in 1876, advocated "the antiseptic incision," and this has been largely used of late.

After either incision or excision it is advisable, in order to obtain complete obliteration of the sac, to scrape gently the surface of the serous membrane, or to rub it over with iodine, carbolic acid, zinc chloride, or silver nitrate, and throughout the healing to keep the wound well drained, and dressed from the bottom with gauze coated with boracic ointment or iodoform paste.

The treatment by seton, whether of silk, silver, or carbolised catgut, has nothing to recommend it, and need not be here further considered.

CONGENITAL HYDROCELE.

This is an accumulation of fluid in the tunica vaginalis and funiculo-vaginal process (or into the process alone) communicating with the peritoneal cavity owing to the non-obliteration of the process. The size of the communication varies from that of a hay-straw, or less, upwards. Though generally met with in infancy and soon after birth, its occurrence may be delayed for a long time, even till adult life.

The fluid in some cases is derived from the peritoneum, and accumulates by trickling from above; in other cases it is secreted by the vaginal sac and process.

Congenital hydrocele is to be distinguished from congenital hernia by being dull on percussion; reducible gradually, and without jerk or thud, and only on steady, continuous pressure; by its translucency, and by not gurgling on manipulation. It has, however, an impulse on coughing and crying.

It is of some danger, because, if owing to any affection of testicle or epididymis, or to injury or other cause, inflammation or suppuration occurs in the sac, fatal peritonitis may be the result.

The *treatment* consists in wearing a truss with the view of obliterating the funicular process; if this fails, the sac should be laid open, removed in part, and its neck ligatured.

The injection treatment is not to be recommended, though it has been employed without harm after a truss has been worn for a short time previously.

INFANTILE HYDROCELE

is not very uncommon; it differs from congenital hydrocele in that it is shut off from the peritoneal cavity by a partial obliteration of the funicular process, and generally as low down as the external abdominal ring. The fluid is, of course, derived from the vaginal sac itself.

It is also distinguished from the congenital hydrocele by the fact that it is quite irreducible, and does not lessen in size in the recumbent position or by elevating the scrotum. From hernia it is diagnosed by its translucency, its irreducibility, and absence of gurgling.

The only *treatment* required in most cases is acupuncture. If this fails, the incision and partial excision treatment will succeed. Jacobson says that in thirty-seven cases he has never known acupuncture fail, and that if this treatment be properly tried no other will be needed in infants. My experience in boyhood and in adults is that the partial excision treatment is best.

BILOCULAR HYDROCELE, OR HYDROCELE " EN BISSAC."

It has been mentioned in the description of the pathological changes of the tunica vaginalis in common hydrocele (page 50) that the vaginal cavity sometimes assumes an hour-glass shape, either from irregular expansion of the tunica or from its constriction by some inflammatory thickening; and to this form some of the French writers apply the term hydrocele *en bissac*. It has also been mentioned that a secondary sac, or a pouch, in communication with the general cavity of the tunica vaginalis, is sometimes found in common hydroceles by distension of the digital fossa between the testis and epididymis (Figs. 14 and 17); and, further, that another variety of hydrocele *en bissac* is produced by globular, oval, or finger glove-like diverticula or processes on the front or sides of the tunica vaginalis. In each of these varieties the two cavities communicate with one another by openings of varying and uncertain size; but the wall of the diverticulum or secondary pouch is generally less firm and less resistant than that of the vaginal sac, and it may, therefore, attain even a greater size than the tunica vaginalis itself. Such pouches are contained within the limits of the scrotum, and are characterised by their rapid development and extreme translucency.

A much rarer form of

BILOCULAR HYDROCELE

has still to be described. It consists of an *infantile* hydrocele with a prolongation of the sac into the abdominal or pelvic cavity.

In these cases the funiculo-vaginal process is unobliterated generally as high up as the internal ring; and it may remain open below as far down as the testis, or only to the top of the scrotum.

As the fluid in the hydrocele in these cases increases, it gradually passes into a pouch, which may attain even much greater dimensions than the funiculo-vaginal sac, and which reaches either upwards between the muscles of the anterior abdominal wall and the parietal peritoneum, or passes downwards between the pelvic peritoneum and the wall of the false or true pelvis.

Villeneuve collected eighteen examples of hydrocele *en bissac* (*Mercredi Médicale*, 6 Aout, 1890); and other cases of this sort have been reported by Syme, Humphry, Lister, M. Bazy (*Arch. Gén. de Méd.*, 1887, lxx. p. 553), and some others.

Symptoms.—There is a separation of the hydrocele into

two parts by a constriction situated in some cases at the external abdominal ring, in others higher or lower. The two parts or sacs communicate with each other by an opening of very varying size. The abdominal portion is usually much the larger, though in one of Kocher's cases it was much the smaller and only the size of a nut.

As the upper pouch enlarges, it presses the parietal peritoneum of the abdomen before it, and thus may rise as high as the umbilicus (Fig. 22), or more commonly presses back into the iliac fossa or descends into the pelvis. Fluctuation is generally communicated from one pouch to the other, and is sometimes obtained by the finger in the rectum. The intra-abdominal pouch has been known to press on the bladder and cause retention of urine, or much difficulty in micturition.

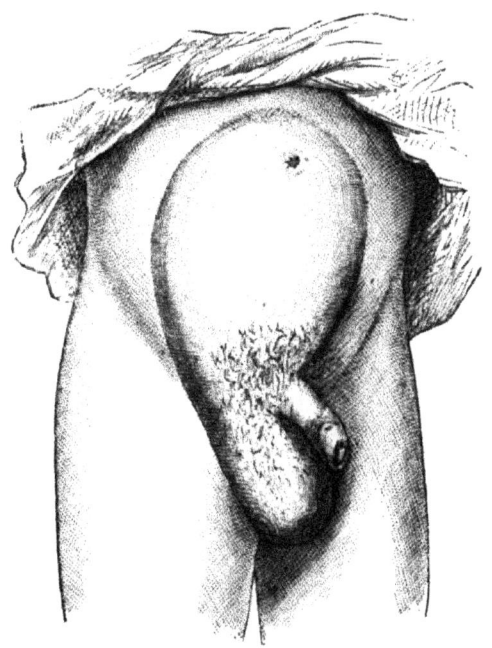

Fig. 22.—Bilocular Hydrocele, or Hydrocele *en Bissac.* (*After Bazy.*)

The best *treatment* is incision followed by excision of as much of the sac as can be readily separated from its connections. Care must be taken in dealing with the upper pouch, as it may have intimate adhesions to the peritoneum.

INGUINAL HYDROCELE

is the name given to common or vaginal hydrocele when the testis is undescended and occupies a position somewhere between the internal abdominal ring and the scrotum; or the testicle may have passed through the external ring and be situated between the aponeurosis of the external oblique muscle and the integuments. It presents itself as a tense fluctuating swelling, irreducible, and giving rise to the peculiar sickening testicular sensation when tightly squeezed, and it has often a slight impulse on coughing. The corresponding side of the scrotum will be unoccupied. If the testicle is found, after tapping, to be small, the best treatment is excision of the testis with the sac; castration is also the treatment if the hydrocele recurs after simple tapping.

FATTY, CHYLOUS, OR MILKY HYDROCELE.

These names are given to hydroceles which contain, in place of the usual straw-coloured fluid, a white fluid like cow's milk. After withdrawal this fluid settles, and becomes denser at the top than at the bottom, the fat floating and forming a layer like cream. In some cases it is a whitish-yellow milky fluid, in others, like pea-soup.

Many theories have been advanced to explain the characters of the fluid; but they can only be alluded to here under the following headings: (1) The parasitic, (2) the traumatic, (3) the lymphatic, and (4) the theory that they are due to fatty degenerative changes in the epithelium of the tunica vaginalis and the fluid of an ordinary hydrocele. (*See* Jacobson, pp. 176 *et seqq.*)

The *symptoms and diagnosis* of ordinary hydrocele are only modified in these cases by the want of translucency. The affection is sometimes double. In this form of hydrocele the blood should be examined for filaria, and the scrotum for incipient elephantiasis or lymph scrotum.

The *treatment* is antiseptic incision, and if leaking lymphatics are found they should be ligatured.

ENCYSTED HYDROCELE OF THE EPIDIDYMIS AND TESTIS.

The encysted hydroceles of the epididymis and testis differ widely in mode of origin from the encysted hydroceles of the cord. The latter are commonly due to the imperfect and irregular obliteration or want of obliteration of the funicular process of the peritoneum; they are described in Chapter XIII., Part I., under Diseases of the Spermatic Cord.

Hydroceles of the epididymis and testis are entirely new formations. The fluid is contained in a cyst distinct from the tunica vaginalis and shut out behind that membrane like the testicle and epididymis themselves. They are often called

Spermatoceles, a term implying that the fluid contained within them is mixed with spermatozoa; and this is true of the great majority, though not of all. In some of the smaller cysts no spermatozoa are found. As a rule, in the larger cysts the fluid is opalescent, milky, or like thin soap and water, owing to the large number of spermatozoa; and, no matter how often the cyst may be tapped, the re-collected fluid will contain these spermatozoa in abundance. Generally, the spermatozoa are lively and active, but in some instances they are quiescent, or even disintegrated, all traces of their tails being lost and only their heads remaining as small nucleus-like bodies.

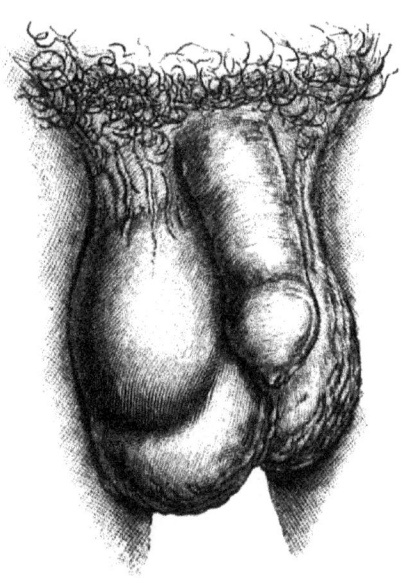

Encysted hydrocele of the epididymis and testis might be appropriately described as cysts or new growths of the testicle.

ENCYSTED HYDROCELE OF THE EPIDIDYMIS

occurs either as *small cysts* varying in size from a pin's head to a pea, frequently multiple, and found usually in persons over forty years of age; and *large cysts*, usually single, varying in size, though

Fig. 23.—Encysted Hydrocele. (From patient in Broderip ward, Middlesex Hospital.)

rarely containing more than two or three ounces, and met with generally in men between twenty-five and fifty years of age. They make their first appearance usually before the forty-fifth year.

The *small* cysts are unimportant clinically if they do not give rise to severe neuralgic pain in the testicle or scrotum or perinæum, though this they sometimes do. They project from the outer or free aspect of the head, body, or tail of the epididymis. They rarely occur till after middle life, but then become very common, being present, according to M. Gosselin, in two-thirds of the testicles examined. They may be sessile, or pedunculated, and they sometimes become detached and

F

form the "loose bodies" occasionally found in the tunica vaginalis. These cysts have a distinct fibrocellular wall and are lined by epithelium. They can be easily shelled out from their surroundings. The contained fluid is usually clear, limpid, and transparent, but if spermatozoa are present, which is rare, the fluid is of a turbid character. Spermatozoa are found in about eight per cent. of the cases, according to Lewin.

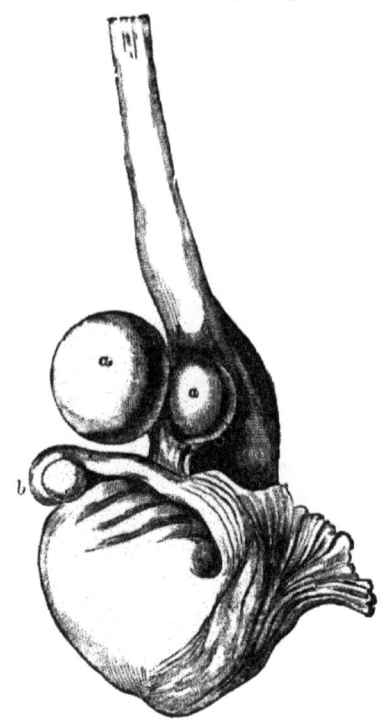

These small cysts originate either (*a*) in distension of traces of Müller's duct (especially the hydatid of Morgagni), which have not been obliterated (Figs. 24 and 25); or (*b*) as involution cysts connected with changes taking place in the epididymis of advancing life. According to this latter view (MM. Monod and Arthaud), they arise in ampullary dilatations of the ducts of the epididymis produced by the unequal dragging and compressing effects of sclerosis of the inter-tubular connective tissue. In this respect they resemble the cyst formations in the kidney, and the cystic degeneration of the mammary gland of women past middle life.

Fig. 24.—Spermatic Cysts. (*Jacobson.*)
a, Cysts originating in organ of Giraldes; b, cyst arising in position of hydatid of Morgagni.

The *large* cysts are usually single, though two or three may exist in the same organ. In some instances a cyst is divided into compartments by delicate septa. Both organs are frequently affected. They vary much in size, but do not usually contain more than a few ounces of fluid; but there are cases in which they have by their size obliterated the tunica vaginalis and compressed the testicle, and some few are recorded from which a pint and a half to over two pints of milky fluid rich in spermatozoa have been evacuated (*Med. Times and Gaz.*, 1853, vol. i. p. 629; and Dr. Cameron, *Lancet*, 1884, vol. i. p. 842).

I have recently seen a case under one of my colleagues in which both organs of an elderly man were affected with multiple encysted hydrocele of varying size from a white currant to an exceedingly large lemon. Some of them from time to time underwent rapid enlargement, attended with temporary but considerable heat, redness, and pain of the scrotum. Three or four of the largest of these encysted hydroceles were excised, and were found to contain a thin milky fluid and spermatozoa. Some time afterwards the scrotum became fuller than before, owing to the rapid enlargement of other cysts connected with each testis. Again the largest of them were excised, but many smaller cysts were left behind embedded in the tissue of the epididymis behind the tunica vaginalis.

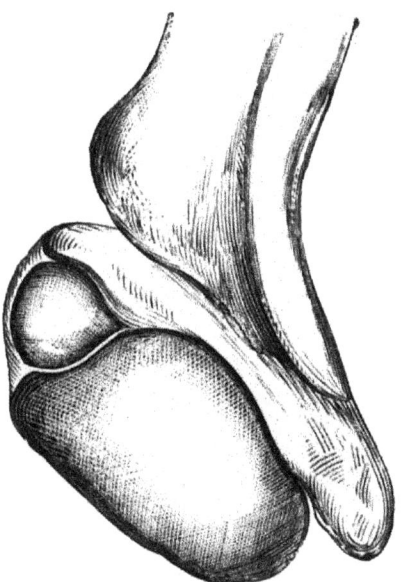

Fig. 25.—Encysted Hydrocele arising in Position of the left Corpus Morgagni. (*Osborn.*)

They are situated outside, *i.e.* behind the tunica vaginalis, though they often project into the cavity of that sac. They contain usually a limpid, colourless, non-albuminous, or nearly non-albuminous, fluid; but occasionally it is brown and mucoid, probably from a former extravasation of blood. The absence of albumen marks these cysts off from vaginal hydroceles, the fluid of which is rich in albumen and contains also fibrinogen.

The fluid of encysted hydroceles, on the other hand, is altogether unlike blood serum and inflammatory *serous* fluids; it is *seroid*, and resembles more cerebro-spinal and hydatid fluids and the aqueous humour of the eye. When it is opalescent or milky, it contains spermatozoa, which are, as a rule, found in the larger cysts in great abundance.

The fluid is alkaline from the presence of sodium chlorides, sodium phosphates, and alkaline carbonates; the carbonates are the cause of the fluids effervescing with acetic acid. The cysts when of long standing are lined with pavement epithelium, though, in recent cases, cubical, columnar, or even ciliated epithelium may be found.

The *large* cysts may be met with at any age after the twenty-fifth year. They originate in various ways. Thus (*a*) as a retention cyst, due to dilatation of a seminal tube owing to some obstruction in the vas deferens or other part of the excretory passages (Liston, Luschka, and others). (*b*) As a new formation in the connective tissue between the tubes of the epididymis subsequent upon the rupture of a seminal tubule and the escape of some drops of seminal fluid. The opening in the duct may afterwards cicatrise, so that there need not persist a communication be-

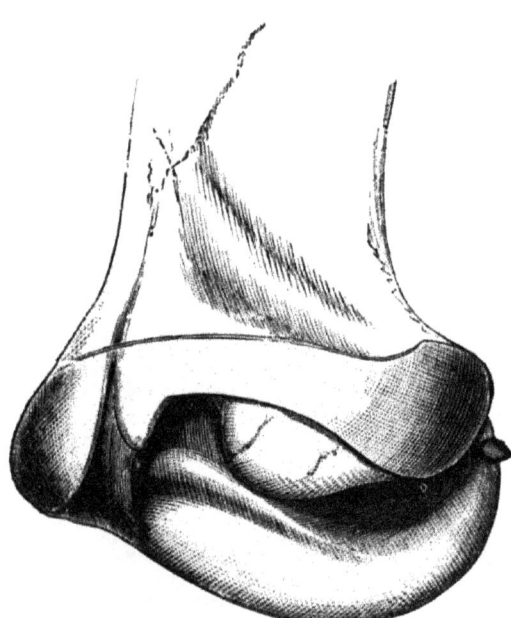

Fig. 26.—Encysted Hydrocele situated between Epididymis and body of Testicle. (*Osborn.*)

tween the duct and the new-formed cyst (M. Gosselin). (*c*) The cyst may be formed originally in the connective tissue, and by gradually enlarging may cause subsequently the rupture of a seminal tubule, and thus the entrance into the cyst of spermatozoa (Curling). (*d*) The cysts may arise from the distension of certain fœtal relics which exist in the neighbourhood of the epididymis, especially near the globus major.

The fœtal structures from which cysts of the epididymis originate are:—(1) The paradidymis, or organ of Giraldes, a minute body, the remnant of the mesonephros or glandular portion of the Wolffian body. This is situated in front of the lower part of the vas and above the head of the epididymis, and behind the upper part of the tunica vaginalis (Fig. 24). Cysts having this origin are situated above the testis and epididymis and extend sometimes a little way along the cord. They correspond to paroöphoritic cysts in the female. (2) The ducts of Kobelt, which are remnants of the tubules of the Wolffian body — situated in the globus major. (3) The vestiges of the duct of Müller, part of which is represented by the hydatid of Morgagni, and another part of the duct can sometimes be traced from the globus major down to the globus minor, along the body of the epididymis in the digital pouch (Fig. 26). Cysts derived from these sources (2 and 3) are situated between the epididymis and testis, most frequently between the globus major and the upper end of the testis. The cysts which are derived from the vasa efferentia and

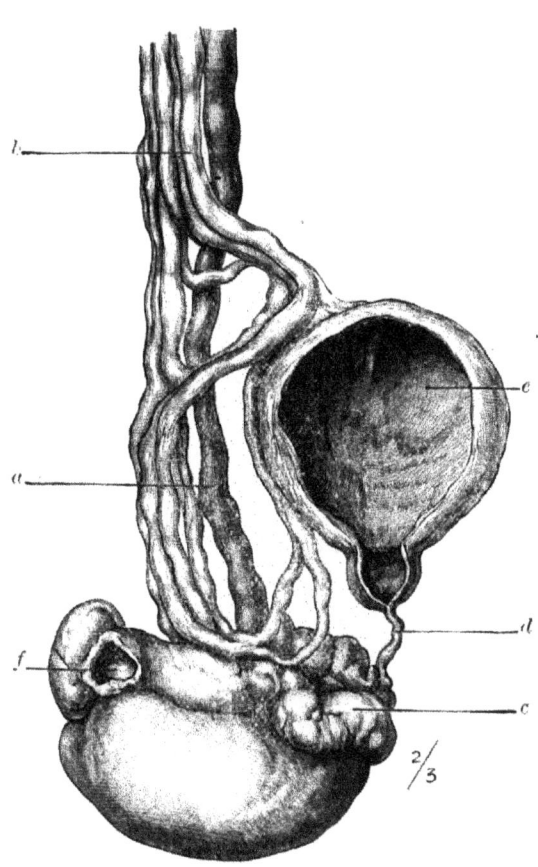

Fig. 27.—Encysted Hydrocele of the Epididymis, consisting of a dilated vas aberrans.

a, Vas deferens ; *b,* spermatic veins ; *c,* epididymis ; *d,* vas aberrans ; *e,* cyst of the vas aberrans ; *f,* cyst of globus major, so-called encysted hydrocele of tunica vaginalis. (St. Mary's Hospital Museum.) (*Pepper.*)

other remnants of the Wolffian tubules are homologous with parovarian cysts in the female. (4) The vas aberrans of Haller, which is a diverticulum of, or a convoluted cæcal tube opening into, the vas deferens close to the lower end of the epididymis ; this also is a part of the remains of one of the tubes of the Wolffian body still in connection with the representative of the excretory duct of that body—namely, the vas

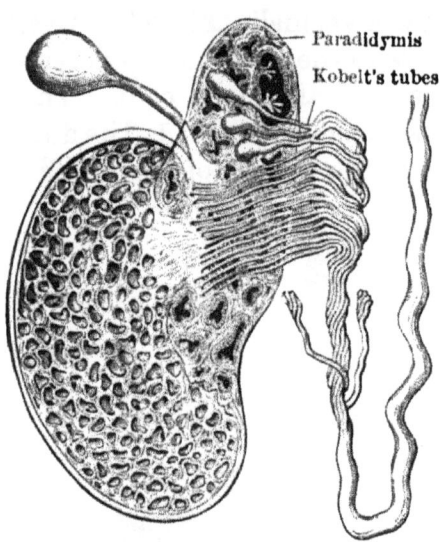

Fig. 28.—Diagram to show the Relation of the Mesonephron and its Ducts to the Adult Testicle. (*Sutton.*)

deferens. It is only rarely a source of encysted hydrocele. Fig. 27 is from a specimen in St. Mary's Hospital Museum, and Luschka describes a specimen in which the vas aberrans was converted into a cyst.

In the accompanying diagram (Fig. 28) the relation of the embryonic structures to one another is seen. The paradidymis is the remnant of the Wolffian body, Kobelt's tubes and the vasa efferentia the representatives of the tubules of that body, whilst the epididymis and vas deferens represent its duct.

ENCYSTED HYDROCELE OF THE TESTIS.

Cysts in these cases are situated between the tunica albuginea and the tunica vaginalis, or in the substance of the tunica albuginea itself. They are usually single, of small size, and so tense as to feel like solid bodies. They usually occur on the front of the body of the testis (Fig. 29), and may attain to the size of a goose's egg or larger. They contain fluid, which has sometimes a greyish-brown colour, and in a case recorded by Mr. Hutchinson there was a quantity of soft intracystic solid growth like granulation tissue. (Path. Soc. Trans., vol. vii. p. 246;

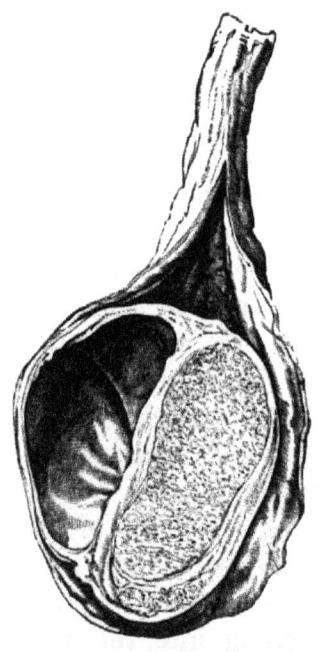

Fig. 29.—Encysted Hydrocele of the Testis. The cyst is situated in front of the body of the testicle proper. (*Curling.*)

Hunterian Museum, No. 4,217). These cysts may arise as new formations in connective tissue spaces, or possibly, as suggested by Mr. Hutchinson, from a puncture of the testis in tapping for hydrocele by the organisation into a cyst of the tissue around an extravasation of blood.

Symptoms of Encysted Hydrocele of the Epididymis and Testis.—The small cysts may give rise to hydrocele of the tunica vaginalis, and be discovered only after emptying this. They can be often felt through the tissues of the scrotum as grape-seed or pea-sized nodules. They have no clinical significance whatever, unless they excite hydrocele, or some neuralgic pain in the testis, scrotum, or perinæum, as I have known them do to a very distressing and disabling degree. Even then they may, from their minute size, be easily overlooked or undetected until a very careful tactile examination is made of the several parts of the epididymis. They may be no larger than small shot, yet be exquisitely tender, and the cause of pain not only in the scrotum, but radiating over the perinæum.

The larger cysts grow slowly and insidiously, giving rise to no pain or sense of dragging sensation, as a rule, though Mr. Curling speaks of severe pain as sometimes being caused by the stretching effect of the enlarging cyst on the epididymis. In their earlier stages they are rounded, and move with the testicle, above or on the outer side of which they are placed; as they grow they may become multilocular and lobulated, or pear-shaped with the large end upwards. They are usually translucent and elastic, if not fluctuating. The testicle is very rarely found behind the cyst; but is below and to the inner side, if not below and in front of the cyst. In doubtful cases the diagnosis will be made clear by tapping and an examination of the fluid withdrawn. It is rare for an encysted hydrocele to extend upwards along the groin, but when large and multiple they may do so.

Treatment.—So slight is the inconvenience which some encysted hydroceles produce that patients often decline having any treatment. A man under treatment for stricture, having a cyst as large as a Tangerine orange, declined to have it tapped, because it caused no inconvenience.

When any treatment is employed, tapping with a fine

trocar and cannula should be first tried, and will often suffice. If simple tapping fails, excision of the cyst is the best form of radical cure.   These cysts are, as a rule, quite easily dissected out entire, and the result is quite satisfactory.   If complete excision should not be found possible without damaging the testis, or epididymis, partial excision, with the application of pure carbolic acid, linimentum iodi, or silver nitrate to the portion left behind should be employed.

The injection treatment is not very satisfactory, being even more apt to fail in encysted than in vaginal hydrocele.

HYDROCELE OF A HERNIAL SAC.

This term is applied when the sac of a hernia emptied of its hernial contents and almost or quite shut off from the general peritoneal cavity becomes distended with serous fluid exuded from its inner surface.   Sometimes after the reduction of its contents, the neck of the sac is obliterated by the pressure of a truss ; or the orifice is completely occluded by a plug of adherent omentum ; or, again, in a third class of cases, the sac still communicates with the peritoneal cavity by a very narrow channel.   This form of hydrocele is often spoken of as extremely rare, but I have operated upon several cases, in some of which there was no communication whatever with the abdomen ; in others a fine probe could be passed along the neck of the sac into the peritoneal cavity, and in another a small plug of omentum effectually shut the sac off from the abdominal cavity.

In all the cases which I have had to treat the hernial sacs have been of the acquired inguinal variety; but Mr. Jacobson has related a case in which the hydrocele seems to have occurred in the unobliterated funiculo-vaginal process, the orifice of which had become firmly plugged with omentum. The fluid is usually straw- or amber-coloured, though it may be more or less blood-stained : it is derived from the vessels of the sac wall, and probably never from the omental vessels : even when the neck of the sac is occupied by this omentum, it is by but a small nodule, which is generally very thickened, and but little vascular.

Symptoms and Diagnosis.—There is usually the history of a hernia and of the wearing of a truss.   There is a swelling

in a common situation of a hernia, generally of an inguinal
hernia. This swelling fluctuates or is elastic, and is frequently
also translucent. It has little or nò impulse on coughing, though
it extends upwards with a sort of pedicle along the inguinal
canal like a hernia. It obscures the cord, but is quite distinct from the testicle. It occurs rather later in life than
encysted hydrocele of the cord, and is of larger size, and
contains a darker and much more albuminous fluid than
those hydroceles do. Encysted hydroceles of the cord appear
about puberty, are small in size, and contain a light-coloured
and but slightly albuminous fluid.

Treatment.—Injections should never be employed, because
of the uncertainty as to whether or no there is a communication with the peritoneal cavity. Simple tapping may be tried,
but if the fluid collects again, the complete removal of the sac
should be the treatment. This is better and quicker than the
antiseptic incision, especially for cases in which there is a
channel of communication with the abdominal cavity.

"**Spurious Hydrocele of the Hernial Sac**" was the
name given by Mr. Curling to cases of scrotal hernia in which
the sac contained a very large quantity of fluid. In most
cases the fluid is formed rapidly, and under the acute
conditions of strangulation of the hernia. But in other
cases it accumulates slowly, and quite independently of
symptoms of strangulation. When a person with ascites
has also a hernia the hernial sac may become greatly distended with ascitic fluid. In some instances the dropsical
fluid has been drawn off from the abdomen by puncturing
the fundus of the sac.

CHAPTER VI.

HÆMATOCELE.

HÆMATOCELE is a collection of blood in the tunica vaginalis or in the scrotal tissues outside the tunica vaginalis.

Cause.—It is nearly always traumatic in origin, and follows suddenly the reception of a blow, kick, or puncture of the testis or tunica vaginalis, as in tapping common hydrocele. In some of the cases following the tapping of hydrocele, and also in those where the hæmatocele comes on whilst coughing, sneezing, or straining at stool, there are good reasons for the opinion advanced and supported by M. Gosselin (*Arch. Gén. de Méd.*, 1851, t. xxvii.), Reclus, and other French writers, that there is a precedent diseased condition of the tunica vaginalis by which it has become the seat of false membranes, and that it is the rupture of the fragile embryonic vessels which traverse these false membranes that brings about the hæmorrhage. The slightest cause, even the engorgement of the vessels in simple congestion, is then, they argue, sufficient to lead to extravasation. But true as this view may be in certain cases, the observation of the tunica vaginalis in men of all ages, and in both the quick and the dead, as well as the results of the treatment of hydrocele, convince one that the tunica vaginalis is prone to inflame infinitely less than other serous membranes, and that false membranes form very rarely upon its surface. Varicose veins and atheromatous arteries predispose to hæmatocele.

Relation between Hydrocele and Hæmatocele.—Hæmatocele may follow tapping of a hydrocele, owing to the wounding of a small vessel of the scrotum, or more rarely of the testicle, in the operation. A punctured wound of the *testicle* is, however, more likely to be followed by orchitis than by hæmatocele. Again, hæmatocele may follow tapping, not as the result of a wound of any vessel, but from the giving way of some weakened vein or capillaries as soon as the hydrostatic support derived from the hydrocele fluid is taken away; just as one sometimes finds hæmorrhage taking place from the surface of the bladder, or pelvis of the kidney, after the rapid evacuation of long-retained urine.

Hydrocele may be converted into a hydro-hæmatocele by a blow or strain, and this will show itself by the sudden increase in the size of the swelling; in these cases the over-tense or thickened tunica vaginalis is usually rent.

Finally, hæmatocele may occur quite independently of hydrocele, either as the result of strain or injury, or in association with malignant disease of the testicle.

Pathological Changes vary with the age of the hæmato-cele. In old cases the *sac* is greatly thickened, partly by layers of false membrane of fibrinous characters, or connective tissue, and partly by sclerosis of its own structure. Both the false membranes and the sclerosed sac may be in places cartilaginous or calcareous. The connective tissue outside the sac is often thickened, and the testis altered in shape, atrophied, or absolutely unrecognisable. These changes in the tunica vaginalis increase the risk of sloughing; and during an operation the attempt to peel away the false-membrane may lead to laceration of the tunica, or, if the hæmatocele be extravaginal, the skin of the scrotum may be torn by the attempt. The contents in old hæmatocele are chiefly solid, and consist either of dirty-coloured clot, laminated as in an aneurysm, or of soft clot devoid of lamination; the fluid blood, if any is present, will be thick, dark, and treacly. In more recent cases fatty matter and cholesterin will be found; the sac is much less changed, and the false membranes, if any are present, are but feebly adherent; the contents are a mixture of fluid blood of a deep red colour mixed with dark blood-clot, some of which will be adherent to the walls.

When hæmorrhage has taken place into a hydrocele, the sac will vary with the history and the duration of the hydrocele, but the contents will be almost entirely fluid and of a lighter or darker colour, according to the extent of hæmorrhage. Some fresh blood-clot will be found mixed with the fluid.

Symptoms.—In the formation of a hæmatocele the tunica vaginalis is filled rapidly with blood after a strain, blow, or other injury, such as tapping a hydrocele; or if a hydrocele already exists, it rapidly increases and becomes more voluminous and tense after an injury. The swelling in either form of the affection has the shape and outline of hydrocele, but is not translucent, feels heavier and firmer, and is often associated with ecchymosis of the scrotum and even of the skin of the groin and upper part of thighs. If it comes on after tapping, free external bleeding may occur through the punctured wound. The testicle occupies the same position as in hydrocele, namely, behind and on a vertical level somewhat below the centre (Fig. 30); it can be made out on manipulation in recent cases by the peculiar testicular sensation. The surface of the swelling is not invariably uniformly smooth and regular; for it may be yielding in some spots, very resisting in others, and bossy or lumpy, or of cartilaginous hardness in others —this especially may be the case in old hæmatoceles.

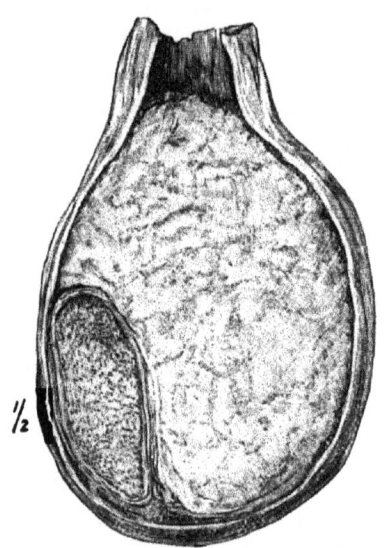

Fig. 30.—Hæmatocele. (Middlesex Hospital Museum.)

It should be borne in mind by the student that occasionally the onset of hæmatocele may be insidious, and its progress slow or irregular.

If acute or chronic inflammation ensues, the swelling will become tense, tender, and painful, and the skin over it may be red and œdematous, whilst the thermometer will register one, two or more degrees of fever.

If suppuration occurs, the tumour will bulge at some part, and the skin will soften over it, and undergo the usual changes in colour prior to sloughing or ulcerating; rigors may occur. The pain will be of a throbbing character until an opening is formed, or an incision made into the tumour.

Diagnosis.—Hæmatocele has to be distinguished from hydrocele, from enlargements of the testicle by inflammation or new growths, and from hernia.

From *hydrocele* by its opacity, greater firmness, want of fluctuation, and its suddenness of onset. In a recent hæmatocele there may be discoloration of skin. An aspirating needle would settle any doubt.

From *enlarged testicle* by the history, rate of increase, the discovery of the testicle of natural size and sensibility at the back of the swelling, by less pain and tenderness than in orchitis and new growths, and by the swelling having a less definite outline of the testicle than exists in either orchitis or the early stage of new growths. In many cases, however, it will only be by an exploratory incision that the distinction can be made.

From *hernia* by the absence of impulse, the better definition of the spermatic cord, and by the swelling commencing in the scrotum—not at the inguinal canal. It is between large hæmatoceles of long standing and irreducible, scrotal, omental hernia that there will be most difficulty in diagnosis ; but in most of such cases of hernia there has been a time in their course when they were reducible.

Treatment will be either palliative or curative. Palliative treatment is applicable in the early stages of hæmatocele, and consists in absolute rest in the recumbent position, with the scrotum well raised on a cushion or in a sling; the constant application of an ice-bag in the robust and of coagulating lotions in the very old or feeble ; and by the occasional use of aperients to keep up a regular and free action of the bowels. If little or no progress in absorption is made, some of the fluid blood should be withdrawn through a cannula, and the same treatment as above described continued. A second or a third tapping may be advisable. When the blood has been well-nigh removed, and if there is no pain or marked tenderness, strapping may be applied with advantage.

Radical Cure.—In hydro-hæmatocele, when the tunica vaginalis is not much thickened, the injection treatment is advised by many, but is not to be recommended, because in many cases the tunica vaginalis will have been ruptured, and thus the injection fluid will probably find its way into, and cause inflammation of, the extravaginal scrotal tissues ; and further, because there are masses of blood-clot in the fluid which may undergo degenerative changes if the injection fluid excites much inflammation of the tunica vaginalis. I greatly prefer the incision and partial excision treatment. The incision into the sac ought to be free, and after all the contents have been turned out, the tunica vaginalis, with any layers of false membrane which may be adherent to it, should be removed, except over the testicle and epididymis —just as in hydrocele; then the surface of the part of the membrane left behind should be well cleansed of adherent clot and false membrane, and treated with carbolic acid, iodine, or nitrate of silver, as in hydrocele. The wound should then be closed, with a drainage-tube *in situ* for a few days. Neither in these cases nor in hydrocele is it, in my opinion, advantageous to stitch the cut edge of the tunica vaginalis to the edges of the skin. If, however, the tissues on the outer side of the tunica vaginalis are condensed and firmly adherent to it, excision of the sac may be impossible. In this condition the surgeon should content himself by removing as much as possible of the false membrane and adherent blood-clot, and, after rubbing the surface of the sac with iodoform or carbolic acid, he should insert a drainage-tube and close the wound.

When the hæmatocele has suppurated, free incision and drainage, after clearing out the sac, are important.

In all cases in which the position of the testicle has not been previously made out, the incision into the sac must be very carefully performed, so as to avoid wounding the testicle.

Castration should be unhesitatingly performed when the testicle is degenerated by fibrous or fatty changes, as is often the case in old-standing hæmatoceles; when the tunica vaginalis is much diseased; when the patient is old and feeble; when the hæmatocele has ruptured, and blood is diffused amongst the tissues of the scrotum; or when suppuration or sloughing is threatened. It shortens convalescence, and diminishes the risk of hæmorrhage, of cellulitis, and of blood-poisoning.

HÆMATOCELE OF THE SCROTUM, NOT OF THE TUNICA VAGINALIS, sometimes occurs as the result of tapping a hydrocele. I have given the account of such a case in Chapter I., on " Injuries and Diseases of the Scrotum."

ENCYSTED HÆMATOCELE.

A hydro-hæmatocele is sometimes formed by extravasation of blood into an encysted hydrocele. Such cases are rare. The swelling has the same position to the testicle as the encysted hydroceles; though there will probably be a history of the swelling following an injury, the patient may be quite ignorant of the preexistence of the encysted hydrocele. Occasionally they attain a large size, and then may be mistaken for vaginal hæmatocele.

When the encysted hæmatocele is not large it may be removed without castrating. Castration should be performed under the same conditions and for the same reasons as in vaginal hæmatocele.

BILOCULAR HÆMATOCELES

have been described as hæmatoceles in a bilocular sac, in which one of the pouches occupies the scrotum and the other is situated within the abdomen. (*Vide* Jacobson, pp. 245–246.) These cases are hydro-hæmatoceles, being formed by extravasation of blood into bilocular hydroceles. They should be treated by incision, followed by carefully-applied pressure to prevent subsequent bleeding and drainage. Professor Annandale has recorded (*Ed. Med. Journ.*, vol. xviii. p. 714) a case in which the sac of a right hydro-hæmatocele ruptured and formed a second pouch in the perinæum.

HÆMATOMA OF TESTIS AND EPIDIDYMIS.

It occasionally happens that extravasation of blood takes place into the substance of the testicle or of the epididymis as the result of a blow or other injury inflicted upon the organ.

It probably sometimes follows the accidental puncture of the testicle in tapping a hydrocele. Probably, too, intratesticular hæmorrhage precedes the orchitis and suppuration of the testis, in some of those cases of chronic and subacute abscesses of the organ not otherwise explained.

These hæmatomata may occur without any sign of extravasation into the scrotal tissues; or, on the other hand, the scrotum may be deeply ecchymosed and swollen. In some cases it has occurred in association with hydrocele, in others quite independently of any such condition. In some cases hæmatocele of the tunica vaginalis, as well as hæmatoma of the testis, has been caused by the same injury.

Symptoms. — Intense throbbing pain, following quickly upon an injury, with a feeling of great fulness and tension of the testis or epididymis, entirely unrelieved by elevation or treatment, would give rise to the suspicion of hæmatoma. The testis or epididymis, as the case may be, will be larger than normal; probably it will be very tender at one spot, but it will not be acutely tender throughout, as in the case of epididymo-orchitis.

The temperature will be normal, and there will be no evidence of increased local heat. The pain immediately and for a long while after the injury may be excruciating, causing the patient to writhe and grasp his genitals in agony.

In some instances in which hæmatocele has coexisted and been incised, the tunica albuginea has given way, and a black mass made up of clotted blood and seminal tubules has protruded through into the cavity of the tunica vaginalis.

In some instances of long standing the testicle has been destroyed and converted into a large, ovoid, smooth, and very painful mass composed of a large cyst containing broken-down and fœtid blood.

Treatment. — When rest, elevation, ice, or other measures employed to promote the absorption of blood have failed, immediate relief from pain will sometimes follow the puncture of the tenderest point of the swelling with an aspirating trocar and cannula. Or a small subcutaneous and antiseptic incision with a tenotomy knife should be made into the most prominent and most painful spot. If the tunica vaginalis is deliberately laid open by an incision, the testis or epididymis may be seen to project or bulge at some spot, and, if so, this should be chosen as the site of puncture. As a consequence of hæmatoma, the patient should be led to anticipate the possibility of a hernia protrusion, or of a degree of permanent hardness and swelling, or of atrophy of the testicle.

Where the testicle or epididymis has been very much disorganised by the extravasation of blood, castration should be performed.

CHAPTER VII.

EPIDIDYMITIS, ACUTE AND CHRONIC.

WHEN inflammation affects the body of the testicle alone we speak of it as orchitis, when it involves the epididymis alone we speak of it as epididymitis, and when it involves both body of testicle and epididymis it is called epididymo-orchitis.

It is very uncommon for inflammation which begins as epididymitis to spread to the body of the testicle. It does not occur in two per cent. of the cases, to judge by statistics given by Dron of Lyons, Hardy, and others.

These affections may be acute, or subacute, or chronic. The two commonest forms of chronic inflammation are the tubercular and syphilitic.

Causes.—Acute or subacute epididymitis and epididymo-orchitis are almost always excited by some affection of the membranous or prostatic urethra, such as gonorrhœa, or gouty or other form of urethritis; the use of instruments upon the urethra; stricture of the urethra, and the changes which take place behind a stricture; by inflammatory conditions of the prostate, prostatic calculi, ulceration of the prostatic urethra; impacted calculus in the urethra; contraction of the meatus; and possibly by the frequent voiding of urine highly charged with uric acid, and by the use of very strong urethral injections. Injury is but a rare cause of this disease.

Various theories have been advanced to explain the frequency of epididymitis in connection with urethritis, prostatitis, and other forms of urethral irritation. Some of these must be mentioned:—

(1) *Metastasis*, or the shifting of inflammation from one part to the other, as in rheumatic fever. (2) *Sympathy.* (3) *Reflex congestion*, brought about in this instance in the same way as duodenal congestion and ulceration are said to be excited by huge superficial burns. (4) *Direct extension* of the inflammation from the urethra along the vas deferens to the epididymis. It is possible that each of these theories is on

G

occasions justified, but in the large majority of cases facts seem to prove that the theory of "direct and continuous extension" is the correct one.

Other causes of epididymo-orchitis are masturbation, excess in coitus, and the opposite extreme ungratified sexual appetite. Cases of epididymitis associated with acute inflammation of the tunica vaginalis have been recorded as occurring during the course of several of the specific fevers, as in smallpox, and scarlet fever.

Pathology.—When the inflammation spreads from the urethra by travelling along the vas deferens the walls of this tube become infiltrated with inflammatory products, are turgid with excess of blood, and the vas sheds its epithelium, and may contain pus; in many cases inflammation spreads from the vas itself to the cellular tissue of the spermatic cord.

The epididymis is chiefly affected at the globus minor, the body and globus major being less involved. The thickening of the globus minor is due to exudation into the cellular tissue between convolutions of the duct as well as into the connective tissue immediately beneath the vaginal tunic. The tubes of the epididymis are in places sometimes dilated into little pouches filled with pus. The testicle is not invaded in more than two per cent. of cases of epididymitis, and then only in the most acute.

The tunica vaginalis is always somewhat inflamed, and some amount of fluid is always effused into its sac owing to the intimate cellular tissue connection between the tubes of the epididymis and the portion of the tunica vaginalis covering them.

The skin of the scrotum is red and œdematous, owing to the inflammation spreading to it from the cellular tissue embedding the epididymis and commencement of the cord.

Some induration may persist in the globus minor for a long time after the attack has passed off, owing to the nonabsorption of the inflammatory products; this, by obstructing the duct, may lead to dilatation and sacculation of the tubules of the body and globus major.

Symptoms.—Aching, then more acute pain, and then swelling of the epididymis, are the leading symptoms. They may come on after the use of a catheter, sound, or lithotrity, but most usually in the course of some affection of the urethra or prostate. The globus minor is the seat of the first marked swelling, but an early and careful examination in many cases of the cord will detect some tenderness or even thickening there ; and some patients refer to a pain in the inguinal or deep pelvic regions.

The swelling increases in the tail of the epididymis and spreads upwards in the body to the globus major, and thus a boat-shaped enlargement and hardness can be detected on the outer and back part of the testicle, if the sickening pain and exquisite tenderness will permit of a careful digital examination. Later this condition may be lost, owing to the effusion of fluid into the vaginal sac and the matting together of the inflamed tissues with the lower part of the testicle. In the very acute cases the amount of fluid poured out by the tunica vaginalis is considerable, and the condition sometimes described as " acute hydrocele " is produced. The scrotum is more or less red, glossy, and œdematous, and assumes the " flat-sided " swelling described by Mr. Hutchinson as being caused partly by the moulding of the œdematous scrotum against the thigh, and partly by the swollen epididymis pushing forward the testicle proper. In many cases the cord is painful and swollen up to the external ring, in rare instances the inflammation may be limited to the cord and not descend to the epididymis—a point which should be remembered, as in this latter case the inguinal swelling, the extreme pain, the vomiting and constipation, will simulate strangulated hernia. The high temperature, the pain preceding the swelling, the gradual though rapid increase of the swelling, and its hardness and excessive tenderness, will serve to distinguish it from hernia.

Rigors may usher in or occur during the early part of the attack, the temperature for several days is usually above normal, a feeling of sickness or vomiting may be present, the bowels are generally constipated, the tongue is foul, and the patient thirsty.

In an acute case the symptoms increase for four or five days, and remain at their height for two or three days more, from which time they rapidly decrease, and the patient is convalescent in from a fortnight to three weeks. Some amount of hardness and thickening of the cellular tissue of the globus minor may remain for months or even become permanently organised. MM. Monod and Terrillon have described blood-stained seminal emissions as liable to occur during convalescence from epididymitis; the source of the blood may be the vesiculæ seminales, they think, as these organs have been found inflamed and enlarged, and by rectal examination are often highly sensitive, during the acute stage ot epididymitis. M. Gosselin has drawn attention to widespread neuralgic pains occurring in epididymitis in neurotic persons, and also to the persistence of neuralgic pains for a long time after the inflammation has ended. When epididymitis occurs in the course of gleet, or urethritis, the urethral discharge will generally cease or diminish during the acuteness of the inflammatory attack, and return again when it is over. Kocher attributes this to the change in the patient's condition wrought by the pyrexia.

Though both testicles may be affected, they are attacked one after the other, never simultaneously; and if a relapse in one takes place during recovery from an attack in the other we have what M. Ricord called the " see-saw " epididymitis. The cases in which the inflammation, arising in connection with urethral irritation, attacks the vas deferens but does not reach the epididymis, afford a strong argument in favour of the " direct extension " theory of Sir A. Cooper to explain the connection between epididymitis and inflammation of the urethra.

The Complications and Terminations of Epididymitis. —As a rule to which happily the exceptions are very few, epididymitis and epididymo-orchitis terminate in resolution. Though a small hard lump of dense fibro-cellular tissue may remain for a long time in the globus minor, this does not often lead to atrophy of the testicle. A similar deposit in the globus major is still less likely to damage the secreting power of the testis, because there, instead of a single convoluted tube, as in the globus minor, the seminal ducts are multiple.

Abscess in the testicle, in the epididymis, or in the course of the vas deferens, occasionally occurs in the unhealthy and debilitated, and also as a part of pyæmia after operations on or suppuration in the deep urethra. Suppuration of the tunica vaginalis and the conversion of an "acute hydrocele" into an abscess is rare, and is most likely to occur when the epididymitis has followed the use of instruments, or gleet, or gonorrhœa. (*See* page 47.)

Sloughing of the epididymis and testis are occasional complications in old or intemperate persons or broken-down constitutions. I have once seen sloughing in a young man in whom an abscess of the testicle requiring incision was followed by hernia testis and sloughing of the herniated portion. As soon as the slough had separated, the herniated stump was scraped and detached from the integuments, the edges of which were freshened, and the wound was closed by sutures. Healing followed, and was rapid and complete.

Peritonitis may be started from the vas deferens or the vesicula seminalis, but very rarely is this the case; it may be limited to the immediate neighbourhood of the genital structures, or spread, become general, and end fatally. Inflammation attacking an undescended testicle thus becomes a special source of danger.

Treatment.—The patient should remain in bed, have the scrotum well raised, and for the first three or four days keep an ice-bag or an iced evaporating lotion constantly applied. A full dose of calomel should be given at once if the bowels are constipated, and a saline mixture composed of nitrate of potash, spirits of nitrous ether, and carbonate and sulphate of magnesia should be taken every eight hours. If the patient is healthy or plethoric, it will be well to add twenty drops of antimonial wine to each dose of the medicine; and if there is acute pain, and there nearly always is, eight or ten minims of tincture of opium should be also added. The diet should be light, and consist only of milk, beef-tea, and light puddings. An extra dose of morphia or opium may be required at night. Of late years anemone pulsatilla has been highly recommended by several excellent authorities; two or three drops of the extract of pulsatilla every four hours is said to rapidly subdue swelling, heat, and pain. After the acuteness of the inflammation has subsided a mixture containing potassium iodide and bicarbonate will assist the absorption of the inflammatory products, and the testicle should still be kept well elevated. At the end of a fortnight, if all pain and tenderness have vanished, the testicle should be strapped and the patient allowed up, still, however, keeping the scrotum suspended in a well-fitting suspensory bandage.

In the early stage, if ice cannot be borne well, or if, owing to the age or feebleness of the patient, sloughing is anticipated, warm fomentations of lead and opium, lead and carbolic acid, or of poppy heads should be applied and changed every two or three hours.

In very robust men and where the inflammation runs high, leeches or venesection of one of the superficial veins of the same side of the scrotum is beneficial; the bleeding following either method can be checked by collodion and cotton-wool. When "acute hydrocele" complicates the case the fluid should be let out by introducing a trocar and cannula into the sac, or by making a small puncture incision with a tenotomy knife. Puncture of the testicle or epididymis is, in my opinion, never justifiable except with the object of evacuating pus.

After the employment of ice for some days, and in cases in which the patient is unable to lie up, marked relief is said to follow painting the scrotum with a solution of nitrate of silver ($\mathfrak{z}$j to $\mathfrak{z}$j). The painting should be repeated at very short intervals of a quarter to half an hour, until a smarting or pricking sensation is excited, but not vesication. This treatment was introduced by Mr. Furneaux Jordan, and is spoken of most favourably by Mr. Jacobson. Strapping may be applied a day or two after the application of the silver nitrate solution.

CHRONIC EPIDIDYMITIS.

Chronic inflammation may be a sequel of the acute or subacute form; or some of the products of acute or subacute inflammation may be left behind and remain for a long while in the epididymis, especially in the globus minor, and cause obstruction in the seminal passages. When chronic epididymitis continues, or recurs at short intervals, it is nearly always because there is some mischief persisting in the deep urethra. Owing to the immediate proximity of the orifices of the ejaculatory ducts, there is, so long as the urethra is not in a healthy state, a great tendency for inflammation to extend to one vas deferens and epididymis as soon as it has subsided in the other, and then after a time to recur in the first as soon as the second has nearly recovered. In this way is brought about the "see-saw" epididymitis referred to on page 84, and in this way may be formed those small fibrous masses in the tail of the epididymis which, persisting, may result in sterility. Sterility, though it has existed a year or more, may be cured by the absorption of the deposits which obstruct the passage of the semen. Mr. Jacobson writes:—"If the patient persist in treating this relic of his attack as an unimportant matter, he should be warned that if it become bilateral and permanent—though there be all the signs of virility, with desire and power of copulation and emission—there is likely to be no impregnation in consequence of the absence of spermatozoa in the fluid emitted." He quotes the investigations of M. Liégois to show that the absence of spermatozoa is much more frequently found in cases of bilateral epididymitis arising from blennorrhagic causes than when caused by injury. Knowing this, the surgeon should insist upon continuance of treatment until the urethral trouble is cured and the deposits in the epididymis are absorbed. Whether there be stricture, gleet, prostatic calculi, or some other cause of deep urethral irritation, it ought to be submitted to appropriate treatment, medicinal or operative; whilst the continued use of a suspensory bandage, the daily application to the testicle of some absorbent ointment such as the iodide of lead or potassium, and the internal administration of perchloride of mercury or iodide of potassium should be insisted upon. Tonics and sea air, especially a sea voyage, are very beneficial.

CHAPTER VIII.

ORCHITIS AND EPIDIDYMO-ORCHITIS.

In describing epididymitis, I have stated that the inflammation may spread to the testicle itself, and so produce an epididymo-orchitis.

In studying orchitis it must be understood that inflammation, beginning in the testicle, may spread to the epididymis, and thus epididymo-orchitis be brought about, but in the inverse order.

But there is this difference—that, whereas it is rare for the inflammation to reach the testicle proper when the epididymitis has been caused, as it is most usually, by some prostatic or urethral irritation or disease, it is quite common for inflammation of the testes, from whatever cause arising, to extend to the epididymis.

Causes.—Orchitis may occur alone, as the result of injury, of cold, of congestion from unfulfilled function, or of some constitutional or bacterial condition. It may be acute, subacute, or chronic. The chronic forms are generally, though not always, either the sequel of the acute or subacute, or else are of syphilitic origin.

Orchitis occurs in gout, and less frequently in rheumatism, and is met with as a complication of many infectious diseases —namely, mumps, typhoid fever, small-pox, scarlet fever, influenza, malaria, and tonsillitis. The inflammation of the testicle behaves somewhat differently, according to its cause.

When due to *mumps*, the testicle alone is commonly affected, the epididymis rarely. It begins about the sixth or eighth day of the illness, attacks boys and young adults, and is unknown in childhood and old age. The course of the orchitis is rapid, the testicle attaining twice its size in a day or two; it is attended by fever, more or less pain, and tenderness. The pain, sometimes slight, is in other cases very severe, and radiates along the groin to the hypogastrium and loins. The constitutional disturbance at the outset of the attack may be severe, even alarming; intense fever, delirium, epistaxis, and diarrhœa, or collapse may usher in the orchitis, but generally disappear when the orchitis is established. The testis preserves its smooth and natural outline, and is less hard than in some other forms of orchitis. One testicle after the other may be involved, but it is rare for both to be affected simultaneously. After the fourth day the local inflammation begins to subside, and the disease ends usually in resolution. Atrophy of the testicle is reported by foreign surgeons to have occurred in some epidemics, and that, too, even in mild cases.

When due to *typhoid fever*, the epididymis is rarely—some observers say never—affected, unless the inflammation is set up by the irritation of catheterism, and then the epididymis only may be attacked. One testicle only is affected. The onset is commonly sudden, but may be gradual; it occurs during the height of the fever, or during convalescence therefrom. The pain is not so great as in other forms of orchitis; or, possibly, less attention is drawn to it during the delirium of the fever. The inflammation is not generally severe; the attack lasts from six to ten days, or it may be even much more transient; it ends usually in resolution, but suppuration, or atrophy, or persistent induration follows, though very rarely. Cases of inflammation of the body of the testicle have been reported as occurring in the course of *small-pox, scarlet fever,* and *influenza.*

Orchitis occurs in persons subject to *malarial fever;* it follows or accompanies the fever, but generally at a late period of the disease, and yields readily to quinine. It comes suddenly, lasts two or three days, during which the testicle may swell to three or four times its natural size, the testicle and epididymis being completely blended in the hard, smooth mass. The scrotal veins swell, the skin is œdematous, and there is generally a little fluid poured out into the tunica vaginalis. Pain is severe, and may be paroxysmal; it passes off when the temperature falls. The swelling may take three or four weeks to disappear, and the testicle may be left atrophied, or the epididymis enlarged and hard.

M. le Dentu is of opinion that, besides this, the inflammatory form, there is also a form of orchitis the result of malaria, akin to elephantiasis of the scrotum, with which it may or may not be associated ; he regards this " elephantiasis of the testis " as a chronic lymphangitis of that organ—an intra-testicular lymphangitis. The enlarged testicles found on tapping the hydroceles of men who have lived in the Tropics, and also seen in cases of chylous hydrocele, in M. le Dentu's opinion, show that " elephantiasis of the testis " may exist independently of scrotal elephantiasis.

Gouty Orchitis.—Under epididymitis it has been mentioned that gout may give rise to an urethral discharge, and this to epididymo-orchitis. The more frequent affection, however, is orchitis proper, which occurs in persons with a mild form of gouty constitution, and in whom gout does not show itself in the characteristic manner.

It commonly affects persons over fifty who are subjects of bronchitis, laryngitis, dyspepsia, or arthritic pains of gouty nature. It occurs more rarely in men of typically gouty constitution, or during or just before an acute attack of gout. The inflammation is acute, and may, though rarely, spread to the epididymis; there is a good deal of pain and swelling, the body of the testicle being uniformly smooth and hard. It is often a very obstinate affection, and may end in suppuration. Even when the inflammation is chronic from the outset, it may end in suppuration. Gouty orchitis often affects both testicles, one after the other so closely, that both organs are involved simultaneously. It is frequently brought on by fatigue or over-exercise.

M. Verneuil and Dr. Joal (*Arch. Gén. de Méd.*, 1857 and 1886) describe orchitis as occurring in association with acute tonsillitis. It affects boys after puberty, and young men under twenty-two who are suffering from follicular tonsillitis. It usually comes on as the tonsillar inflammation is passing off, but may precede it. It is unilateral, usually limited to the testicle proper ; lasts from fifteen to twenty days, and usually ends in resolution. Atrophy and abscess have, however, been known to follow.

Treatment.—The treatment of acute and subacute orchitis, if of traumatic origin, is the same as for epididymitis. (*See* p. 85.) Some modifications are required, according to the cause of the orchitis, when occurring in the course of other diseases, or as the outcome of some constitutional condition. In orchitis due to mumps, or typhoid fever and the other infectious diseases, warm boracic or lead and opium lotion should be applied to the scrotum instead of ice; or ointments of opium, conium, and belladonna should be spread over it beneath fomentations. A dose of Dover's powder or morphia should be given at night, and the scrotum should be kept well raised from the first and throughout the attack, the patient being confined to bed the while. Gentle laxative medicine will be required at the beginning of and during the orchitis, but no lowering aperients or other measures are suitable. A saline mixture, followed in a day or two by one of quinine, or acid and bark, or ammonia and bark, and a nutritious diet are the other adjuncts of treatment required.

In orchitis with ague quinine should be given. In orchitis from gout or rheumatism the general treatment is that appropriate to gout or rheumatism itself; the local application should be ice in the robust, but warm sedative lotions in the old or feeble.

The Pathological Connection between Orchitis, Epididymitis, and the Infectious Diseases.—The view expressed by Mr. Jacobson in 1882 ("Syst. of Surgery," vol. iii. p. 517) with reference to the nature of orchitis in mumps, namely, "that the inflammations of the salivary glands, testis, etc., are different localised manifestations of one pyrexial condition, probably due to a special organism," seems to me to explain best the occurrence of orchitis also in typhoid fever and the other continued fevers, in influenza, and in acute tonsillitis.

The typhoid bacillus has been found in the testicles of patients with typhoid fever, and it is highly probable that the action of these upon the testicle is the exciting cause of the orchitis. It is highly probable also that bacteriologists will before long discover a specific microbe for each of the other infectious diseases, and will be able to prove that orchitis occurring in the course of them is but a local manifestation of an infective specific disease. There are good reasons for rejecting the time-honoured theory of metastasis by which, as Kocher expresses it, the inflammation is supposed to "leave one organ to go to another, like an unclean spirit."

It must be borne in mind that in any disease in which

the use of the catheter is required, the urethral irritation may be the cause of the inflammation of the testicle; also that slight injury during the tossings of fever and delirium may explain the origin of some cases; and, thirdly, that phlebitis of the spermatic veins may follow féver and start an inflammatory action in the epididymis or body of the testis.

In ague the orchitis, whether of the inflammatory kind or of the elephantiasic or lymphatic form described by M. le Dentu, is the result of the malarial poison.

In gouty and rheumatic orchitis the inflammation is the local expression or outbreak of the gouty or rheumatic diathesis, just as are the articular, fascial, or tendon affections in those diseases.

CHAPTER IX.

SUPPURATION AND ABSCESS OF THE TESTICLE AND EPIDIDYMIS: FUNGUS OR HERNIA TESTIS.

SUPPURATION in the testicle, epididymis, and cord, though comparatively uncommon, except in the advanced stages of tubercular disease and in tertiary syphilis, is more frequent than the accounts usually given of it would lead us to expect. All the forms of inflammation of the testicle and epididymis described in the preceding chapter end sometimes, though infrequently, in abscess and diffuse suppuration.

The most frequent cause of suppuration is the use of instruments on the urethra and bladder; thus it occurs after operations for stricture, lithotrity, or the passage of a calculus along the urethra.

I shall refer in the chapter on Diseases of the Cord to a case of suppuration along the cord after the use of Holt's dilator. I have known it occur in association with pyuria due to renal calculus; though no stone was ever passed, so far as is known, and no sound or other instrument had been used for about three months prior to the testicular abscess. In this case the abscess healed rapidly after it was opened, but many months later the patient died from a large peri-nephric abscess.

In inflammation of gonorrhoeal origin abscess is much more rare than after the use of instruments.

In pyæmia and the infectious diseases, especially typhoid fever, in gout, and orchitis and epididymitis from injury of any kind, suppuration sometimes occurs. Mr. Sheild was unable to find records, or to learn from the medical officers of public schools of England, of a single case of suppuration after mumps.

Abscess occurs, too, in infancy, without any assignable cause. The amount of pus varies, but is sometimes large. Its characters are very often foul and mixed with threads of slough.

Suppuration sometimes extends from the epididymis some way along the cord; in other cases, diffuse suppuration, or a succession of abscesses first occurs along the cord, or pus may form simultaneously in cord and testicle.

Suppuration is more likely to occur in those of weakly and unhealthy constitutions, and does not follow the most acute and intensest forms of inflammation. It is met with in chronic orchitis as well as terminating acute and subacute inflammation. In a case published in the *Lancet*, June 16, 1894, I have recorded the notes of an elderly man in whom chronic inflammation of both testicles, of uncertain origin, ran on to suppuration in one of his testicles, the other getting well slowly by resolution. Mr. Jacobson explains the rarity of suppuration by the remarkable development of the lymphatics of the testis, and their origin in wide lacunar passages between the seminal tubules whereby the products of inflammation are readily and easily absorbed.

When pus forms in the testicle, and is not let out by an incision, it may find an exit through an ulcerated fistulous opening; or when in the body of the testis it may spread beneath the tough tunica albuginea, destroying the testicle entirely, and burst, giving rise to several fistulous openings. When circumscribed, the pus may remain shut in until its fluid part is absorbed and the leucocytes cretify; or, like an abscess in bone, it may have periods of quiescence, alternating with attacks of pain and renewed inflammation.

After an abscess has been opened either by incision or ulceration, true hernia of the seminal structure may follow, as in a case of suppuration of gonorrhœal origin which I recorded in the *Lancet*, June 16, 1894.

Another sequel is sloughing, by which, after the formation of only a very small quantity of pus, the greater part of the whole testis may be lost. It should be borne in mind that gangrene may follow orchitis without previous suppuration and unattended by pain; this has been observed after long-standing prostatic irritation, the passage of calculi, and in association with hæmatocele.

Suppuration in the cavity of the tunica vaginalis either secondary to or independent of acute hydrocele is, like testicular abscess, an occasional sequel of the use of instruments on the urethra and bladder, and must not be confused with suppuration of the testicle. The two conditions are, however, sometimes met with together. Abscess in the scrotum and in the cellular tissue of the cord is not to be mistaken for abscess of the testicle or epididymis. Mr. Marmaduke Sheild, after a careful review of the whole subject of the suppurative affections of the testicle and epididymis, says he has not been able to find a single case of abscess of the testicle complicating urethrotomy, and remarks: "It seems that so far as orchitis and abscess after catheterisation are concerned, such cases are apt to present themselves in those who have long suffered from chronic irritation of the urethra, prolonged gleet, constant catheterisation, or prostatic irritation. It is usually agreed that the cause is the spread of inflammation along the seminal duct. In some cases, and especially after operations, a septic factor may be introduced and thus produce suppuration. Or this latter termination may occur in the aged, feeble, or intemperate, whose tissues are more prone to suppurate than healthily repair. I believe that cases of orchitis of this nature are more frequent than the published records of them would lead us to believe." (Med.-Chir. Trans., vol. lxxiv. p. 75.)

As regards orchitis and abscess of testicle in typhoid fever, Mr. Sheild says: "One can hardly doubt but that this complication is of a pyæmic nature, occurring in feeble individuals whose health generally is shattered and undermined by the prolonged ravages of an acute and dangerous malady" (*op. cit.*, p. 82). In this respect suppuration of the testis after typhoid is like necrosis, abscesses of joints, and other sequelæ of the eruptive fevers.

Symptoms.—When the testicle suppurates it does so with more or less pain, or it may be merely with a sense of discomfort; the temperature usually rises, but not always or necessarily; there may or may not be one or more rigors. Though the pus may for a time or altogether remain within the tunica albuginea, it usually ulcerates through this tissue into the tunica vaginalis, and sets up suppuration in that cavity, or, what is more usual, adhesions form between the testicle and the scrotum, the scrotum swells and becomes œdematous, red, glazed, hot, painful, and tender over the affected area, and thus in one or more places ulcerates, and thereby exit is given to the pus. Following the opening, as also after the pus has been let out through an incision, hernia testis may occur; or the whole or greater part of the organ may slough away or have to be excised.

Treatment.—It is of great importance to open the abscess early so as to relieve tension and save the seminal tubules from disintegration or sloughing. As a rule, healing follows at once on the evacuation of the pus. If hernia testis takes place, it will be in some cases successfully treated by sprinkling the powdered red oxide of mercury night and morning over its surface; it then dries up and falls off, and cicatrisation follows. Or the parts should be pared, the testis freed from the scrotum, and the edges of the skin sutured. Should these means not succeed, or if the testis is in a gangrenous or sloughing state, castration will be required.

FUNGUS OR HERNIA TESTIS.

This may occur either as the result of an abscess of the testicle, or in the second stage of tuberculosis, or in the tertiary stages of syphilitic orchitis; or after sloughing from injury, fever, extravasation of urine, and other causes; or in the progress of malignant disease.

In malignant disease—sarcoma or carcinoma—the protruding mass (fungus hæmatodes) is new growth, not testicular tissue. In the other two forms of fungus—the tubercular and the syphilitic—the protrusion may consist of glandular tissue and granulation material, or of granulation and inflammatory material only. The fungus may spring from the scrotum, tunica vaginalis, tunica albuginea, or from the tubular structure of the testicle or epididymis.

The tubercular fungus is generally situated on the outer side of the testicle, and in connection either with the epididymis or testis proper, and usually springs from the cavity of a tubercular abscess. Sometimes, however, in what is called the superficial variety of fungus, it starts from a broken-down caseous nodule situated in the scrotum or in the tunica vaginalis; then the testicle may be involved secondarily, the tunica albuginea becoming thickened and adherent, and the underlying part of the testicle inflamed, until in time it generally breaks down, even if it does not project through the ulcerated opening of the scrotum. In the deep glandular or parenchymatous variety of fungus testis, the projecting tissue is always continuous with the tubular structure through an ulcerated opening of the tunica albuginea, and the fungus may increase until the greater part of the organ is external to the scrotum.

Even in this latter variety the presence of seminal tubules cannot always be made out by the microscope, because the caseating process which has caused the hernia may have completely destroyed the gland tissue at the part from which the fungus springs.

The syphilitic fungus begins in the breaking-down of a gumma of the body of the testis; or of a thickened, gummatous condition of the tunica albuginea; or, very exceptionally, in a gumma of the scrotum. In either case the tunica albuginea becomes inflamed, and the tunica vaginalis adherent to the scrotal tissue, so as to obliterate the vaginal cavity around the fungus. When the breaking-down gumma is situated on the tunica albuginea, or in the structures of the scrotum, the tunica albuginea may not be perforated—at any rate, not at first,—but granulations springing from it form the superficial variety of syphilitic hernia testis.

Symptoms and Course.—The size of the protrusion varies from a pea to the whole substance of the testis, but, as a rule, it is not much larger than a cherry or a strawberry. The tubercular fungus attains a larger size than the syphilitic. It is painless, firm, reddish yellow, and moist, being covered with sero-pus, sometimes mixed with slough. Around it there is 'a ragged ulcerated edge of skin and dartos, altered by inflammation, often undermined, and later tending to contract like a collar or ring upon the peduncle of the fungus. When tubules can be unravelled from the protruding mass, or when spermatozoa are found in the discharges, or when there is a well-marked stalk or peduncle, it is certain the fungus is of the deep variety; but the absence of tubules and spermatozoa is not proof that the fungus is superficial.

Treatment.—The superficial form sometimes disappears under local and constitutional treatment—namely, iodoform dusted over the fungus, and tonics, good diet, and cod-liver oil in the tubercular variety; red oxide of mercury powder

H

locally, and mercury and iodide of potassium internally, in the syphilitic form. Strapping may be applied with advantage in some cases. In other cases the herniated tissues should be excised, together with the edges of the opening in the scrotum. These tissues are then completely detached from their adhesions around the peduncle of the fungus; the peduncle is scraped clean away, and dusted with iodoform; pressure with iodoform gauze is maintained for a few minutes, and then the scrotal tissues are united by sutures over the testicle. This treatment has occasionally given me excellent results. In severe or obstinate cases of tubercular fungus, castration is the only remedy, and should not be long deferred.

CHAPTER X.

SYPHILIS OF THE TESTICLE.

THE testicle is affected with syphilis both of acquired and congenital origin. Syphilis of the testicle, as commonly met with, occurs in the intermediate and tertiary stages of the disease, and in two forms—(1) as diffuse or interstitial orchitis, (2) as gummata. Both these forms are spoken of as syphilitic sarcocele.

SYPHILITIC EPIDIDYMITIS.

Syphilis affects the epididymis, though rarely, in the early secondary stage, and then occurs as a localised nodular mass, the size of a pea, in the globus major. The testicle proper is not generally involved, but syphilitic orchitis has been associated with the epididymitis in two out of sixteen cases observed by Dr. Dron, of Lyons (*Arch. Gén. de Méd.*, 1863, tome xi.). Syphilitic epididymitis has been proved to occur quite independently of any gonorrhœal disease; it is painless, slow in progress, and the enlargement is never great. Hence it is rarely looked for, and consequently has not been commonly described. Both epididymes may be affected simultaneously. The period of attack is, on an average, three and a half months after the primary sore. The disease rapidly yields under mercury, and, like other forms of secondary syphilis, tends to spontaneous cure if not treated.

The co-existence of other and more obvious syphilitic lesions and the rapid good effect of mercury make the diagnosis clear.

HEREDITARY SYPHILIS

is seen in the form of orchitis or sarcocele, and M. Gosselin met with a case of hernia testis from congenital syphilis in a child ten months old.

Congenital sarcocele, in its pathology, is usually of the interstitial form ; gummata are rare ; but there is not unfrequently a combination of the interstitial and gummatous forms. The

epididymis may be, but is not often, involved. Both testicles
are often simultaneously attacked. The organ is as hard as
scirrhus, may be nodular, is not painful nor tender, and
may become the seat of hernia testis. The enlargement is
not great, and may be, especially in the earlier stages, masked
by hydrocele. Atrophy of the organ is prone to follow.

Dr. Carpenter (*Practitioner*, September, 1892) points out
that it is only in a small percentage of cases that congenital
orchitis can be detected by physical examination; that for
its detection the microscope is frequently needed; that it
occurs in an inflammatory form akin to congenital syphilitic
hepatitis; and that when an atrophied testis is found in a
natural scrotum, and with a natural vas and vesicula seminalis,
and in the presence of other evidences of congenital syphilis,
the cause of the atrophy of the testis is at once suggested.
The treatment required for congenital syphilis in other
phases of its existence is that which is appropriate to
syphilitic orchitis of hereditary origin.

SYPHILITIC SARCOCELE OF THE ADULT.

This is an affection of the late secondary and of the
tertiary stages of syphilis. It occurs in the two forms
mentioned above, but in many instances they are combined.

Pathology.—(1) *The interstitial orchitis* is a chronic inflammation of the intertubular connective tissue affecting more
or less of the organ, but generally leaving some areas of it
free. When the inflammation proceeds unchecked the cellular
products, which are grouped in irregular mass or diffused in
lines along the intertubular septa, are converted into fibrous
tissue, and this, in turn, is followed by contraction, resulting
in scarring, puckering, and, finally, atrophy of the organ.
The walls of the vessels and tubules, and the tunica albuginea
participate in the same changes as the intertubular connective
tissue. If atrophy ensues, it is generally a slow and gradual
process, although cases have been witnessed in which the
testis has shrivelled to the size of a haricot bean in the
space of only a few months.

On section a syphilitic testicle in the early stage looks
redder and feels harder than normal, and the tubules do
not readily unravel; in the second or fibrous stage it looks

paler, but has lost its natural yellow, soft appearance, and the intertubular septa look thickened and tough—like scar-tissue in the rete testis, and like radiating bands extending from the thickened tunica albuginea to the mediastinum testis in the body of the organ. When the testicle is atrophied the fibrous tissue is increased out of all proportion to the tubular, until, when the atrophy is complete, nothing but a hard irregular little mass of fibrous tissue at the end of the vas deferens remains.

(2) *The gummatous Orchitis.*—This is probably only a legacy of a previous diffuse inflammation, or it may be a localised inflammation started in the coats of a spermatic vessel or tubule, as suggested by Lanceraux. The nodules which occur in this form of orchitis are at first minute, but, blending together, may at length form large masses or gummata the size of marbles or much larger. The gummata are usually multiple. They result from the formation of imperfect connective or fibrous tissue out of the embryonic cells, which are collected on limited areas instead of being dif-fused throughout the testicle, as in the interstitial form. There is a great tendency for them to caseate and

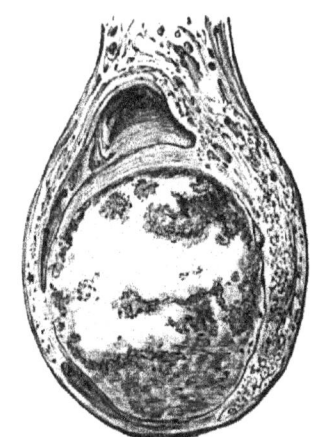

Fig. 31.—Syphilitic Disease of the Testicle. (London Hospital Museum.) (*J. Cantlie.*)

break down, and in this respect, as well as in general structure and character, they resemble gummata in other textures and organs of the body. An uneven surface is often given to the testicle, partly owing to the puckering and thickening of the tunica albuginea, and partly to the nodular swell-ings of superficially-placed gummata. The diffuse form of orchitis is often largely combined with the gummatous, the former being an earlier stage of the gummatous form (Fig. 31).

Associated with both these forms of orchitis there is generally much irregular thickening of the tunica albuginea; and in the earlier stages there is a small degree of hydrocele, but as the disease advances the fluid is absorbed, and tough fibrous adhesions form between the surfaces of the tunica vaginalis until at length complete obliteration of the vaginal cavity is the result. The epididymis and cord are usually unaffected. The scrotal tissues may become adherent to some part of the testicle as a necessary forerunner of hernia testis. In very exceptional cases the spermatic cord has been thickened, and even nodulated. When the vas deferens is thickened, search should be made for any urethral irritation which may have acted as an exciting cause of the orchitis.

Prognosis.—Syphilitic orchitis, especially when treated early, ends usually in resolution ; and it is very remarkable how rapidly a large testicle, in some instances, returns to its natural size under the influence of mercury. The function of the testicle is recovered after proper treatment. Impotence and sterility only result from advanced disease in both organs. Atrophy, the breaking down of gummata, and hernia testis are occasional terminations. Atrophy is the ordinary consequence of neglect of treatment ; the breaking down of gummata and hernia testis occur, but rarely, in the weakly, the intemperate, the strumous, and the untreated. My own experience goes to support Ricord's statement that syphilis of the testis never ends in suppuration.

Symptoms.—The testicle slowly and insidiously enlarges until perhaps it reaches the size of a pear or an orange. It is either pyriform or rounded in shape, smooth or irregular or nodular on the surface, painless, heavy, and resistant to the touch, and generally quite devoid of the ordinary testicular sense. The scrotum is unaffected except when hernia testis is threatened. There is often slight hydrocele. One testicle only may be affected, or both may be so either consecutively or simultaneously ; the second testis may be attacked whilst the patient is under specific treatment for the first. If the disease is not treated, and is thus allowed to take its course, the function of the testicle is impaired or lost. When an injury has immediately preceded and excited the attack the onset may be quite sudden and painful, and the symptoms may resemble those of acute epididymo-orchitis. These acute symptoms, however, last only a few days.

Diagnosis.—Syphilitic orchitis has to be distinguished from chronic orchitis, tubercular disease, new growths of the testicle, and, when it is excited by an injury, from the acute inflammatory affections of the testicle. From all these diseases the history of the case, the physical characters of the enlargement, the frequency of bilateral affection, the co-existence of other evidences of syphilis, and the undoubted improvement under mercurial treatment when continued for a few weeks, will suffice to prove the specific nature of the orchitis.

Treatment.—This should be both local and constitutional. The local consists in removing any hydrocele fluid by tapping, and then strapping the testicle with simple soap or mercurial plaster. The constitutional treatment should be the avoidance of alcohol, the discontinuance of sexual connection, and the administration of mercury alone, or mercury combined with small doses of iodide of potassium.

In the greater number of cases, and especially in those in which the orchitis occurs within two years of the primary disease, mercury alone is the best drug; even in cases in which the orchitis is present in the more advanced tertiary period, mercury alone is sometimes better than iodide of potassium alone or combined with mercury. The larger doses of iodide so often given in late syphilis have a very lowering effect upon these patients, who are generally much debilitated already by the disease, and by their habits of life, and perhaps by hardships and exposure. The mercury may be given as a pill in the form of one grain of the green iodide, of calomel, or of hydrargyrum cum cretâ combined with a sixth, a fourth, or a third of a grain of opium three times a day; or as a mixture composed of a drachm of the perchloride solution combined with decoction of sarsaparilla, or a simple bitter infusion, three times a day. When iodide is employed it should be given in the smallest doses which are found to affect the disease: three or five grains combined with a drachm of the liquor hydrargyri perchloridi in a bitter infusion will be found generally enough, and it is a combination which has long had the test of experience.

In syphilitic orchitis, as in all other forms of syphilitic disease, the treatment should be continued for two or three months, or even more, after the disappearance of the enlargement of the testicle.

CHAPTER XI.

TUBERCULAR DISEASES OF THE TESTICLE.

CHRONIC tubercular disease of the testicle may be either (*a*) primary, or (*b*) secondary to tubercular deposits in some other part or organ of the genito-urinary apparatus, or (*c*) the testicle may be affected with acute tuberculosis as part of a general disease, but this is very rare (Fig. 32).

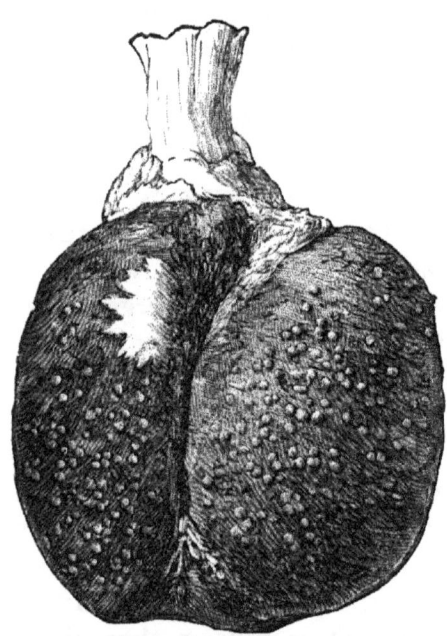

Fig. 32.—Miliary Tuberculosis of Testis. (St. Thomas's Hospital Museum.) (*Osborn.*)

The discovery of the bacillus tuberculosis by Koch, and the fact that tubercular disease of the testicle is precisely of the same nature and tendency as tubercular lesions of other organs, make it unnecessary to dwell at any length on the pathology of the disease. It will be sufficient to point out how the bacilli gain access to the testicle, and briefly what are the naked-eye and microscopical changes which take place in the organ.

Pathology.—There are three possible channels of infection along which the bacilli can pass, namely, the lymphatics, the blood-vessels, and the vas deferens. When the testicle is primarily affected the bacilli, no doubt, reach the organ in most cases by the spermatic artery; in some rare instances it is probable that they may be conveyed through the vas deferens during coitus.

When the disease of the testis is secondary to tubercle of the urethra, prostate, or bladder, the bacilli find their way along the vas deferens to the epididymis. When once the disease is started in the epididymis, the bacilli probably spread by way of the lymphatics as well as by the blood-vessels and seminal tubules.

The explanation given of the frequency with which the epididymis is the first part affected, is the small size and the great tortuosity of the blood-vessels of the epididymis as compared with those of the testicle and vas deferens, and the fact that the spermatic artery divides opposite the epididymis into two main branches: one for the epididymis and the other for the testicle proper.

The channel of the vas deferens is supposed to offer a means of direct infection during coitus, both of the male by the discharges of the female and of the female through the semen, in either of which fluids the bacilli can be conveyed from the deep parts

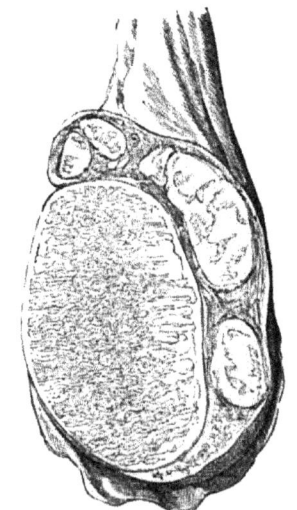

Fig. 33.—Epididymis containing several cretifying Masses of Tubercle. The body of the testis appears sound. (*Curling.*)

of the sexual organs of the one sex to those of the other.

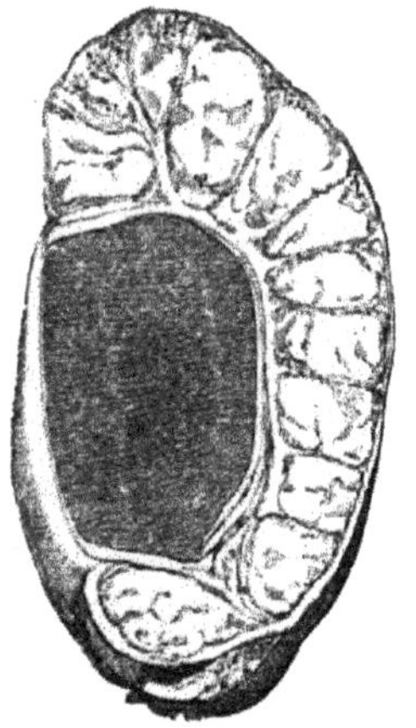

In the earliest clinical stages of tubercular testis a small nodule is present in the head of the epididymis, followed in time by similar nodules in other parts of the epididymis. By degrees these nodules may coalesce until the whole epididymis is converted into an irregular, hard, boat-shaped mass (Figs. 33 and 34). At a later stage the tubercular mass softens and breaks down in one or more places, and, after ulcerating through the tissues of the scrotum, a fistulous opening or a hernia testis may result.

Fig. 34.—Tubercular Disease of the Epididymis. The testicle is small, but appears healthy. The patient died of phthisis. (*Curling.*)

When the body of the testicle is involved, tubercular granulations spread irregularly through the testicle in lines radiating from the corpus Highmorianum; or caseous masses are deposited, as in the epididymis (Fig. 35), which masses may soften and make a way through the tunica albuginea and scrotum, forming fistulæ or hernia testis.

The tunica vaginalis is the seat of chronic inflammation, and by the formation of adhesions between the visceral and parietal portions, the cavity becomes partially or entirely obliterated (Fig. 35). When these adhesions are not universal, they sometimes limit collections of fluid of a serous or sero-purulent or thick purulent nature in which the tubercle bacilli have been found to be present. Tubercular granulations are sometimes seen scattered on the tunica vaginalis, and this membrane may be thickened and velvety, like a pulpy synovial membrane.

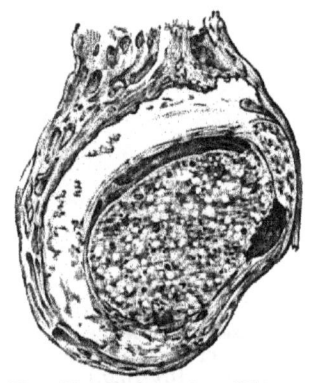

Fig. 35.—Tubercular Disease of the Testicle. (London Hospital Museum.) (*J. Cantlie.*)

The vas deferens is frequently thickened and indurated, its walls being infiltrated and its cavity stuffed with the products of the tubercular inflammation. This thickening may be regular and continuous for an inch or two, or irregular nodules may be dotted along the cord.

The parts of the vas deferens generally affected are its two extremities, so that frequently, when it feels to be normal, at the upper part of the scrotum and in the groin, one or other or both its extremities may be much diseased.

In association with disease at the prostatic end of the vas deferens are similar changes in the vesiculæ seminales and prostate, and these organs ought always to be examined with the finger in the rectum before expressing an opinion as to the limitation of the disease or the advisability of castration.

Histological Characters.—The essential component elements of a tubercle nodule are (*a*) leucocytes, (*b*) giant cells, (*c*) epithelioid cells, (*d*) reticulum, (*e*) tubercle bacilli. In the ordinary form of tubercle, as it is met with in the testicle, the epithelioid cells and the leucocytes are found in the meshes of a well-defined reticulum, composed of pre-existing connective tissue and a delicate network of branching giant cells. The tubercle bacilli are found here and there amongst the areas of small round cells, and in some of the giant cells.

Whilst many of the seminal tubes are quite healthy, others have their walls infiltrated with small, round cells; and within the tubules are masses of degenerating, desquamated, and coalescing endothelial cells mingled with leucocytes. The inter-tubular connective tissue around these masses becomes affected, and takes a share in the formation of caseous nodules.

The bacillus of tubercle sets up tissue proliferation when brought into contact with fixed tissue cells susceptible to its action, and a special form of chronic inflammation is established which results in a typical tubercle nodule.

The earliest microscopic evidence of the formation of a tubercle nodule is a small cell infiltration like embryonal cells—the product of tissue proliferation by karyokinesis from connective tissue, endothelial or epithelial cells. The epithelioid and giant cells are developed later by transformation of the small cells; the giant cells occupy the centre of the nodule; around them are the epithelioid cells, and amongst the giant and epithelioid cells and about the periphery of the nodule are found the leucocytes, the smallest cells of all, which reach the part through the inflamed walls of the capillaries in the immediate neighbourhood.

Each tubercle nodule increases in size by the growth of new cells from pre-existing tissue, and by the migration of leucocytes ; and as the bacilli multiply in the peripheral part of the nodule, and are carried into the surrounding tissue, they start new centres for the formation of fresh tubercle nodules. Subsequently, large masses are formed by the coalescence of the individual nodules.

The centre of each nodule of the confluent mass is a focus of caseation, and as the caseating process extends into the outer zone of the nodules, these several foci blend to form large broken-down cavities, containing filamentous shreds and cheesy, solid material, which are composed of the products of cell necrosis. It is not an ordinary fatty degeneration, but a coagulation necrosis of the cells. The early death of cells is the characteristic pathological feature of tubercle, and distinguishes the tubercular from all other forms of chronic inflammation. This necrosis begins in the giant cells, and the epithelioid cells in the *centre* of each nodule, and spreads outwards, for two reasons—first, because there are no bloodvessels in these tubercle nodules, and the central cells are the most remote from vascular supply; and secondly, because these central cells have been longest exposed to the action of the bacilli and their ptomaines, the specific action of which is to cause coagulation necrosis.

This cheesy material does not afford a suitable medium for the life and development of the bacilli; hence, they die of starvation, so that no bacilli are found in this material. But the spores of the bacilli are more durable and resisting, and remain in an active state for an indefinite time; hence, successful inoculations can be made with this cheesy material. So long as a cheesy mass remains solid, it may be latent and harmless; but as soon as it liquefies the spores of the bacilli which it contains can be conveyed far and wide by the bloodvessels, and acute general tuberculosis may thus result.

In this way, tubercular complications affecting the lungs, liver, kidneys, peritoneum, bones, joints, and membranes of the brain may be brought about. The kidney may also be affected by direct extension upwards from the prostatic urethra or bladder, to which the bacilli may have been conveyed along the vas deferens.

The tubercular process may be arrested by the destruction and disappearance of the bacilli, and the conversion of the cells into tissue of a higher type. The masses may then become encysted by surrounding interstitial simple inflammatory products.

Another way of checking the local extension of tubercle is calcification of the tubercular product. This change is always secondary to caseation, and is a substitution of inorganic calcareous material for the cheesy material.

Causes of Tubercular Testis.—The essential cause is the entrance of the tubercle bacillus into the system of an individual whose testicular structures are susceptible to its pathogenic action. The predisposing causes are hereditary taint, injury, venereal excitement, and gonorrhœa.

There are a few cases on record of tubercular testis in the new-born child; but by hereditary taint is generally understood lowly-vitalised tissues unable to resist, still less to eliminate, the tubercle bacillus. Possibly, the bacilli or their spores may be actually inherited, but remain dormant till brought into activity by some slight injury or an attack of gonorrhœal or other form of inflammation.

The alteration brought about in tissues by slight injuries will lead to the determination of the localisation of the bacillus, or may start into activity and development the bacilli previously existing, but in a dormant state, in the system.

Venereal excesses may predispose to tuberculosis by weakening the individual and lowering the resisting power of the tissues, or if the disease already exists, it may hasten its progress and development.

Gonorrhœa and other forms of inflammatory affections of the testis may, by impairing the resisting power of the tissues, render them more assailable to the bacillus. Possibly, too, the patient may become the recipient of the tubercle bacillus at the same time that he acquires the microbe of gonorrhœa.

Symptoms.—The early stage of primary tuberculosis of the testis will almost certainly be unrecognised by the patient, or he will detect it by chance as a small, painless nodule in the upper part of the epididymis.

The course of the disease has been artificially divided into three stages. The first may be called the stage of deposit; the second, the stage of caseation; and the third, the stage of fistulæ or of fungus testis. The first stage of primary tuberculosis of the testis is almost certainly unnoticed by the patient because the onset and progress of the disease are painless. When detected in this stage by the surgeon it presents itself as a nodule, or as nodules, in the epididymis, and generally in the upper part of the epididymis. These nodules are at first hard and well defined, and devoid of any symptom of inflammation. By degrees the whole of the epididymis may be involved, either uniformly or as a string of nodules (Figs. 33 and 34). As a rule, the nodules are larger in the head and tail than elsewhere. The testicle itself usually remains unaltered for a time, then softens, and becomes more diffluent than elastic, and small, round, shot-like bodies may be felt near the hilum.   In rare cases the body of the testis, as well as the epididymis, may be affected simultaneously, and, enlarging, form a swelling the size of a hen's egg, or larger, in which there is no distinction between epididymis and testis proper (Fig. 36).   There may be some hydrocele fluid in the general sac of the tunica vaginalis or in a cyst-like space of the sac.   The fluid may subsequently undergo changes towards pus, or may become absorbed and leave the vaginal cavity more or less obliterated.

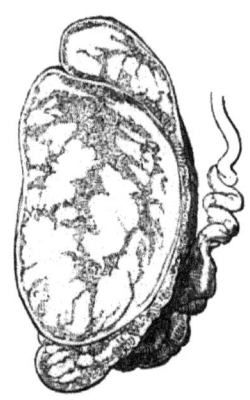

Fig. 36.—Testis as well as Epididymis affected with Tubercle.   The patient died of phthisis. (*Curling.*)

In the second stage the tubercle nodules soften into a caseous mass in a slow, insidious, and painless manner. Over one of these softening nodules the tunica vaginalis and, later, the skin become adherent; the skin becomes red, then bluish, and, later, still darker in colour, and fluctuation is detected.   The period at which this second stage sets in varies, in different cases, from several weeks to some years.   It is generally not till after several months.   It is hastened by sexual excitement, intemperate or careless living, and by any exercise which shakes or is liable to injure the testicles.

The third stage is marked by the ulceration of the skin over the adherent and discoloured parts and the discharge of a puriform fluid with curdy or cheesy flakes.   Later, the discharge becomes thin and watery, and fistulous openings are established, the orifices of which have ragged edges and are surrounded by thin, purplish, cold skin.   Or a large ulcerated opening on the skin may be soon followed by a large mass of prominent granulation-tissue, sprouting from the tunica albuginea or tissue of the testicle, thus forming a fungus testis. It is rare for these fistulæ, when once established, to become permanently healed; if they cicatrise for a time, which they do not often do, they will pretty surely break open again in circumstances of impaired health or of injury.

It is very common for tubercular disease of the prostate, vas, or vesiculæ seminales to be associated with tubercle of the testicle, and the general health and aspect of the patient are generally indicative of the tubercular diathesis. This is not by any means an invariable rule, for tubercular testis does sometimes affect the vigorous and healthy-looking, and men of good physique.

Not infrequently both testicles are infected, either simultaneously or within a short time of one another.

When the disease in the epididymis becomes latent, which it rarely does, the infection may still extend to the testicle or along the vas deferens.

The *diagnosis* is rarely a matter of any difficulty. The small hard nodules which are sometimes left behind after an attack of acute epididymitis are distinguished by being in the globus minor rather than in the globus major, by following an acute inflammation of the organ, by having no tendency to suppurate, break down, or become adherent to the scrotum, and by not being associated with signs of tubercular affection of the prostate, vas deferens, or vesiculæ seminales.

The disease with which tubercular testis is most likely to be confounded is tertiary syphilis of the testicle, this mistake being possible when the epididymis and the body of the testicle are alike involved in the tubercular process. But the tendency of tubercle to soften and break down, its irregular nodular outline, its tendency to become worse, not better, under the anti-syphilitic treatment, and the result of inoculation experiments with the discharge from the fistulæ or fungus, or even with the fluid of an accompanying hydrocele will serve to clear up any doubt.

Sarcoma and other **malignant growths** generally will be distinguished by their affecting the body of the testicle, first and chiefly by their greater weight and painfulness, by their more rapid growth, and by being confined to one organ, whilst tubercle is prone to attack both testicles. Examination per rectum will not discover any enlargement of the prostate or vesiculæ.

It must not be forgotten, however, that tubercular disease may grow to a great size, and with much rapidity, and may quickly extend along the structures of the cord, in these respects resembling malignant growths.

Mr. Walsham has recorded a case in which in history, course, and clinical symptoms the tubercular testis closely simulated sarcoma; and another in which the tubercular disease imitated very nearly the diffuse orchitis of tertiary syphilis. (*Brit. Med. Journ.*, vol. i., 1884, p. 855.)

Course and Prognosis.—The kidney and other and anatomically quite unconnected organs and structures, such as the lungs, joints, bones, spine, pleura, or peritoneum, may become secondarily affected from tubercular testis.

The rate of progress of tubercular disease of this organ varies much in different cases. In the first stage it may remain long localised to the epididymis, or may rapidly extend to the testicle proper; in the second stage the rapidity and multiplicity of points of softening are equally variable, and so, too, is the liability of the disease to affect both testicles. In some cases, after a prolonged period of quiescence in one stage, the disease rapidly advances, and that either by extension in the same stage or by transit from one stage to a later.

Whether the disease runs a slow or a rapid course, it sooner or later tends to a fatal termination, either by extension to the urinary part of the genito-urinary apparatus, or by setting up secondary tubercular disease in some other tissues or organs.

Whilst the disease is not very likely to become permanently quiescent, or to undergo a natural cure, there is, on the other hand, no justification of the doctrine that tubercular testis any more than tubercular kidney is always and necessarily a fatal disease; or that it is a mere local expression of a general affection of the genito-urinary organs. By early recognition, the disease, when primary, may be in some cases checked by change of residence to a suitable climate; in others it may be eradicated by well-timed surgical treatment.

When the disease is secondary to, or associated with tuberculosis of some other part or organ, life may still be prolonged and rendered more comfortable in cases of suppurating fistula or hernia testis, by castration.

Treatment.—This will be either medical and palliative, or operative. The medical treatment consists in good air, good diet, cod-liver oil, tonics, stimulants in the shape of a moderate quantity of good port wine, and, in fact, everything which will improve the health and hygienic condition of the patient, so as to enable him to resist and overcome the inroads of the tubercle bacilli which have localised themselves in the testis. A residence in Australia or some other warm and dry climate may check or cure the disease when in an early stage, and especially before softening of the tubercle nodules has commenced; sea voyages or a residence at the sea-side has proved very beneficial. Some surgeons, though the number is diminishing, approve of prolonged trial of these medical means, either because they deem the disease curable, or for the other extreme reason, because they regard it only as part of a necessarily fatal affection. But if improvement does not soon follow upon general, hygienic, and climatic treatment, some surgical operation will be requisite, and should be undertaken without further loss of time. This consists either in removing the deposits, or in scraping out the fistulæ, or in castration.

Medical treatment should be tried as long as the deposits are small and hard; but as soon as caseation has commenced operative treatment should be employed.

The testicle should be treated in the same way as bones, joints, cervical glands, and as I have treated kidneys affected with softening tubercular deposits, i.e. every softened area should be opened, the contents well scraped out, then the cavity well rubbed with iodoform. It is surprising how rapidly wounds in organs so treated heal. Though it is believed that such treatment leads to atrophy, yet this is a lesser evil than extension and diffusion of tubercle. When erasion has failed, when the fistulæ persist or are numerous, when there is fungus with a small wasted testis, and when the whole or greater part of the organ is invaded, castration is the only treatment. Castration may be done for two different classes of case; first, as a curative operation for advanced cases where the disease is limited to one testicle, and has not extended too high along the cord, and when the bladder, prostate, and vesiculæ seminales are unaffected, and where, therefore, the whole disease can be removed; and, secondly, as a means of prolonging life and giving relief from a source of great discomfort and of exhausting discharges, even when the general state of the patient's health, or the existence of disease in the other testis, or in the prostate, vesiculæ, or some distant organ, such as the lungs, renders a cure impossible.

It is, however, only in exceptional cases of the latter kind that the operation should be resorted to. As a rule medical and hygienic treatment only should be employed in cases in which advanced pulmonary phthisis or tubercular disease of a large joint co-exists with tubercular testis. In castration for tuberculosis, the tunica vaginalis should be removed with the testicle, and so, too, should any portions of adherent or ulcerated scrotal tissues.

In cases in which operative treatment is not considered necessary, every care should be taken to prevent the lighting up of fresh active mischief by injury, urethritis, sexual excitement, or intemperate or unhealthy living.

The treatment recommended by Professor Verneuil in 1871 by the actual cautery as a substitute for erasion and castration has not, in my opinion, any strong claim for adoption.

ACUTE TUBERCULOSIS OF EPIDIDYMIS AND TESTIS.

This has been described by M. Duplay (*L'Union Medical,* 1860, and article by Reclus) as galloping ("galopante") tubercularisation of the testis. It is rare, and begins, like gonorrhœal epididymis, suddenly and with acute symptoms. There is pain in the testis radiating to the groin and loins, the scrotum is œdematous, there is effusion into the tunica vaginalis, and the testicle enlarges to two or three times its natural size. There may have been some previously existing tubercular nodule in the organ, but, if so, it is rarely noticed by the patient. In some cases tubercular nodules have been found in the opposite testis, or lesions have existed for a longer or shorter time in the cord, prostate, or vesiculæ seminales ; or an urethral purulent or sero-purulent discharge may have preceded the outbreak in the testis. As the swelling increases, the epididymis becomes more prominent, and suppuration is often established in about three weeks from the commencement.

This urethral discharge sometimes contains the bacilli of

tubercle, and their presence, together with co-existing tubercular nodules in the prostate or elsewhere, and perhaps the scrofulous aspect of the patient, will serve to distinguish the rapidly-enlarged testicle of acute tuberculosis from malignant disease.

The acute form may attack men of any age.

TUBERCULOSIS OF THE TESTICLE IN INFANTS,

according to some French writers, is not so rare as was once thought, but has been overlooked owing to the slow and painless way in which the disease sets in and advances in an organ which at this age is in a functionless condition. The left organ is somewhat more frequently affected than the right; the disease may be either chronic or acute ; it often follows, or is followed by, tubercular peritonitis, probably through the passage of the bacilli along the open processus funiculo-vaginalis. The testicle proper is more often affected than the epididymis. The cord, vesiculæ, and prostate are rarely attacked.

The *diagnosis* must be made from congenital syphilis and from sarcoma.

Syphilis more frequently affects both organs, is associated with other evidence of the constitutional disorder, has no tendency to suppurate, and improves under specific treatment.

Sarcoma occurs in otherwise healthy children, grows much more rapidly, and attains a very much larger size than tubercular testis.

CHAPTER XII.

NEW GROWTHS, SOLID AND CYSTIC, OF THE TESTICLE.

THE clinical forms of new growths of the testicle are far less numerous than the histological or microscopical elements which are found in them. So mixed are these elements that in the same tumour we find fibrous, myxomatous, sarcomatous, and cartilaginous tissues blended. Nor is it possible to draw a sharp distinction between innocent and malignant growths of the testicle, because in this organ there is a tendency for so-called simple tumours, such as cystomata, myxomata, and chondromata, to be followed, like sarcomata and carcinomata, by secondary deposits in the lumbar glands and elsewhere.

The varieties of solid tumours of the testicle which have been described are (1) carcinoma, (2) sarcoma, (3) lymphadenoma, (4) chondroma, (5) fibroma, (6) myxoma, (7) myoma, and (8) osteoma.

CARCINOMA

occurs in the *medullary* form : scirrhus is well-nigh unknown —no well-authenticated case being on record. The medullary cancer of the testis is very soft, being composed of very delicate and highly vascular fibrous tissues, the alveoli of which are filled with cells like those of the seminal epithelium. The new growth starts in the glandular epithelium of the tubules in the centre of the organ near the rete testis. It at first is confined within the tunica albuginea, and so long as this is so the testicle, though much and rapidly enlarged, is ovoid in shape and regular in outline ; but as the disease progresses nodular projections form on the surface, and at length the tunica albuginea gives way, the skin becomes involved, and a fungus hæmatodes results.

On section the tumour is creamy-white, pinky-white, or fawn-coloured, very soft, and its cellular substance is readily washed away by a gentle stream of water, leaving a flocculent filamentous membrane behind. Extravasations of blood commonly occur into the substance of the tumour, and other changes are apt to occur in it, such as colloid, caseous, and mucoid, fatty, and cystic degenerations.

There is rarely any proper testicular tissue left in these tumours, such as there is in adenomata and cystomata of the testis, which also begin in or near the rete testis.

The tunica vaginalis becomes wholly or in part obliterated by inflammatory adhesions; any unobliterated portions are filled with blood-stained serum. Mr. Jacobson mentions cases in which blood has been extravasated into the vaginal sac from the surface of the new growth, thus forming a malignant hæmatocele.

The epididymis is usually lost in the mass. The structures of the cord become infiltrated by the growth; and the pelvic and lumbar glands are invaded by propagation along the course of the lymphatics. By extension from these glands the spinal column and spinal cord, or the mesentery, peritoneum, abdominal viscera, and lungs, may become involved.

What are called *mixed carcinomata* of the testis are cancerous tumours in which the fibrous stroma, instead of forming alveoli, develops into cartilage, bone, or fatty tissue.

SARCOMA

occurs as a soft, round-celled medullary tumour, with very little intercellular substance; or as a firm, fleshy tumour composed of spindle and mixed cells, and having an abundant fibrillar stroma—the fibro-sarcoma. When the matrix is more mucous and elastic, or granular, than fibrous, the growth is called myxo- or granulo-sarcoma. The round-celled or medullary sarcoma is the one most often met with in the testicle in an unmixed form. The fibro-sarcoma, myxo-sarcoma, and granulo-sarcoma are often combined with other tissues of the connective tissue type, such as cartilage, muscle, or fat tissue. Conversely, a myxoma or chondroma may after a time become sarcomatous by conversion of connective tissue elements into spindle or round cells.

The sarcomata are usually described as originating in the connective tissue between the tubules, or in that contained in the wall of the tubules. In naked-eye appearances, in rapidity and mode of growth, and in the mode of extension of the disease to the lymphatic glands and other organs, the sarcomata resemble the carcinomata. Sarcoma is more apt to attack both testicles, and to be associated with multiple secondary deposits in the skin, than is carcinoma.

Myo-sarcomata of the testis have been recorded by Neumann and Ribbert in Virchow's *Archiv.* They are largely composed of striated spindle cells, and affect the testes of boys from infancy to puberty or later (Fig. 37).

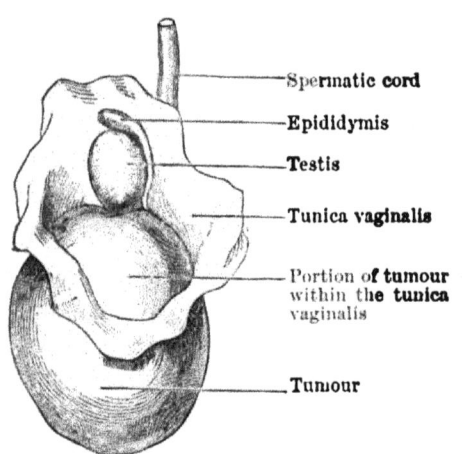

Spermatic cord
Epididymis
Testis
Tunica vaginalis
Portion of tumour within the tunica vaginalis
Tumour

Fig. 37.—Myo-sarcoma of Testis. (*Neumann.*)

Lympho-sarcomata occur in boys and young men, and may affect one testicle after the other. They grow rapidly, and terminate fatally by secondary growths in distant organs. Hutchinson (Trans. Path. Soc., vol. xl. p. 193) has reported a case in a man aged seventy, both organs having been involved.

The Clinical history of carcinoma and sarcoma shows that their exciting cause is frequently some form of injury. They mostly occur between twenty-five and forty-five, carcinoma being almost unknown in infancy and boyhood, though sarcoma is met with in childhood as well as in young adult and middle life. Both forms of disease develop rapidly and often painlessly, and as long as the tunica albuginea remains intact, the tumour, though of great size, retains the normal shape of the testicle; thus, unfortunately, mistakes in diagnosis are frequent, the disease being regarded as inflammatory, and castration delayed till too late to be of much benefit. In other cases the consistence of the swelling is so soft that the new growth is apt to be mistaken for hydrocele or hæmatocele. In other cases, if seen in an early stage, the testicle feels firmer at the part in which the disease is commencing. As a rule, the growth is firm at first, and becomes softer as it increases.

A feeling of weight and dragging is complained of, but not usually of pain; though neuralgic pains, not relieved by rest or support, are felt in the testis, groin, and down the thigh by some patients. Growth progresses steadily, as a rule; if, however, the swelling ceases to increase for a while, or seems to diminish somewhat owing to the absorption of hydrocele fluid, the lull is but very temporary. The coverings of the testis stretch greatly, then yield, and ultimately, if castration is not performed, a fungus hæmatodes is developed, and rapidly increases and readily bleeds.

The cord enlarges at first from turgescence of its blood-vessels, subsequently from infiltration of the tissues by new growth. The veins of the scrotum swell, and the lower extremities may become œdematous from pressure by the affected pelvic and lumbar glands upon the iliac vein and the inferior vena cava. The patient usually dies from the marasmus and pain caused by the invasion of some of the abdominal organs, from lung complications, or occasionally from the exhaustion induced by the discharges, sloughing, and hæmorrhages which attend a fungus hæmatodes.

In the firmer forms of sarcoma the rate of growth is for a time not rapid, and at the end of twelve months the tumour may not have attained a size greater than a goose's egg. Subsequently its increase is sudden and rapid, and it softens in parts of, if not throughout, its bulk.

Diagnosis.—Carcinoma and the soft varieties of sarcoma are not distinguishable except by the microscope. As a rule, carcinoma more quickly invades the cord and scrotum than does sarcoma. Carcinoma does not occur in infancy and childhood; sarcoma may.

Tubercular disease beginning in the testis and rapidly advancing to a great size may be mistaken for cancer or sarcoma, as in a case reported by Mr. Walsham (*Brit. Med. Journ.*, 1884, vol. i. p. 855). There is a risk that some of the forms of orchitis may be mistaken for one of the firmer and more slowly growing sarcomata; but the history of syphilis in some cases, the antecedent symptoms of inflammation in others, and the chronic indolent nature and uniformly hard character of the swelling in other forms of orchitis, will assist towards a correct diagnosis.

Hæmatocele will be distinguished by the sudden formation of the swelling following an injury; and old hydroceles by their history, duration, and the use of the aspiratory needle.

Prognosis and Treatment.—The only prospect of cure or prolongation of life lies in early castration. It is unhappily the common case for recurrence to take place in the lumbar and pelvic glands within a year, more or less, after castration; but there are on record some most encouraging instances of patients living several years after the operation without any return of the disease.

The other forms of solid new growths enumerated above are very rare and of little clinical importance. The several structures of which they are composed are seldom met with *alone* in tumours of the testicle; but in combination with one another, with cysts, or with cancer and sarcoma they are not uncommon.

Of these different tumours the *chondromata* are the least rare. They occur (1) in a pure and uncombined form, consisting usually of hyaline, and more rarely of more or less fibrous cartilage; and (2) as mixed chondromata in which the cartilage elements are combined with cysts or sarcomatous material. Both forms have a tendency to spread and invade distant parts and organs; but the mixed chondromata are much more malignant than the unmixed.

Early castration is the proper treatment for all these solid growths.

CYSTIC DISEASE OF THE TESTICLE.

Under this heading are included the " cystic fibromata " or simple cystomata; and the " cystic sarcomata " of the testicle. The former are innocent, the latter malignant; but between these two typical forms there are all grades of intermediate varieties.

Some tumours consist (1) of numbers of minute cysts interspersed with other cysts of considerable size (Figs. 38 and 39); (2) some of very firm dense fibrous tissue, in which are numerous cysts of varying size; and (3) in others the cysts are small and unequally distributed, and the stroma consists of round-celled sarcoma tissue.

In the cystic fibromata the cysts are the leading prominent feature, and the intercystic stroma is composed of simple fibrous or fibrillar tissue. The contents of the cysts vary, being sometimes clear and limpid, at others thick and glairy, sometimes colourless or clear yellow, at others opaque, white, curdy, or brownish, like coffee grounds. In the cystic

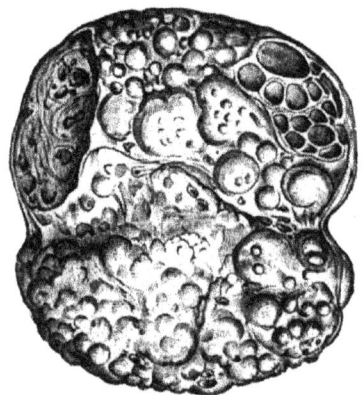

Fig. 38.—Cystic Disease of the Testicle. (London Hospital.) (*J. Cantlie.*)

sarcomata the cysts are much smaller, fewer in number, and less uniformly distributed, and contain papillomatous, sessile, or pedunculated masses; whilst the intercystic stroma is more

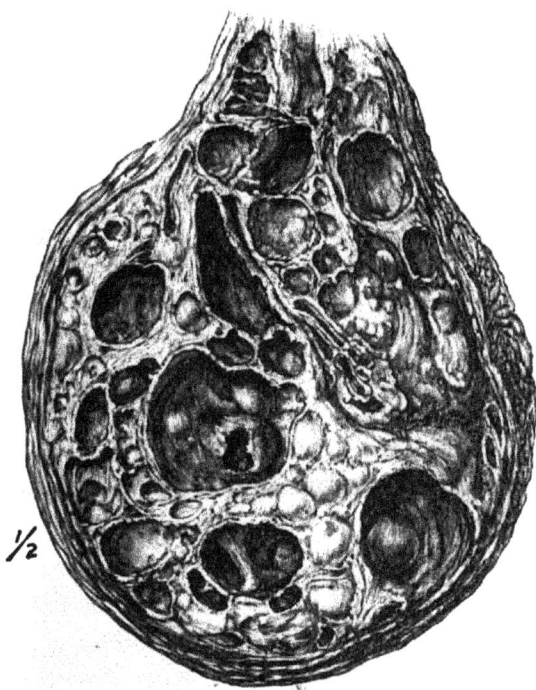

½

Fig. 39.-- Cystic Testicle, composed of a congeries of cysts varying in size from a pea to a small walnut. Some contain small solid growths, others secondary cysts. The cysts are separated by fibrous septa, which contain small nodules of cartilage. The cysts are lined with epithelium, and some contain clear straw-coloured fluid; others gummatous matter stained with blood. (Middlesex Hospital Museum.)

mixed, and consists of myxomatous, round- and spindle-celled sarcomatous, fibromyxo-sarcomatous, or myomatous tissues. These tumours are grouped by Sutton as "testicular adenomata."

In both forms of disease, but more abundantly in the cystic fibromata, a varying amount of cartilage (Fig. 39), arranged in rods or nodules, may be found embedded in the stroma; in both the testicular tissue is found, in a large number of cases, expanded over the

upper and front part of the new growth (Fig. 40); in both
the disease starts in or near the mediastinum testis; and in
both relapses and metastases may occur. Several theories
have been advanced as to their mode of origin by Curling,
Malassey, Sutton, and Shattock; but both forms probably
originate, as Mr. Eve ("Erasmus Wilson Lecture on Cystic
Disease of Breast and
Testicle") has suggested,
from rudiments of the
Wolffian body—not from
the tubular remains of
that body, but from
numerous groups of cells
derived from the epithelial
columns of the body em-
bedded in the hilum of
the normal testis.

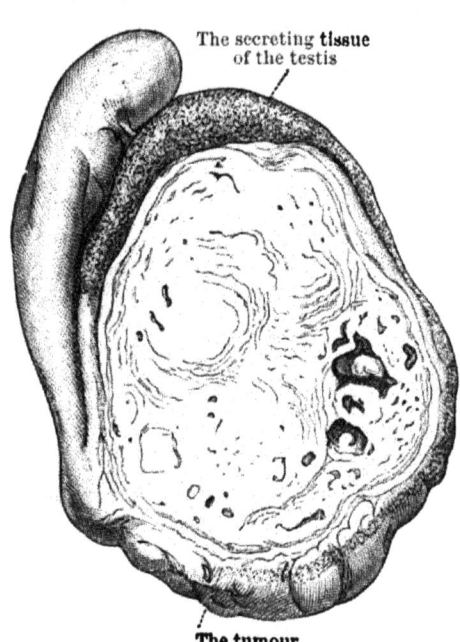

The secreting tissue
of the testis

The tumour

Fig. 40.—Adenoma of Testis. (St. Mary's
Hospital Museum.) (*Sutton* on "Tumours,
Innocent and Malignant.")

Symptoms and Course.
—They may affect the
testicle at any age be-
tween birth and old age.
They grow insidiously and
painlessly.   The more
innocent forms may attain
slowly, even through a
period of many years, to
the size of a turkey's egg
or larger.   They are smooth, uniform, and ovoid; but, as they
enlarge, careful palpation may detect some spots softer and
more elastic than others. The spermatic cord and lymphatic
glands are unaffected; the general health is not impaired;
they rarely affect children or old men, but are mostly met
with in the middle period of life. I have met with fibro-
cystic disease in a boy under ten years of age, however.

The more malignant grow much more rapidly, and may
attain to a much greater size in the course of a comparatively
few months.   They feel more elastic to the touch, and as they
grow they tend to become uneven on their surface, and to
throw out bosses or nodules (still covered by the tunica
albuginea) into the cavity of the tunica vaginalis.

Prognosis is grave in the cystic sarcomata, and uncertain in the cystic fibromata, as recurrences or metastatic deposits may take place in any form of these tumours.

Treatment.—Castration is the only remedy, and ought not long to be delayed, especially if the tumour is growing rapidly.

TERATOMATA.

In connection with cystic disease mention must be made of Teratomata. These are (1) congenital cystic growths containing fragments of bone, teeth, nervous tissue, or intestine, or (2) the more ordinary forms of dermoid cysts containing epithelium, hair, or sebaceous material. Both kinds are met with outside the testicle, near the junction of the testicle and epididymis. Their mode of origin is uncertain. They are always congenital, and are in some cases noticed immediately after birth, but in others they have not been detected for many months. They may remain quiescent, or may become inflamed and suppurate, and burst.

Prognosis.—They tend to cause atrophy of the testicular structure, and may possibly develop into malignant disease.

Treatment.—They should be operated upon early ; either they should be incised freely, and their contents evacuated with scoop, forceps, and sharp spoon, and then drained; or castration should be performed. In all cases where complete obliteration of the cyst does not follow its evacuation, or where proliferation of the lining membrane of the cyst occurs and persists after scraping, castration should be performed. Any attempt completely to excise the cyst, and prolonged efforts to remove solid contents, are apt to be followed by destruction of the testicle.

GROWTHS OF THE TUNICA VAGINALIS.

Scattered throughout modern surgical literature are rare instances of new growths beginning in the tunica vaginalis and forming tumours in which the testicle and epididymis take no share, or only a subordinate one.

Mr. Jacobson has collected several, and described them under the heads of " Lipoma," " Fibroma," and " Sarcoma."

He points out that, like the teratomata, the fibromata may

exist for years and attain a great size, but, unlike them, are never congenital. They are with difficulty distinguished from an old orchitis or hydrocele.

Only one case of lipoma is known (recorded by Dr. Park, of Buffalo, "Annals of Surgery," May, 1886, p. 365), and in that instance the testicle was crowded into a small space above the fatty mass which filled the scrotum. The testicle was incorporated with the fat by fibrous trabeculæ and blood-vessels. The growth was supplied with blood by the vessels of the cord and testicle. Castration was performed.

Castration should also be performed for sarcoma of the tunica vaginalis.

As fibromata of the tunica vaginalis grow to a large size, may slough and bleed, or become sarcomatous, they should be excised early, so as to save the testicle, if the relations of the growth to that organ will allow.

CHAPTER XIII.

INJURIES AND DISEASES OF THE SPERMATIC CORD.

INJURIES OF THE CORD.

INJURIES may be inflicted upon the vas deferens or the blood-vessels, or both. They may be either subcutaneous injuries or open wounds. The causes of them are blows, sprains, bites of animals, gunshot and machinery accidents: and sometimes they are self-inflicted. Contused, lacerated, and gun-shot wounds are all very rare. Incised wounds are often made by the surgeon; and during such surgical operations as removal of the sac in the radical treatment of hernia, or in the course of the excision of an encysted hydrocele of the cord, the vas deferens may be torn across, and atrophy or even gangrene of the testicle may be the consequence. This risk ought always to be borne in mind during operation on the spermatic cord and testis.

Contusions.—What is described as *diffused hæmatocele* and hæmatoma of the cord is an extravasation into the meshes of the cellular tissue. It arises from falls astride, direct blows, strains by suddenly and violently abducting the lower limb, falls from a horse, violent coughing, etc. It is much more likely to occur in young adults the subjects of varicocele than in others, but it has happened in boys of only eight years of age.

The extravasated blood may either be widely diffused in the cellular tissue, or be collected within a limited space so as to form an elongated, cylindrical, or sausage-shaped swelling; or the two conditions may exist together.

When a circumscribed and fluctuating collection forms, the question always arises whether it is not contained within an unobliterated portion of the funiculo-vaginal process of peritoneum, and whether the blood is not derived from some ruptured vessels of that membrane.

Kocher made some experiments by injecting glycerine under the fibrous tissue of the spermatic cord, and found he could produce a sausage-shaped swelling extending from the testicle along the inguinal canal to the iliac fossa, where the injected fluid spread out more widely into the tissues.

These blood tumours sometimes attain a great size, reaching from the scrotum high up into the abdomen.

Violent coughing has been known to cause rupture of one of the veins of a varicocele. The symptoms were a sharp crackling noise at the moment of rupture, soon followed by swelling in the scrotum and inguinal and iliac regions, and a sense of deep-seated fluctuation. Some days later ecchymosis was evident, and then all traces of the effusion gradually disappeared. In a case recorded by Cousin (" Des Inflammations en Masse du Cordon Spermatique," *Thèse de Paris*, 1887), a fall on the perinæum was immediately followed by violent pain and a hard, smooth, cylindrical swelling of the cord, which extended all along the inguinal canal and was of the size of small intestine ; the fold of the groin and the testicle of the same side were also much swollen. Inflammation and prolonged suppuration of the hæmatoma resulted in this case.

Treatment consists of rest in the recumbent position and the application of ice or cold lotions. If the swelling tends to increase, or if absorption does not take place satisfactorily, the swelling should be laid open, the blood-clot turned out, any bleeding vessel ligatured, and the wound antisepticised and closed by sutures. A drainage tube had best be retained for twenty-four or thirty-six hours.

Rupture of the Vas Deferens.—This is a rare accident, and is not generally referred to in surgical works. It is most likely to occur at that part of the vas which is between the internal abdominal ring and the ureter, and is caused by a violent blow on the lower part of the abdomen, by the passage of a cart wheel, or by a sudden strain as in slipping or falling with the legs wide apart.

The symptoms of the injury are a sudden and violent pain in the groin, gradually extending over the lower part of the abdomen ; the discharge of blood from the urethra ; the absence of blood in the urine, which is withdrawn from the bladder by catheter ; some swelling and tenderness of the testis of the injured side ; and some degree of fever, and perhaps the signs of localised traumatic peritonitis. After the lapse of a few weeks the testicle atrophies. The bleeding from the urethra is not considerable and soon ceases; the blood is derived from the artery of the vas deferens or from the torn walls of that tube, and it enters the prostatic urethra through the ejaculatory duct. Mr. Hilton has left the records of three cases (published by his colleague Mr. Birkett in the article on "Injuries to the Pelvis" in "A System of Surgery" by Holmes and Hulke, vol. i. p. 934) which occurred in his own practice, and in which he diagnosed the injury. He has further given us the report of a *post-mortem* examination of another case in which he found the testis excessively atrophied and the vas ruptured and closed at each end. The ends of the ruptured vas were two inches apart, the upper being near the internal abdominal ring and adherent to the surrounding tissues; the lower lying near the spot at which the vas crosses the ureter. The vesicula seminalis of the same side was smaller than its fellow.

Diagnosis.—This accident is likely to be mistaken for a contusion or slight rupture of the urethra, especially if the cause of the injury is a direct blow upon, or the passage of a wheel over, the groin. In the case of slight injuries to the urethra, only a slight bleeding from the urethra may occur, and the urine drawn off by catheter will be free from blood; moreover, the catheter may pass quite easily. There is no extravasation of urine, and the patient may be able to micturate at will, though probably with some pain. Thus at first the symptoms of the two injuries will be very much alike; but later there will be no tenderness or swelling of the testis in lacerated urethra as there will be when the vas deferens is ruptured, but there will be some thickening about the injured area of the urethra and some obstruction to the introduction of a catheter after the first twenty-four or forty-eight hours.

Treatment.—This consists in the patient keeping his bed, and in the application of cold lotion or an ice-bag to the groin to check further extravasation and prevent the onset of inflammation. If inflammation occurs, hot fomentations and leeches and saline medicines will be required. If suppuration follows, an early incision above Poupart's ligament will be required.

INFLAMMATORY AFFECTIONS.

It is rare for any of the structures of the spermatic cord to be the seat of inflammation.

The vas deferens, with the cellular tissue around it, may become acutely inflamed owing to the extension of inflammation spreading along it from the urethra. Gonorrhœa, an urethral stricture, or an operation in the urethra, may be the starting-point. I have in one instance seen acute inflammation along the vas deferens followed by a deep-seated abscess in the cellular tissue near the external abdominal ring, as an immediate sequel to the use of Perréve's dilator for stricture of the urethra. Mr. Hutchinson (*Med. Times and Gazette*, vol. i., 1879) has recorded a case in which, after lithotomy, the patient had a succession of abscesses in each iliac region, which, he had no doubt, had their starting-point in the inflamed vas deferens. In my own case the abscess was single and uncomplicated except for a widespread inflammatory induration surrounding it. In Mr. Hutchinson's there was no evidence that the abscesses were pyæmic.

Mr. Jacobson (" Diseases of Male Organs of Generation," p. 498) gives a case in his practice in which a purulent urethral discharge associated with a stricture four inches from the meatus was followed by a slight epididymo - orchitis, together with considerable inflammation and swelling of the vas deferens, which near " the globus minor was of the size of the barrel of a stylographic pen, while the cord from the external to the internal ring was of the size of two adult fingers, standing out in distinct outline beneath the skin of the groin."

Inflammation may spread from the vas deferens to the peritoneum.

Another form of inflammation of the cord affects the cellular tissue without involving the vas deferens.

In a case under my care of very obstinate suppuration, starting in the glands in the groin, the suppurative process spread along the cellular tissue of the cord to the scrotum in one direction, and to the inguinal canal and the planes of fascia between the abdominal muscles at the groin in the other.

Inflammation starting in the skin and subcutaneous tissue, whether of simple or erysipelatous nature, may spread along the cord, either by the connective tissue, or more directly by the peritoneum, if the funiculo-vaginal process is patent, and thus set up fatal general peritonitis.

Yet another way in which acute inflammation of the cord may arise is by phlebitis of the spermatic veins, whether the veins are varicose or not. Inflammation of a varicocele is, however, a very rare occurrence.

Gosselin ("Clin. Chir. de la Charité," p. 379) refers to two cases in which, after gonorrhœa, a vas aberrans was inflamed and formed a very painful swelling, the testis and epididymis and cord being intact.

What has been described as "acute hydrocele of the cord," is in all probability an acute inflammation of the remains of the unobliterated funiculo-vaginal process of peritoneum, the result of sprain or other injury, or possibly of a rheumatic inflammation of this serous membrane.

Treatment.—The treatment of acute inflammation of the cord should be directed to the cause of the inflammation. The local treatment should consist in the application of ice or evaporating lotion to the groin and scrotum in the early stages, and of antiseptic fomentations in the more advanced. Pus should be evacuated by early and deep incisions, for in some cases the matter is very deeply placed. The constitutional treatment should be directed to the free and daily action of the bowels, and to a properly regulated diet.

The vas deferens is, though very rarely, the seat of gummata, and the cord has been found by Lanceraux enlarged and swollen in several places in a case of syphilitic sarcocele.

HYDROCELE.

Hydrocele of the cord is an accumulation of serous fluid either within a distinct cyst, or diffused amongst the cellular tissues of the spermatic cord.

There are four varieties, only one of which is at all common, and that is (1) the encysted variety. The other three are (2) the hydrocele of the unobliterated funicular process of peritoneum, (3) a rare form of hydrocele along (though not of) the cord, namely, hydrocele of a hernial sac, and (4) the diffused hydrocele of the cord.

(1) **Encysted Hydrocele of the Cord.**—In this form the fluid is contained in one or more distinct cavities or cysts, which are formed (*a*) by the imperfect or irregular obliteration of the funicular process of peritoneum (Fig. 41). These are much more common on the right side than on the left,

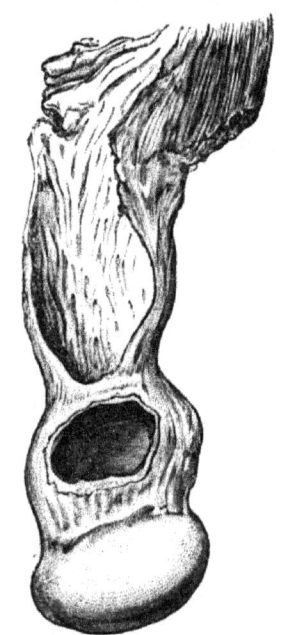

Fig. 41.—Encysted Hydrocele of the Cord. (London Hospital Museum.) (*J. Cantlie.*)

owing to the fact that the closure of the funiculo-vaginal process takes place earlier and more completely on the left side. In some instances there are as many as four or five cysts arranged linearly along the cord, in others there may be only a single cyst. If these cyst spaces become distended with fluid, one or more encysted hydroceles are formed. They vary in size from a pea to a hazelnut or larger, and may be situated within the inguinal canal, or at any spot between the external abdominal ring and the testis. They are often associated with congenital hernia, when the upper end of the funicular process is patent. Being of congenital origin, they are often seen in childhood; but, on the other hand, young adult, middle, or advanced age may be reached before the cysts become distended with fluid. (*b*) Much less frequently encysted hydrocele may result from the formation and distension of a cyst space in the cellular tissue of the cord quite independently of any want of proper obliteration of the funiculo-vaginal process of peritoneum.

(2) **Congenital and Tubular Hydrocele.**—In certain cases the process of peritoneum which is prolonged in front of the testis in its descent to the scrotum, and which normally is obliterated between the top of the scrotum and the internal abdominal ring, is closed only at the top of the scrotum and at the internal ring, but remains unobliterated throughout

the space between these points. If then the whole of this cavity becomes distended with fluid, a large elongated swelling occupying the length of the cord is formed, instead of one or more small globular swellings, as in the above-described "encysted" variety. This is what I have called Tubular Hydrocele of the cord, and has by some authors been spoken of as Diffused Hydrocele. Into such a hydrocele an acquired inguinal hernia may be protruded (Fig. 42). In some cases the upper end of the tubular process is not completely closed, and then the hydrocele communicates with the general peritoneal cavity. This is the congenital hydrocele of the cord.

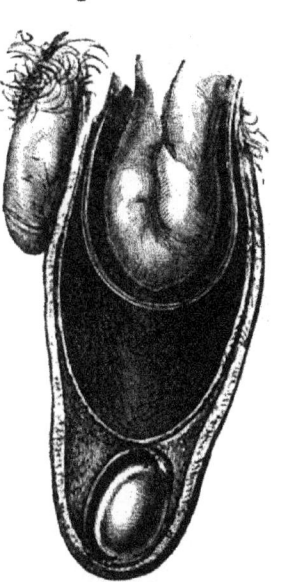

(3) **Hydrocele of a Hernial Sac** is said to be of very rare occurrence, but is less unfrequent than is supposed. Such cases have been described by Bryant and some of the French surgeons, and I have met with several. On one occasion I operated upon three cases within a few weeks of each other. In one a small lump of omentum plugged the neck of the sac; in a second there was much thickening and contraction of the neck of the sac, but a probe could be passed along it into the general peritoneal cavity; and in the third case the neck of

Fig. 42.—Hernial Sac containing Ilium. The sac dipped into an encysted hydrocele of the cord. (*Curling.*)

the sac was completely closed by adhesion of its walls. In another case the mouth of the sac was closed by omentum, a long tag of which was hanging loose in the fluid. It is extremely difficult, unless there is a clear history of rupture (and not always then), to say whether the fluid is contained within an unobliterated process of peritoneum or in an acquired hernial sac. Without a free dissection of the parts this distinction cannot always be made.

Symptoms and Diagnosis.—The swelling varies in shape and size, according to its mode of origin. It is round (Fig. 43), or oval, or oblong in form, defined in outline, uniformly smooth on the surface, painless, often translucent, and moves freely with the cord if it be of either of the first two varieties.   By pulling upon the testis the swelling is made to descend; by pressing the swelling upwards it will partly or entirely disappear within the inguinal canal, but it cannot be reduced completely beyond the abdominal walls, and it gives rise to no gurgling sound as it recedes.

Fluctuation is by no means distinct; percussion generally, but not always, gives a dull note; and when the swelling is

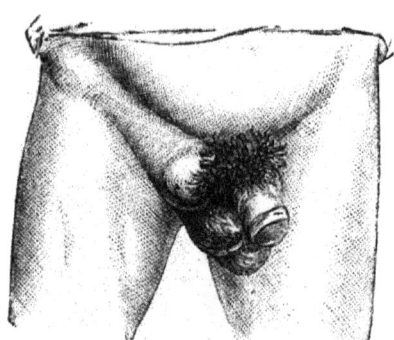

Fig. 43.--Encysted Hydrocele of the Cord. (*Bryant.*)

entirely below the external ring there is no impulse whatever on coughing.   Translucency cannot be made out if the patient is very fat, or if the swelling is confined between the external and internal rings. When of long standing, the cyst wall often becomes very thick, and blood may be effused into the cyst cavity, whether the swelling has been previously tapped or not.

Treatment.—In very young children discutient lotions, such as the chloride ammonium, spirit or lead lotions; or counter-irritants, such as tincture or ointment of iodine, may disperse the swelling. Acupuncture has also succeeded in the very young. Injections are to be avoided, as they may reach the peritoneal cavity if used in either the second or third variety. Setons are unnecessary, as where they succeed repeated acupuncture will do the same.   The best treatment is the radical cure, *i.e.* the excision of the cyst or cysts in the encysted variety; of the funiculo-vaginal process in the second variety; and of the hernial sac in the third variety. When the second or third variety communicates with the abdomen, the constant wearing of a truss may succeed. If the cyst-wall be calcified and firmly adherent to the vas deferens, castration has been recommended; but I think it much better to deal with it as in excision of the sac of a hydrocele of the testicle and cut away all the parts not adherent to the cord, and without interfering with the cord itself.

(4) **Diffuse or Infiltrated Hydrocele of the Cord.**—This is only œdema, and Percival Pott described it as "the hydrocele of the cells of the tunica communis" ("Pott's Surgical Works," vol. ii., 1808, p. 256). This so-called tunic is the cellular tissue or fascia which contains the spermatic vessels; it is continuous above with the cellular tissue between the abdominal muscles, and has the cremasteric fascia spread out upon it. This form of hydrocele does not affect the tunica vaginalis, but is confined to the cellular tissue. It is very rare, Pott and Scarpa being almost the only surgeons who have recorded well-authenticated cases of the kind.

Symptoms.—It causes little or no trouble; the scrotum, testis, and epididymis are unaffected; the spermatic cord is increased in size, has a pyramidal form with its broader part below; it recedes gradually on pressure, but swells again on ceasing pressure. If the swelling extends along the inguinal canal, it dilates the abdominal rings and produces to the touch and to the eye a semblance of omental hernia. The size attained may be great; in one case Pott drew off 11 Winchester pints of fluid.

Treatment.—When small, Pott remarks, it is not an object of surgery, and few persons would choose to submit to an operation to get rid of it; but when it is large and causes deformity, or is inconvenient because of its weight, it must be radically cured by an aseptic incision, and packing or drainage. Pott records one case of a gentleman aged thirty-five who died of exhaustion from the enormous drain of fluid after operation.

HÆMATOCELE.

Hæmatocele of the cord may be either diffuse or encysted, but, unlike hydrocele of the cord, the diffuse is less rare than the encysted.

Diffuse Hæmatocele of the Cord is brought about by rupture of one of the blood-vessels of the cord, usually one of the spermatic veins, whether varicocele exists or not, followed by the more or less rapid extravasation of blood into the cellular tissue of the cord. A blow, kick, or hard straining at stool may be the cause of the rupture, and Jacobson met with a case in which the hæmatocele was produced by the patient's endeavours to reduce a large scrotal hernia. If the blood escapes slowly an elongated swelling forms, if rapidly, it is apt to break through the cellular investment of the cord into the subperitoneal tissue, so that it is impossible to distinguish the cord at its exit from the abdomen. (*See* Injuries to the Spermatic Cord.)

Symptoms and Diagnosis.—After some violence, the patient feels a sudden pain in the groin, immediately followed by a swelling. The shape of the swelling may be oblong or rounded; it may be limited to the cord between the external ring and the top of the testis, or it may occupy the whole cord, and more or less completely conceal the testis. Its outline is smooth, its consistence uniformly solid, and the skin covering it may or may not be ecchymosed. It occurs with equal frequency on the left and right sides. When the skin is not discoloured, the swelling may be mistaken for an omental hernia; but the suddenness of the onset, the absence of constitutional symptoms of rupture, and the irreducibility and want of impulse on coughing, will distinguish hæmatocele.

The duration of diffuse hæmatocele before it undergoes either absorption or any progressive unfavourable change is very uncertain. Bowman records a case of hæmatocele of the right groin caused by a fall from a horse, which remained about the size and shape of a hen's egg for seven years, then became suddenly larger, and went on increasing till it hung down as low as the patella, the testis being distinct at the lowest part of the swelling. After fruitlessly puncturing it, the swelling was laid open, and treacly blood and masses of old blood clot were removed. The man, aged sixty, died five days after the operation, from " low irritative fever "—the hæmatocele having existed altogether about ten years.

Treatment.—If rest, with ice, or evaporating lotions, followed by absorbent ointments and well-adjusted pressure, do not succeed in effecting absorption, or if the tension of the swelling from the first is very great, an incision should be made, the clots and fluid blood turned out, and any bleeding vessels searched for and tied. The lining membrane of the space, if it cannot be readily peeled off, should be well rubbed with iodoform, a drainage tube inserted, and the wound sutured and dressed with antiseptic materials. Castration may be necessary, and in elderly men is certainly the best treatment.

Encysted Hæmatocele.—Either of the forms of encysted hydrocele above described (page 130 *et seqq.*) may be transformed into hæmatocele. This transformation may not occur for many years after the formation of the hydrocele, and may take place either spontaneously or follow puncture of the cyst. Its size and shape vary as do the size and shape of encysted hydrocele, but it may increase after its transformation by extending either towards the scrotum or abdomen ; downwards, it may encroach upon the testis. The vas deferens is usually behind and connected with it. The integuments, though more or less stretched over it, are not usually discoloured. As in encysted hydrocele, a hernia may co-exist above and a vaginal hydrocele of the testicle below.

Treatment.—The cyst should be removed entirely when possible ; if intimately adherent to the vas it should be laid open and cut away as completely as can be without injury to the cord, and the part left behind should have its surface well scraped, and rubbed over with crude carbolic acid. The wound should be drained, its edges united, and dry antiseptic dressing used. The quantity of blood-stained serum, which drains away after operation upon any form of hæmatocele, is sometimes very considerable.

SOLID TUMOURS OF THE CORD.

Except the lipomata, of which many have been recorded, solid new growths of the spermatic cord are very rare. After the lipomata, sarcomata are the next most frequent. Examples of myxoma, myxo-sarcoma, myxo-lipoma, fibroma, and myoma, or fibro-myoma arising in the muscular and fibrous tissue of the vas deferens, have been recorded. Carcinoma of the cord has never, to my knowledge, been recorded except as an extension of, or secondary to, cancer of the testis.

Lipomata, as a rule, originate in the subperitoneal fat, and are little by little protruded through the abdominal rings; occasionally they are developed from fatty lobules contained within the coverings of the spermatic cord.

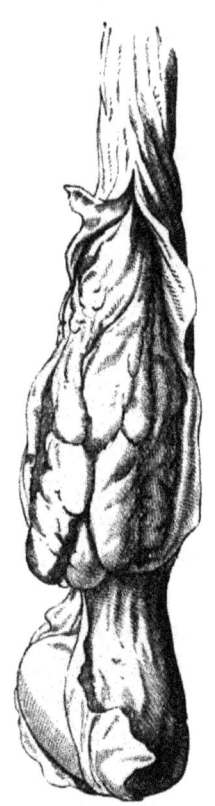

In a specimen dissected by Mr. Hutchinson, jun., the fatty mass which hung down half-way to the testis could be followed up to the fat on the sigmoid flexure, and in a case recorded by Mr. Curling, of recurring lipomata of the left spermatic cord five times excised, there was probably the same anatomical connection, for the tumour used to become tense and painful before each evacuation of the bowels. The left side seems to be much more frequently affected than the right. Out of twenty-five cases collected by Mr. Hutchinson (Path. Soc. Trans., vol. xxxvii. p. 452), the situation of the fatty tumour is stated in eighteen of them; it was thirteen times on the left, three times on the right, and twice on both sides.

Fig. 44. – Lobulated fatty Growth surrounded by thickened Sheath of the Spermatic Cord resembling Omentum in Hernial Sac. (*Curling.*)

When of subperitoneal origin the lipomata tend to draw down in their descent pouches of peritoneum, and thus, as Tillaux and Hutchinson suppose, are predisposing to hernia. Mr. Hutchinson says, "in one case that I dissected, a large fatty outgrowth extended down the entire cord, and in its upper part an empty pouch was found some four inches in length. I found a similar combination in another specimen."

Symptoms and Diagnosis. — Lipomata form painless elongated swellings, sometimes soft, almost to fluctuating, like fatty tumours in other parts of the body; they are distinct from the testicle; not reducible within the abdomen, and give little or no impulse on coughing; though in some exceptional cases they have appeared suddenly, they generally increase slowly and by degrees; pulling upon the testis causes them to descend, which is not the case with an omental hernia (Fig. 44). They are situated within all the coverings of the cord, but are external to a peritoneal pouch, if any such exists. The capsule of the tumour in some cases closely resembles peritoneum, in others is so thin as to be scarcely detectable. The component fat is in larger lobules than in the fat of the omentum, and the lobules are not connected together in the same way by a distinct membrane. They occur in the thin as well as the stout, and may be associated with lipomata in other parts of the body. I have met with a case of lipoma of the cord associated with malignant disease of the testis, and a limited hydrocele of the tunica vaginalis. Clinically, however, and before the parts are exposed in operating, it is often almost impossible to distinguish them from omental hernia.

Myxo-lipomata of the spermatic cord may reach from the abdominal cavity into the scrotum, and be a source of inconvenience and pain from their great size and weight. They are soft, semi-fluctuating, not translucent, and yield nothing on puncturing. Such, at least, is the description given by Mr. Targett (Path. Trans., vol. xl. p. 282) of a tumour which measured vertically 12 inches, and had been growing in the right side of a man aged thirty-five, for five years, at first slowly, but more rapidly during the last two years. An encapsuled myxomatous mass infiltrated with fat globules was situated in the midst of this adipose tumour.

Mr. E. Watson recorded (*Lancet*, 1885, vol. i. p. 838) a case of **fibroma**, the size of a large pear, the stalk end passing up into the inguinal canal, whilst the large end occupied the scrotum. It was successfully removed without sacrificing the testis or cord. The tumour, which was hard and solid throughout, was composed of fibres separated here and there by little masses of fat.

Sarcomata have been met with in the cord as primary new growths; they increase rapidly and tend to infiltrate the neighbouring structures—namely, the peritoneum, omentum, abdominal viscera, and the lumbar glands. They are sometimes multiple along the cord, and may attain a large size, even to several pounds in weight.

Treatment of **Solid Tumours.**—As lipomata generally tend to increase in size and become a source of real inconvenience, though not of pain ; and as, when of subperitoneal origin, they predispose to hernia; and, finally, as in time they contract firm adhesions to cord, testis, and peritoneum, it is best to remove them at an early period. Most of these reasons apply even with much greater force to the other forms of solid tumours. It may be necessary for the complete removal of the growth, or for the purpose of examining the parts thoroughly before removal, to slit up the inguinal canal for a part or the whole of its extent, and then to drag down the cord as far as possible. Castration may be necessary on account of the connections of the tumour to the vas or testis. The divided structures should be carefully brought together by sutures. Drainage may be advisable, and dry antiseptic dressings should be applied.

CAVERNOUS VENOUS ANGEIOMATA OF THE SPERMATIC CORD.

The following are the notes of a case which, so far as I know, is unique, of cavernous venous nævi undergoing cystic changes in the cellular tissue of the cord. The patient, a young Spaniard aged 20, from South America, consulted me in October, 1884, on account of several hard painful lumps along the left spermatic cord. He had been conscious of their presence for some few years, and they had of late been causing inconvenience from weight, dragging, and aching sensations, which had increased as the lumps grew larger.

There was situated in the upper part of the cord, near the external ring, a cystic swelling the size of a large Spanish olive, or small walnut, which had all the clinical characters of an encysted hydrocele of the cord. Below this and between it and the top of the scrotum were four other tense cyst-like bodies among the structures of the cord on its outer and posterior aspect.

On making an incision over the uppermost swelling, it was found to be a cyst, containing clear fluid, embedded amongst numerous spermatic veins, to several of which it was adherent. Its walls were quite thick, especially on its deep aspect, where numerous small cavernous-looking spaces, from which clear fluid escaped, were cut through in removing it. A second cyst, more deeply situated and also containing translucent fluid, was next removed; this was situated in relation to veins like the first, and similar cyst-like spaces, with firm, tough, but thin walls, had to be cut through during the operation.

The incision was prolonged downwards at the back of the cord and the other three lumps were excised. As seen *in situ*, they resembled black grapes in colour, and looked like small vesiculæ seminales into which venous hæmorrhage had taken place. From each of the two larger lumps there was a cystic offshoot containing clear translucent fluid like that in the two first removed.

On section, these masses were cavernous in structure, black in colour, being filled with dark blood, and one of them contained three small rounded, smooth, sand-coloured calculi, the size of grape seeds. These were small phleboliths.

During the operation no vessel of any size had to be divided. The tunica vaginalis was not opened, nor was the testis seen.

The patient made a good recovery. Microscopic examination showed these structures to have the fibrous structure and endothelial lining of venous nævi which were undergoing cystic changes. These changes were in different stages. In the first two the cystic condition predominated, and the cavernous structure formed only a thick wall on one aspect of the cyst. In the other the cavernous spaces were still filled with venous blood, but cysts with clear fluid contents were developed on one side of the pouched and loculated masses.

Such a condition as the above forms a sort of link between the solid tumours of the spermatic cord and varicocele.

VARICOCELE.

The veins of the external genital organs of the male are often varicose. It is by no means uncommon to see those of the scrotum meandering in large size over its whole surface;

the dorsal vein of the penis is still more frequently in a varicose condition; while the milder forms of varicocele are especially common.

Varicocele, with which alone we are now concerned, is the name given to the varicose conditions of the veins in the spermatic cord. Some of these veins surround the vas deferens and accompany the artery of the vas, others and the larger sets are situate more in front of the vas, and frequently

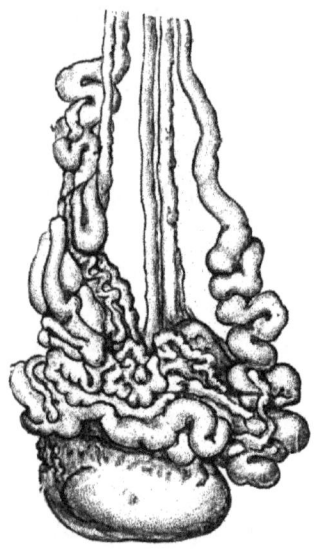

surround the spermatic artery. The latter veins form the pampiniform plexus, and are generally involved in varicocele. They begin in the body of the testicle, enter into the formation of the tunica vasculosa inside the proper fibrous tissue (tunica albuginea) of the testis, are joined by veins from the epididymis, and communicate with the dorsal vein of the penis and the external and internal pudic veins. They unite into five or six tortuous trunk veins which divide and anastomose so as to form the pampiniform plexus. In the inguinal canal the veins of this plexus unite into two or three veins

Fig. 45.—Varicocele. (*J. Cantlie.*)

(Fig. 45), and these, again, before leaving the companionship of the vas deferens, join into a single vein (the spermatic) which, lying on the psoas muscle and behind the peritoneum, accompanies the spermatic artery. The right spermatic vein terminates obliquely in the vena cava; the left in the renal vein, at right angles to that trunk. Cruveilhier and Mr. Bennett have pointed out that the spermatic vein communicates with the portal system; the latter has shown that the left vein receives one or more branches from the veins of the descending colon—the colico-spermatic branches—which communicate with some radicles of the portal system, but vary greatly in size in different persons. Mr. Bennett thinks that the liability to varicocele is increased by these colico-spermatic branches through which any engorgement or obstruction of the portal circulation would cause increased pressure in the spermatic veins.

Varicocele is an affection of puberty and young manhood. In more than half the cases the affection begins between the fifteenth and twenty-fifth years; eighty per cent. are first noticed before the thirty-fifth year. The varicosity ceases in most patients after middle life, and is very rarely seen in old men. The left side is affected from twenty-five to thirty times oftener than the right, and in about seven per cent. of cases both sides are affected.

Pathology. — The veins of the pampiniform plexus are dilated, elongated and tortuous, and their walls,. though for the most part thickened, are elsewhere thinner than normal. The dilatation is in some places cylindrical or fusiform, in others sacculated. The thickening of the walls is in part due to inflammatory formation of fibrous tissue; in part to muscular hypertrophy; and in part, in some instances, to an exceptional thickness of structure of congenital origin (Fig. 46). Phlebitis and thrombosis occur rarely, suppuration still more

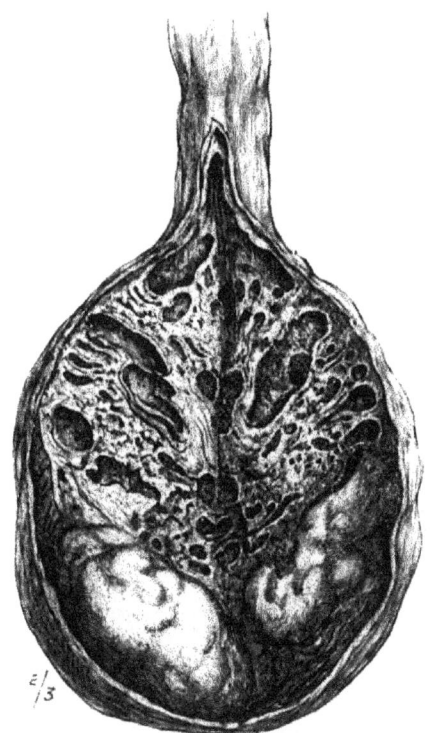

Fig. 46.—Section of a Varicocele.
(Middlesex Hospital Museum.)

rarely, and rupture of a vein is of only occasional occurrence. The varicose state is most marked from just above the testicle upwards to the level of the symphysis pubis; it rarely affects the veins in the inguinal canal, and still more rarely the trunk of the spermatic vein upon the psoas muscle. In very large varicoceles the loops of the varicose veins sometimes hang around and conceal the lower end of the testis; and sometimes the veins of the testis, where they lie upon the outer surface of the tunica albuginea, are varicose (Fig. 47). Opinions differ as to whether varicocele leads to wasting of the testis—in a very few cases of large and neglected varicoceles this may be the case, but in the majority atrophy is unknown. It is probable that the nutrition and function of the organ may be temporarily lowered, but even if both sides are affected, varicocele will not destroy the virility of the individual. Nor

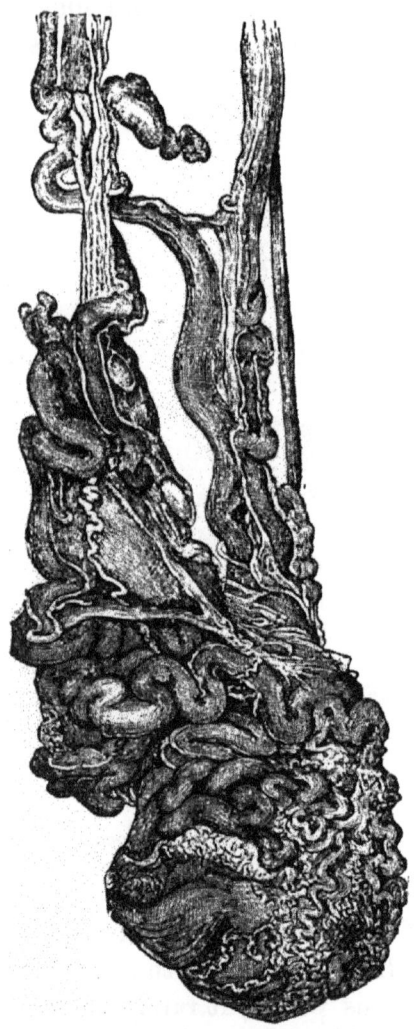

is there any reason, from analogy, to suppose that atrophy would occur; varicose veins of the leg do not lead to wasting of the muscular or other structures of the limb, nor to appreciable impairment of function if due attention is paid to the mechanical support of the veins by elastic stockings or bandages. Even in long-standing and neglected cases, which have been subjected to injuries and in which the skin of the leg has broken down into an ulcer, the muscles, bones, and nerves of the limb are unaffected.

Causes of Varicocele.— Many have been assigned but few are proven. Some of the assigned causes are (*a*) congenital abnormality in the spermatic venous plexus (Bennett); (*b*) persistence of fœtal veins, which are the veins of the Wolffian body and duct; (*c*) venous hypertrophy or primary growth of venous

Fig. 47.—Varicocele, showing a great number of small Veins investing the Testicle below. (*Osborn.*)

tissue (Gould); (*d*) prolonged standing, lifting heavy weights, straining at stool or in passing water, and the constant action of the abdominal muscles (Gaujot); (*e*) chronic meso-phlebitis (Monod and Terrillon); (*f*) the absence or defectiveness of valves in the spermatic veins, and at the junction of these veins with the cava and renal vein: (*g*) masturbation and excessive sexual indulgence. It is probable that varicocele, occurring as it does most frequently at or soon after puberty, is brought about through the rapid developmental changes in the sexual apparatus acting upon veins which are predisposed to varicosity (1) by their great tortuosity; (2) by their great length and dependent position; (3) by their want of support from the loose tissue which surrounds them; (4) by the constant pressure to which they are subjected by the contraction of the abdominal muscles, and (5) by the very feeble *vis à tergo* force with which the blood circulates through them owing to the great length and small calibre of the spermatic artery.

That varicocele retrogrades spontaneously as manhood advances, and is very rarely seen in old men, are facts which oppose the theory that it is induced by the direct connection of the spermatic veins with the portal system through the colico-spermatic branches; it is precisely at those periods of life when varicocele is so rare that engorgement and congestion of the portal circulation are prone to occur.

Various reasons have been assigned, but with too little proof, for the greater frequency of left varicocele. The pressure of the fæcal-laden sigmoid flexure upon the spermatic vein, the great length of the left vein, its entrance into the left renal vein at a right-angle to its own course, and the greater force and frequency of the contraction of the muscles of the left half of the abdomen in right-handed persons, have each been described as the cause of the greater frequency of varicocele of the left.

Symptoms.—The testicle is usually normal, though, if the veins which surround it are affected, it may be masked by them; the scrotum is more or less relaxed, and may or may not be marked by varicose veins on its surface. When the patient stands, the veins swell to a more or less considerable size, and feel like a congeries of soft, distended, but easily compressed tubes, or, as it is invariably described in books, "like a bag of worms." They are often visible through the thin scrotal skin. On coughing, the veins swell more, and give a slight impulse; on lying down, they slowly and almost imperceptibly empty, very unlike the manner in which a hernia suddenly slips back.   The pressure of a finger on the external abdominal ring will at once cause them to become full and distended.   Though painless in the robust and the healthy, in weak, anæmic, and easily-fatigued men varicocele causes an aching in the testis, cord, the groin, and loins, and gives rise to a sense of weight and dragging, and occasionally even to a severe spasmodic pain along the cord.   In the feeble the testis is sometimes very tender and sensitive; and in delicate young men there is often a considerable degree of mental depression, and a dread lest impaired virility or impotence should be the consequence.   Despondency is more likely to seize upon those who have previously masturbated.   It is only in young men that varicocele is a cause of mental anxiety; with the common sense and confidence begot of riper knowledge, the older subjects of the affection are indifferent to its existence, whilst there is a natural tendency for its spontaneous subsidence as age advances, and especially after the regulated coitus of marriage.   It usually appears at or within five or ten years after puberty, though in most instances it probably exists potentially from birth.   It comes on painlessly and insidiously, and is first noticed as a swelling on account of the testis hanging lower and the scrotum becoming relaxed.   If the veins enlarge before or at puberty the perfect development of the testis may be interfered with, and as a consequence the left may be smaller and softer than the right; if they do not enlarge until some few years after puberty, the growth of the testis is not affected, though the organ may feel less firm and elastic, as its nutrition and function are somewhat impaired by the stagnant condition of the blood within it.   The feeble stream in the long, slender spermatic artery can have but little effect in propelling the large amount of blood in the enlarged pampiniform plexus and the valveless spermatic vein.

A small or atrophied testis may exist with, but not as a cause of, varicocele, and I have met with a few cases of congenitally small right testicle in men who had an unusually large testicle with varicocele on the left side.

Long standing, walking, or riding, or any sudden exertion aggravates the swelling of the veins; hence the increased discomfort often felt towards evening.

Treatment may be either *palliative* or *operative*.   In the large majority of cases palliative treatment alone is requisite. If the patient is a sexual hypochondriac, he must be directed to follow the treatment prescribed for sexual hypochondriasis on page 42. Operative treatment should be avoided in these men. When varicocele is associated, as it may be in later adult life, with neuralgia of the cord or testis, the case should be treated for neuralgia as described on page 37. Operative treatment will be disappointing.

In all cases a well-fitting suspensory bandage should be worn; the bowels should be daily and regularly opened, so as to avoid the effect of straining upon the veins passing through the inguinal canal; and night and morning a cold or chilled bath, or cold sponging about the genitals and groin, should be employed. A tonic will often be of service.

Operative treatment is justifiable when varicocele is a bar to a young man entering the army, or navy, or police force, or from following any active occupation to which he wishes to devote himself. It is beneficial if the varicocele causes much pain or physical distress, and also if by its increase atrophy of the testis seems to be threatened.

There are two chief methods for effecting the radical cure —first, by subcutaneous ligatures; secondly, by excision of the bundle of affected veins.

The subcutaneous ligature may be used alone, or in conjunction with long hare-lip pins. When used alone, the ligature, consisting of stout catgut, fine kangaroo tendon, or silk antiseptically prepared, is threaded into a long needle in a handle, the eye of which is near the point. The needle is made to transfix the tissues of the scrotum behind the veins, and between them and the vas deferens, which is carefully separated by the finger and thumb of the operator's left hand. The needle is then threaded and withdrawn, and one end of the ligature is pulled through the puncture of entrance made by the needle in the skin; the needle unthreaded is again introduced into the original puncture of entrance in the skin, and is insinuated through the tissues immediately beneath the skin, and superficially to the veins, till its point and eye emerge at the original opening of exit. The needle is then threaded and withdrawn, carrying with it the other end of the ligature, which will thus have been made

K

to surround the veins, and both ends will be hanging at the wound of entrance of the needle. This puncture wound should now be slightly enlarged with the point of a scalpel, the ligature

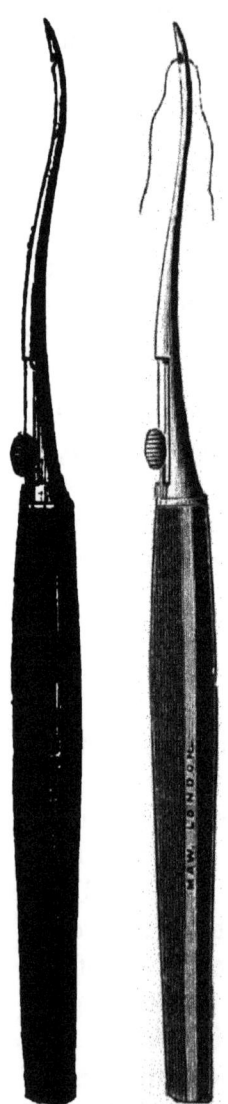

tightly tied, and the ends cut short; the knot will be found to sink into the wound, the edges of which will close over it. Two ligatures, at about one inch apart, are frequently sufficient, but if the veins immediately around the testis and in the lower part of the pampiniform plexus are enlarged, it is safer to apply a third ligature as low down as possible. Having passed as many ligatures as are deemed requisite, the little wounds are sprinkled with iodoform, and then covered with cotton-wool and collodion, and the scrotum is suspended in a T-shaped or triangular bandage. The wounds heal immediately, but the patient should be kept in the horizontal position for a fortnight, to allow of firm consolidation and organisation of the coagula in the veins.

This treatment, which is very simple and quite without risk when performed with due care, has given me completely satisfactory results, and is, in my opinion, to be preferred in most cases either to the combined use of the ligature and pins, or to excision. Fig. 48 is a convenient needle, as it can be readily threaded by opening and closing the eye by a sliding rod and a button.

Fig. 48.—Needles used by the author for Subcutaneous Ligature in Varicocele.

When the hare-lip pins are employed with the ligature, the pins are passed at an interval of one inch from each other behind the veins; a double ligature is then carried between skin and veins by means of a needle which enters and emerges at the same points in the skin as the hare-lip pins. The loop of the ligature is held whilst the needle is withdrawn, and is then slipped under the point of the pin, and the two ends of the ligature are tied tightly beneath the other end of the pin, and the knot slips beneath the skin. The ends of the ligature should not be cut short, and the loop should be withdrawn with the pin on the fifth or sixth day.

Excision of the Veins in varicocele, as in varicose veins of the legs, is the operation which has found undivided favour with many surgeons since the introduction of Listerian dressings and precautions. In the case of varicocele it is performed by making an incision about two inches long over the most prominent part of the veins, and when exposed, without separating them from their fascial investment, two ligatures are passed around them, one at the upper the other at the lower end of the wound, and tightly tied; the intervening portions of the veins are then cut out with scissors, and the stumps are brought together and so retained, either by tying together one end of each of the ligatures, or by passing a suture obliquely through the middle of each stump and tying the ends together, just as in suturing a divided nerve. A few horsehairs may be used as a drain and the wound sutured and dressed in the usual manner.

The plan of suturing or tying together the stumps has for its object the elevation of the testis and the shortening of the cord. It is an improvement on the method of simple excision in cases in which the tissues are very lax and the testis hangs very low. It was practised by Mr. Jacobson in 1887; and special attention was drawn to it by Mr. Bennett, who ably advocated it in 1891 (*Lancet*, February). It has been adopted by many surgeons both in Great Britain and America. Mr. Jacobson and Mr. Mansell-Moullin (*Clinical Journal*, April, 1894) consider the excision or open method the *only one* which has been proved to be efficient or which should now be employed; but though the most excellent results have been obtained by it (of which I have had good proof in my own practice), yet I am of opinion that the method of complete subcutaneous ligatures has much to recommend it, being equally effective in its results and without the necessity of an open wound in a part not always easily kept aseptic.

Recurrence of the Varicocele may take place after any method if not properly performed, or if the patient is allowed to move about too soon after the healing of the wound.

It is said by the advocates of the open method that recurrence is especially likely to follow the subcutaneous method, but I do not find it so if the ligatures are tied tightly, and if a sufficient number of ligatures are used, so as to control the veins at a sufficiently high point towards the external ring, and sufficiently low towards the testicle, as well as between these points. The risk of transfixing a vein if aseptic ligatures are used is nothing. If a large vein were punctured it would be evident by the flow of blood, and the needle would be withdrawn and inserted farther back. If a small vein be transfixed it is nothing more than the risk run with every suture that is used to close a wound. Abscesses and septic poisoning are not to be lost sight of by any method, but are unlikely to occur with the modern precautions of surgery.

As Mr. Jacobson observes, "Insecure knotting of the ligature, or not using reliable material, may, of course, lead to recurrence after any method in which ligatures are used but the veins are not also divided." But why use unreliable ligatures, or tie reliable ones insecurely? It must always be assumed in comparing methods, that each is properly and efficiently carried out. To avoid risk of recurrence, as well as the risk from detachment of imperfectly organised coagulum, two weeks ought to be allowed for convalescence ; and a patient ought not to be allowed to resume his ordinary avocations and exercises in less than three weeks from date of operation.

CHAPTER XIV.

DISEASES AND INJURIES OF THE VESICULÆ SEMINALES.

INJURIES to the vesiculæ seminales are especially rare. They have been, however, produced by firearms, fracture of the pelvis, particularly of the ischia, and in the course of surgical operations.

In wounds of the vesiculæ by firearms or fracture of the pelvis, the bladder or rectum or both have been at the same time wounded. In perinæal cystotomy, and in the bilateral and recto-vesical and transverse perinæal operations on the bladder the vesiculæ have been wounded.

Fistulæ of vesiculæ seminales, attended by the discharge of the vesicular fluid, either at the perinæum or rectum, have resulted from the same kind of wounds, as well as from tubercular and simple inflammatory diseases of the vesicles.

Surgical wounds are less likely than formerly to occur, now that calculi of the bladder are removed, as a rule, either by lithotrity or supra-pubic cystotomy.

ANOMALIES AND ATROPHY.

The vesiculæ seminales are sometimes absent, but they are not invariably so, even when the testicle, epididymis, and lower part of the vas deferens of the corresponding side are wanting. In persons who have neither testis, epididymis, nor vas deferens there may be ejaculatory power, the ejaculated fluid being merely the secretion of the vesicula unmixed with spermatozoa.

Atrophy is a result of inflammation and of old age; but castration is by no means constantly followed by wasting of the vesicula seminalis.

INFLAMMATION

may be acute, subacute, or chronic, and may be caused by gonorrhœa and other forms of urethritis, by stricture, catheterisation, impure or excessive coitus, or by extension of inflammation from prostate or bladder.

Mr. Jordan Lloyd (*Lancet*, 1891, vol. ii. p. 975) believes it to be probably a more common result of gonorrhœa than epididymitis. Velpeau, in 1850, expressed the opinion that inflammation of the seminal vesicles often arose from gonorrhœa. It is generally overlooked through want of proper rectal examination, and is sometimes mistaken for prostatitis.

The inflammation affects mainly the intertubular connective tissue. The disease usually ends in resolution, but it may run to suppuration, and in some cases suppuration of the vesiculæ has occurred without any antecedent urethral disturbance or disease.

Symptoms.—Sometimes the disease begins insidiously; generally, however, there has been for a few weeks a urethral discharge, followed by pain of varying intensity in the groin of the side affected, in the hypogastrium and perinæum. Pain may also be referred to the sacrum, and the hip, and is then likely to be mistaken for the pain of hip-joint disease, or to the loin when it excites suspicion of renal calculus. The pain varies in character as well as in degree, and is aggravated by defæcation and micturition. Micturition in many cases is frequent, and accompanied by straining. There may be retention of urine, or rectal tenesmus with diarrhœa, and discharge of blood and pus from the urethra. Blood and pus may be mixed with the first ounce or two of urine, or may escape by itself from the urethra. In some instances persistent priapism, or frequent blood-stained seminal emissions occur.

On rectal examination, one or both vesicles are felt as hard, elastic, fluctuating, or soft and worm-like (not unlike a varicocele), extending obliquely upwards from the upper edge of the prostate.

The swellings are more distinctly made out when the bladder is full, or a sound is passed into the bladder.

Several complications may arise if the inflammation runs on to suppuration, such as (*a*) burrowing abscesses between rectum and bladder; (*b*) peritonitis from extension of inflammation or by bursting of the abscess into the peritoneal cavity; (*c*) pyæmia; (*d*) irritability of bladder.

Diagnosis must be made from prostatitis; from inflammation of the deep urethra from cystitis; from renal calculus and tubercular kidney and from hip-joint disease.

The frequency of micturition, the presence of blood and pus in acid urine, and of pain in the groin and loin, are very likely symptoms to excite suspicion of stone or tubercle in the kidney. The only way to clear up the diagnosis is by digital examination by the rectum.

Treatment of acute and subacute inflammation consists in frequent hot hip baths, fomentations to the hypogastrium and perinæum, a restricted, unstimulating diet of soup, milk, and light puddings, and the internal administration of mild saline aperients and anodynes, such as belladonna, opium, or morphia. Leeches to the perinæum are of much service in the early stage. If retention of urine occurs a soft catheter should be passed.

As soon as suppuration has occurred as shown by the intensity of the local and general symptoms, and probably by rigors, the pus should be evacuated, either by an incision from the perinæum with a long narrow bistoury introduced one inch in front of the anus and a little to one side of the middle line, and guided by the left index finger in the rectum ; or by an incision through the rectum.

Chronic Inflammation, which is generally the result of an acute or subacute attack, is best treated by the regular and gentle action of the bowels ; the avoidance of all causes of local congestion, such as sexual excitement, sitting in hot rooms on soft-cushioned seats, and the use of alcohol, and horse exercise. The hot and cold douche to the perinæum, the internal administration of tonics, and, if it can be obtained, a sea voyage, or failing that, frequent salt-water bathing, are useful.

DILATATION AND CYSTS OF THE SEMINAL VESICLES.

These conditions, due to obliteration or obstruction of the excretory ducts, may arise from chronic inflammation. In some cases the vesicle is dilated into one large monolocular cyst ; in other cases, namely, those in which there are obstructions at the openings of several of the smaller ducts, instead of in the main duct, there is an aggregation of cysts instead of a single cyst. The single cystic dilatations cause larger swellings than the multilocular, but either may give rise to irritation of the bladder and obstruction to the urine, as an enlarged prostate does. The cysts contain mucoid fluid of various colours, and often well-formed spermatozoa may be found in the same vesicles. They have sometimes attained a great size and caused large pelvic swellings. Dr. Ralfe has recorded (*Lancet*, 1876, vol. ii.) a case of large cystic swelling, probably due to dilatation of the left vesicula seminalis, reaching upwards to the umbilicus and three and a half inches on each side of the middle line; the urine was passed naturally throughout the greater part of the time, but the patient seems to have died of intestinal obstruction from the pressure of the swelling.

Dr. N. R. Smith, of Baltimore (*Lancet*, 1872, vol. ii.), also recorded a case of pelvic swelling reaching higher than the umbilicus, in all probability due to dilatation of the left seminal vesicle. It caused irritability of the bladder. The swelling was tapped per rectum, and ten pints of brown serous fluid were drawn off. After four weeks it refilled, and was tapped again without recurrence.

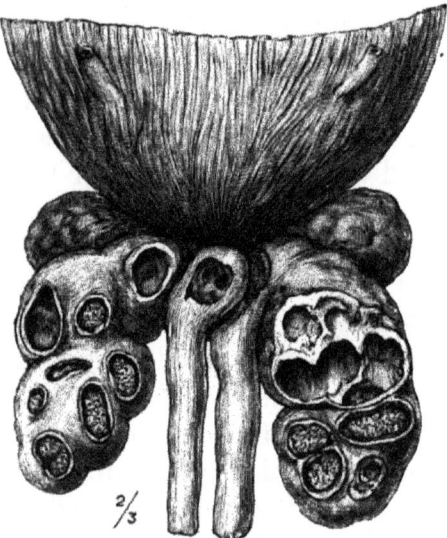

Fig. 49.—Concretions in Vesiculæ Seminales.
(Middlesex Hospital Museum.)

CONCRETIONS

form occasionally in the seminal vesicles. They are at first soft and whitish, and consist of masses of mucus, spermatozoa, and epithelium; after a time they become yellowish-brown, or brownish-black, and they may be coated by deposits of phosphates and carbonate of lime. They are usually multiple (Fig. 49), and may occur at any period of manhood. They are one cause of organic aspermia, and are produced either by obstruction to the ducts or by undue viscidity of the contents of the vesicles.

Symptoms.—The symptoms they cause have reference to the bladder and rectum—severe pain during coitus and defæcation, painful micturition, deep-seated pain in the perinæum, sexual irritation, and perhaps tenesmus of bladder or rectum, or both. A rectal examination will probably reveal one or more nodules in the vesicle. The *treatment* consists in dragging the calculus into the prostatic urethra with the finger in the rectum, or in breaking it up between the finger in the rectum and a sound passed into the bladder.

TUBERCULAR DISEASE OF THE VESICULÆ SEMINALES

· is rare as a primary affection, but occurs more commonly as a sequel of tuberculosis of the epididymis and testis, or of the prostate. The invasion of the seminal vesicle is effected by the tubercle bacillus passing along its duct from the vas deferens or from the prostatic urethra.

The disease begins in the mucous and submucous tissue, and subsequently caseates. It gives rise to a nodular and bossy, or to a doughy and plastic, or to a soft and fluctuating feeling on rectal examination. These variations of resistance to the finger depend upon the stage of the disease in the seminal vesicle. If the so-called abscess stage is reached, the matter may burrow and open into the rectum by sinuous fistulous tracks. In some cases the seminal vesicle enlarges to the size of a man's fist, feels uneven to the finger in the rectum, and is very tender on pressure. Miliary tubercles may follow in the liver, kidney, and hollow viscera, and thus kill the patient.

Treatment.—As the disease is generally secondary to tuberculosis elsewhere, the only available treatment is palliative. But in primary disease, removal of the affected seminal vesicle might be accomplished through a semilunar incision in the perinæum made in front of the anus, with the convexity backwards, and then dissecting the rectum from the prostate, this proceeding being assisted with a sound in the bladder.

I have for several years advocated and practised on the cadaver, this method for prostatectomy, and Ullmann of Vienna has recently and successfully employed it for excision of the vesicula seminalis.

NEW GROWTHS.

Carcinoma and sarcoma have been met with in the vesicula seminalis, but very rarely. They have, certainly, in most instances been secondary to, or actual extensions from, similar disease in the prostate or bladder. Even in the cases in which it has been inferred that the disease was primary, there have been multiple and similar deposits in lungs, liver, peritoneum, omentum, intestine, or heart.

Part II.

GENITO-URINARY ORGANS.

In this part are included the affections of those organs which are concerned with the functions both of generation and the excretion of urine.

   I. *Of the Penis*, as the organ of intromission, and as forming the spongy portion of the urethra.

  II. *Of the Urethra*, as the channel through which both the seminal fluid and the urine pass as they leave the body.

 III. *Of the Prostate*, which is concerned with both the generative and urinary functions, because (*a*) through it pass the common ejaculatory ducts conveying the semen, and because (*b*) it secretes a fluid which is added to and dilutes the semen at the time of ejaculation; because (*c*) it surrounds the first part of the urethra, and because (*d*) it acts like a collar at the neck of the bladder.

CHAPTER I.

INJURIES OF THE PENIS.

The penis may be wounded in many ways, and the injuries may be either quite superficial, or involve the corpora cavernosa, or the urethra. They may occur during erection or otherwise.

Contusions and Contused Wounds have been caused by blows, kicks, the passage of wheels, the falling of a window-sash during the act of micturition through an open window, the catching of the penis in a closing drawer, and by someone falling on to the knees of, or suddenly and forcibly embracing a man whose penis is in a state of erection or semi-erection.

The *symptoms* are ecchymosis, or a blood-tumour beneath the skin, with, possibly, sloughing of the bruised tissues. The discoloration from extravasation of blood may be so black as to simulate gangrene. The ecchymosis or blood-tumour is likely to be very considerable if the dorsal vein of the penis is ruptured, as it has been in some recorded cases. If the contusion is accompanied by an open wound, there will be a free loss of blood instead of a hæmatoma. If the cavernous structure is damaged, the hæmatoma will be situated within the sheath of one of the erectile bodies. When the penis is caught in machinery, the skin may be torn off the body of the penis as well as from the scrotum and front of the pubes and may be left hanging in front of the organ like the finger of a glove.

Contused and lacerated wounds are sometimes inflicted by the bite of an animal. Stricture of the urethra may be a result of these lesions.

The *treatment* should be perfect general and physiological quietude, cold application, gentle elastic compression, and, in cases of wound, strict antiseptic precautions. If a large subcutaneous hæmatoma is formed, it would be proper to lay it open, turn out the blood-clot, antisepticise the cavity, and suture the lips of the incision. Plastic operations will in some cases be necessary to cover in the exposed cavernous bodies.

Punctured Wounds of the Penis are less frequent than contusions. They have been caused by foil and sword thrusts, by knives, and by falls upon nails and other sharp-pointed bodies.

If the dorsal vein is wounded, there may be a considerable loss of blood, and a double ligature may have to be applied. If the urethra is penetrated, blood may flow from the meatus and urine may be passed through the wound, though if the vulnerating body is very fine neither of these symptoms may be present. If the corpus cavernosum is wounded, a large hæmatoma may form within its sheath. Should the weapon be a blunt one, the wound it inflicts will be of the contused variety, and sloughing may follow. A dirty weapon will give rise to a septic wound followed by inflammation, troublesome suppuration, or, may be, to sloughing and pyæmic infection.

The *treatment* is to check bleeding, lay open and cleanse any dirty wound or any suppurating track, and to apply an antiseptic dressing.

Incised Wounds are the most frequent of all. They may be merely superficial, or, being deep, may cause either complete or incomplete division of the penis. The superficial incised wounds involve only the skin and perhaps the superficial vessels. If the larger superficial vessels are divided, they may be difficult to seize and ligature because of retraction within their sheaths; but bleeding having been controlled, the edges of the wound should be brought together by fine sutures.

Wounds of the glans penis have been known to occur during coitus from the presence of a foreign body such as a fragment of a vaginal injection syringe. They are comparatively unimportant; the bleeding, which may be free, is easily stopped by elastic compression, ice, or styptics, and the wounds heal under rest and antiseptic dressings.

Incised wounds which completely divide the penis are veritable amputations, and require to be treated as such. They are self-inflicted by maniacs, and by the Skoptzi, a Russian sect of male and female religious enthusiasts who regard their reproductive organs as the key to the bottomless pit, and excise them as a means of obtaining their salvation; many similar wounds have been inflicted by jealous wives and concubines.

There is great loss of blood, but the amount of bleeding depends upon whether the section of the penis is made during erection or flaccidity. When inflicted during erection bleeding is violent, when during flaccidity it has been described in some cases as slight. Still, our experience of ordinary amputation of the penis, which of course is performed in the flaccid state, would lead us to expect a considerable flow of blood. As in amputation of the penis, so in these self-inflicted or revengeful mutilations, precaution must be taken against retraction and cicatricial contraction of the divided urethra. An immediate symptom of these wounds, if neglected, is dysuria from retraction and spasmodic contraction of the urethral wall; a later symptom is obstruction due to cicatricial stricture. The Skoptzi are quite aware of this danger, and as the cultivation of urethral stricture forms no part of their redemption, they wisely introduce a plug into the divided end of the urethra so as to prevent its obliteration.

The *treatment* consists in ligaturing the divided arteries, stitching the cut end of the urethra to the cut edges of the skin around the corpus spongiosum, and covering the divided corpora cavernosa with a cold antiseptic compress.

Incised wounds which incompletely divide the penis less frequently involve the corpus spongiosum, and therefore the urethra, than the corpora cavernosa. In the treatment of them, every effort should be made to unite the cut surfaces, bringing the several structures respectively together and retaining them so by means of buried and deep sutures, and covering the whole with carbolised-oil lint or some other antiseptic dressing. A catheter should be passed into the bladder and retained during the healing of the urethra, so as to obviate retention and prevent extravasation of urine. Penile fistula and inconvenient distortions of the penis may follow, but will probably be recovered from in the course of a few months, so that neither urinary nor sexual inconveniences will be permanent.

Gunshot Wounds are not very rare in warfare. Otis collected 305 cases which occurred during the war of the American Rebellion. Many of these were complicated with wounds of the scrotum, testicles, bladder, and pelvis. Some of these wounds were quite subcutaneous, the bullet passing between the skin and fibrous sheaths of the cavernous bodies; others were deep, and the bullet traversed the corpora cavernosa without wounding the urethra, or remained lodged in their tissues. The urethra seems to be rarely wounded. Otis does not mention a single case amongst his 305. Dupuytren and Larrey each mention a case in which the whole penis was ploughed off from the front of the pubes.

The *symptoms* of these accidents are swelling of the penis; secondary, but rarely primary, hæmorrhage; retention of urine even when the urethra itself is not directly involved and, later, suppuration and the loss of tissue by sloughing. After the healing of the wound there may be imperfect or distorted erection, for which a plastic operation may be required in order to restore the proper axis of the penis. An encysted bullet, and still more a bullet recently entered and retained in the penis, should be extracted, and the wound should be irrigated and then enveloped in antiseptic dressings.

Fracture of the Penis is caused by the forcible pressure and sudden incurvation of the penis against some resisting surface. The sheaths of the cavernous bodies are thus ruptured. The accident may occur either during coitus or otherwise. Most frequently it is during coitus or attempted coitus, either by forcible attempts to enter the narrow vaginal orifice of a virgin or, on the other hand, by the body-weight and pressure of a too vivacious or lascivious spouse. Guyon reports a case in which rupture occurred without violence of any sort in a man with several strictures of the urethra. This case has been thought to favour the view of Demarquay, that fracture of the penis is predisposed to by a pathological change in the sheaths of the erectile bodies of the penis.

The *symptoms* are a sudden acute pain, followed, it may be, by syncope. This pain is most intense at the level of the fracture, but radiates to the pubes and thighs. It is instantaneous, and accompanied by a dry crackling sound and an immediate cessation of erection. After a while the organ swells enormously, and the skin of the penis becomes darkly mottled, from extravasation of blood into, and superficial to, the cavernous tissues. Sometimes rupture of the urethra complicates the fracture of the cavernous bodies, and dysuria and infiltration of urine follow.

When the swelling subsides and the penis has regained its natural size, it will be found that erection is no longer natural. Either the part of the penis behind the fracture becomes turgid and the part in front remains entirely flaccid, or the anterior portion stiffens some time after the erection of the posterior part is complete. These physiological digressions result from the organisation of blood-clot and the formation of sclerosed tissues.

The *treatment* should be directed against these after-consequences. With this object in view it is best to make an ,incision, to turn out the blood-clots, to ligature any bleeding vessels, and, after antisepticising the wound, to unite the parts by sutures and apply an antiseptic dressing around the penis.

Dislocation of the Penis.—Some five or six cases have been recorded in which the glans and body of the penis have been stripped of their coverings, which have remained in position looking like blown-out goldbeater's skin, whilst the penis has been lodged beneath the scrotal tissues, or in front of the pubes, or on the crease of the groin. The urethra in .one case was ruptured, and urinary infiltration followed. Accórding to Brun and Monod (*Dict. Encycl. des Sciences*

Méd., 2nd series, t. xxii. p. 550, 1887), for this accident to happen there must be a rupture of the fibrous sheath of the penis at its attachment behind the corona glandis.

Treatment must be to endeavour to replace the body of the penis, and to treat the rupture of the urethra, if such has occurred, according to general rules. (*See* page 158.)

Strangulation of the Penis by foreign bodies such as rings, elastic bands, string or tape, etc., has been caused in children in play or in injudicious attempts to stop incontinence of urine ; and in adults by lewd or erotic intention.

Symptoms.—Great œdema, congestion and strangulation are present, the foreign body becomes deeply buried in a sulcus in the tissues, micturition is made difficult and then prevented entirely, and sloughing in places or *en masse* of the end of the penis, and extravasation of urine occurred; and urinary fistulæ are likely to follow.

The *treatment* consists in removing as soon as possible the constricting body. If it cannot be slipped off, a tape bandage should be applied so as to compress the œdematous part in front of the ring, or the ring should be cut with scissors or a file. A gold ring may be dissolved by mercury, or a copper ring by mercury and spirits of nitre. Permanent loss of erectile power may follow if the constriction has been long-continued and considerable.

CHAPTER II.

CONGENITAL DEFECTS AND MALFORMATION OF THE PENIS. PHIMOSIS. PARAPHIMOSIS.

Absence of the Penis.—In the rare instances of entire absence of the penis, the urethra has opened on the anterior wall of the rectum, or just outside the sphincter ani. The scrotum and testes may be well developed and natural. In some cases, umbilical or inguinal hernia, spina bifida or talipes, have coexisted. In a few cases in which the penis was apparently absent it has been found beneath the skin in the lowest part of the abdomen, and in a rudimentary state.

The prepuce may be congenitally absent altogether; or there may be a division, complete or incomplete, in it, situated either on one side or in the middle of the dorsal aspect. When the division is complete—*i.e.* extending quite back to the corona—a plastic operation has been performed, and the freshened edges have been united; but such an operation is not to be recommended, as it is much better to remove the foreskin entirely.

Sometimes the frænum is unnaturally short and may then be ruptured during coitus. Occasionally the rent has extended to the meatus or into the substance of the glans, and very large hæmorrhage has been the result.

The *treatment* for a very short frænum is to divide it transversely, and to pack the little wound with iodoform gauze till it has healed up from the bottom.

Congenital Defects.—The penis may be defective in size and shape. One or both corpora cavernosa may be absent, or very imperfectly developed, the penis thus feeling like a tube of skin. A webbed condition between the penis and scrotum (what the French call *pénis palmé*) has occasionally been met with. The inferior part of the penis alone may be adherent to the front of the scrotum, or the whole penis except the glans may be enclosed by the scrotal skin. Hypospadias may complicate the webbed penis.

The following case is interesting because of the association of ill-developed penis and testes and scrotum with a condition of the integuments resembling the mons veneris and external labia of the female.

A young gentleman aged twenty-two consulted me in November, 1884, as to the probable development of his external genital organs, and the question of marriage. He was of medium height and had a well-proportioned figure, and a bright and confident manly manner, but a voice slightly squeaky and effeminate. His penis, testes, and scrotum were all in miniature. The penis was not larger in circumference than a child's " little finger," and looked to be barely an inch long. It had its glans and pre-puce, and it could be elongated nearly an inch by simply pressing upon the very abundant and prominent fat which covered the symphysis pubis. The testes were about the size of small cherries, but each was differentiated into epididymis and testis proper. There was a pea-sized cyst of the epididymis in the right organ. The scrotum was very small; and the testes, though easily made to descend into it, were usually resident near the external abdominal rings—sometimes even in the lower ends of the inguinal canals. There was a little hair upon the pubes, but what was most striking was the large, soft, prominent cushion of fat in this situation, resembling the mons veneris of the female, and also a soft cushion of fat on each side, extending downwards towards the perinæum along the arch of the pubes. Except-ing for the presence of the hair on the pubes, the condition resembled the organs of a boy seven or eight years of age, with the well-formed mons veneris and diminutive labia majora of a young girl. He told me he had only once, and that not long before I saw him, had sexual connection, and then obtained a smart gonorrhœa. He had never emitted any semen or anything resembling seminal fluid, though he was subject to nocturnal lascivious dreams and had frequent sexual desire. He had masturbated for a short time as a boy twelve years of age, but not since. The only illnesses besides the attack of gonorrhœa were an abscess near the elbow when fifteen years of age and severe mumps when about thirteen years old. This want of development must, I think, have antedated the masturbation and the attack of mumps; how

far either of these illnesses prejudicially affected the growth
of the sexual organs I cannot say.

Torsion of the Penis sometimes complicates hypospadias
and epispadias. It sometimes occurs independently of either
of these urethral defects. The urethra may turn spirally round
one of the corpora cavernosa, or the whole penis may be
twisted on its own axis. Torsion of the penis is perhaps
explained by the outgrowth of one of the genital folds, causing
the genital tubercle or eminence to deviate on one side and
thus twist on its own axis. In a case under my care
(Fig. 50) the penis was of great size, and was bent with the

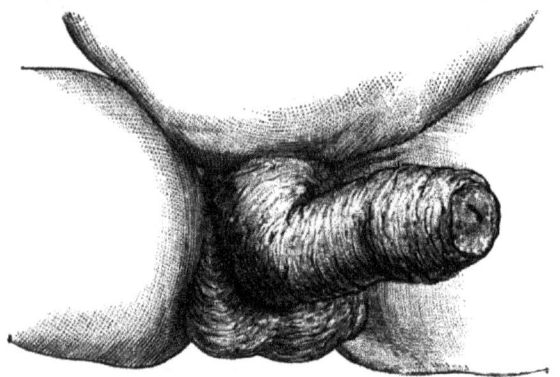

Fig. 50.—Twisted Penis.

convexity to the right, and twisted a quarter of a circle
on its own axis, causing a spiral sulcus on the surface of
the organ. The condition was associated with dilated urachus
and ureters and pelves of the kidneys (Fig. 51).

Double Penis is very rare. A few cases have been recorded
where there has been a third limb, wasted and deformed indeed, but consisting of thigh, leg, and foot, situated between the
thighs. The penes have been well formed, have occupied the
natural position, and have been either quite separate from one
another, or enclosed in a common covering of skin up to the
glans penis. There has been a separate scrotum for each
testis. Urine has been discharged simultaneously from each
urethra. In two adult cases recorded by Mr. Ernest Hart,
and by Van Buren and Keyes, the subjects were healthy men
having sexual desires, erections, and emissions ; both penes
became erect, and in one of the men semen was discharged
simultaneously from each.

Congenital Fistula of the Penis.—Cases are described in which a minute fistula opened either behind the corona or just in front of the pubis, or in a single or in multiple orifices near the urethral orifice in the glans. These do not communicate with the urethra. Some of the fistulous tracts

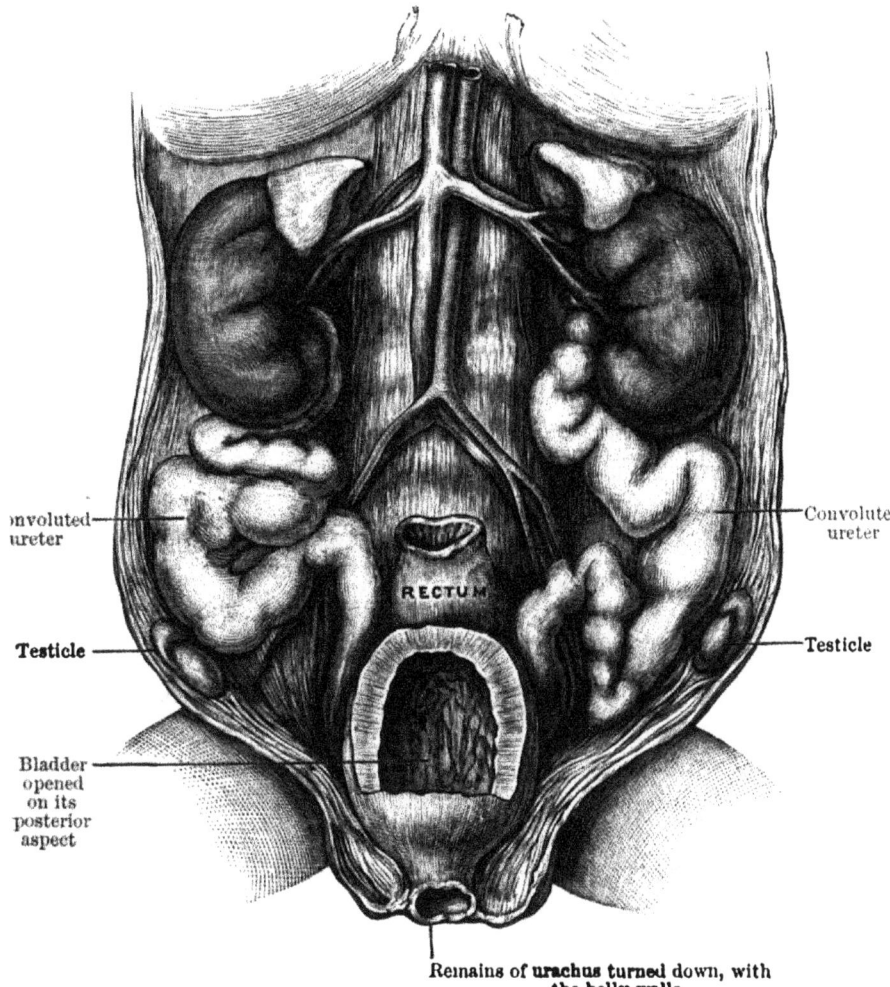

>nvoluted
ureter

Convolute
ureter

RECTUM

Testicle

Testicle

Bladder
opened
on its
posterior
aspect

Remains of urachus turned down, with
the belly walls

Fig. 51.—Dilated Urachus, Ureters and Hypertrophied Bladder (from same child as
Fig. 50). (*Lancet*, June 8th, 1895.)

were very short; one has been traced back along the dorsum penis to a gland lying on the penis, and connected by elastic tissue with the prostate and the bladder (Luschka's case); another ended blindly beneath the os pubis, and nearly joined a small funnel-shaped prolongation running forwards from the bladder just above the vesical orifice. They may give rise to trouble if involved in gonorrhœa. (*See* Double Urethra.)

Phimosis may be either congenital or acquired. The congenital form results from a too narrow preputial orifice, or from the persistence of the natural epithelial adhesion which exists at birth, and for some time later, between the prepuce and the glans penis.

Another condition which aggravates either of the above and may of itself be a cause of phimosis, is a too elongated prepuce. At birth there is a natural adhesion between skin and glans, which, as a rule, spontaneously disappears in a year or more.

Symptoms.—Children with a very narrow preputial orifice, or a very long or unduly adherent prepuce, suffer from frequent micturition, incontinence, pain and difficulty in passing water, and sometimes from retention. The prepuce is frequently dilated or ballooned by the urine during micturition, and the straining to pass water often gives rise to hernia and to prolapsus ani. It is remarkable how soon after circumcision the hernia disappears in some of these cases.

If the phimosis persists, the constant and forcible efforts of the bladder to expel urine in time cause hypertrophy and fasciculation of the bladder-walls, and dilatation of the ureters and kidneys. There is a specimen in St. Bartholomew's Hospital Museum showing extreme dilatation of ureters and kidneys from phimosis, very like to Fig. 68, page 233. Other results of phimosis are preputial calculus, balanitis, thickening and hypertrophy of the prepuce, premature sexual excitement, and masturbation, convulsions, epilepsy, simulated or actual hip disease, talipes, interference with due development, and peevishness and loss of appetite.

In the adult, paraphimosis, rupture of the frænum, balanitis, atrophied and ill-developed glans, epithelioma, and difficult and imperfect coitus are consequences which may arise from congenital phimosis.

Treatment.—If the foreskin is not unduly long and the orifice not contracted, it suffices—by means of a probe, director, or the fingers and a little oil—to detach the adhesions between the prepuce and the glans penis, and then daily dress the parts with a little boracic ointment or white vaseline. But if the prepuce is disproportionately long, if the preputial orifice is very small, if the adhesions cannot be separated, or, having been separated, are allowed to re-form from carelessness, or tender-heartedness on the part of the nurse; if œdema or troublesome cracks and fissures follow the detachment of the adhesions, and if balanitis or hernia complicate the phimosis—circumcision ought to be performed.

This operation, insignificant as it is deemed to be, yet requires care and judgment in its performance; otherwise one of several complications may occur. Insufficient removal of either skin or mucous membrane leaves the patient in as bad a state after as he was before the operation. I have had to operate on several occasions where a mere ring of skin only had been cut away by a previous operator, leaving the narrow orifice of the prepuce just as it was before the operation.

This untoward result occurs to inexperienced operators, who, instead of dissecting the contracted preputial orifice and the mucous membrane, with which it is continuous, off from the glans penis, to which they are often toughly adherent, cut away the loose skin of the prepuce only, and then stitch the cut edge of the skin of the penis to the cut ring of the preputial opening.

There may, on the other hand, be too free a removal of skin, so that the penis becomes curved by the subsequent contraction of the cicatrix.

Cellulitis and erysipelas may follow, unless scrupulous attention is paid to asepticity before, during, and after operation, and unless the patient is placed in good sanitary surroundings. Sir James Paget has recorded a case in which, owing to defective sanitary surroundings, sloughing of the integuments of the penis and scrotum followed the division of the phimosed prepuce.

Infection of the wound with syphilitic or with tuberculous virus has again and again been conveyed by the saliva of the priest when the operation is performed as practised by the Jews, or from the use of impure instruments or dressings. Hæmorrhage is a great source of risk if the operation is done on a member of a family of "bleeders"—*i.e.* the subjects of hæmophilia.   Hæmorrhage from an unsecured vessel ought not to occur, nor ought any damage to be done to the penis or urethra.

ACQUIRED PHIMOSIS.

Men with a slight degree of congenital phimosis, and those with an elongated prepuce, are prone to get an aggravation of the condition following repeated attacks of balanitis, gonorrhœa, or chancre.   The cracks and excoriations which result from over-acid urine in men past middle life, and from diabetes, and the œdema of the prepuce which results from thrombosis of or pressure upon the prostatic venous plexus, bring about a phimotic condition which requires circumcision or constant palliative treatment.

Treatment.—When the phimosis is partly caused by inflammatory œdema, it will be much reduced, if not removed entirely, by frequent bathing and syringing with lead or boracic lotion, keeping the prepuce enveloped in lint soaked in the lotion, and the penis supported against the abdominal walls.

Where there are chancres beneath the foreskin, and the prepuce requires to be slit up or removed, every care should be taken against inoculating the cut surfaces with the virus of the chancres.   To this end, the glans and foreskin should be thoroughly syringed with weak carbolic or mercuric lotion, and the cut surfaces treated with strong nitric acid applied on a glass rod at the time of the operation.   The wound should be subsequently dressed with iodoform and vaseline, to which 5 per cent. of cocain may be added to relieve pain.

PARAPHIMOSIS.

This name is given to the irreducibility of the prepuce after it has been retracted behind the glans penis.

It occurs during masturbation, coitus, or when a prepuce with small orifice is pulled back for the purpose of washing the parts.

It may produce symptoms of an acute, subacute, or chronic kind.   When acute or subacute, the condition is serious, and, unless relieved by the surgeon, must end either by ulceration of the constricting ring of the prepuce, or by mortification of the strangulated glans penis. The latter is less frequent than the former. The strangulating ring may be situated immediately behind the corona, and consist of the mucous fold of the prepuce. It is most marked on the under aspect, but surrounds the organ like a purplish-red œdematous collar; or it may be situated farther back, and will then consist of the preputial orifice. The glans penis swells often to a very great size, and looks œdematous and dusky red or purplish black in colour.

In the chronic form there is no inflammatory swelling, and but little œdema; it may occur as the result of the subacute variety or independently.

The treatment consists in reducing the prepuce, after well oiling the parts, by dragging it forwards between the index and middle fingers of both hands, made to enclose the penis, one pair of fingers in front of the other, and then by squeezing and pressing backwards the glans penis with the thumb. In performing this operation, Mr. Jacobson wisely cautions the surgeon to guard himself against possible infection from chancre, if he has any breach of skin surface about the nails or elsewhere.

If this does not succeed, the constricting band or bands should be thoroughly divided by a sharp scalpel in the axis of the penis, and on the dorsal aspect after well washing the parts with antiseptic lotion. After freeing the glans of all constriction, punctures should be made into the œdematous prepuce, and the whole organ should be wrapped in lint soaked with antiseptic lotion and elevated upon the abdomen.

CHAPTER III.

DISEASES OF THE PENIS.

PREPUTIAL CALCULI.

WHEN phimosis exists, concretions can be lodged within the sacculus formed by the prepuce, and there grow. They are met with most frequently in adults, less so in children, and rarely in old age. They may be facetted and multiple, or oblong or oval, and as large as a sparrow's or bantam's egg, or larger. Some are derived from the urine salts, and are formed originally in the kidney or bladder, pass along the urethra, and thus reach the subpreputial space. Others are formed in this space by deposition of its salts from the urine, retained there owing to a phimosed prepuce. Such calculi are composed partly of uric acid and urates and partly of phosphates.

Other preputial calculi are concretions of smegma, impregnated with lime salts deposited from the urine which is retained behind a phimosed prepuce. Such concretions are soft and easily crumbled, and consist of epithelium, cholesterin, and lime salts.

BALANITIS AND BALANO-POSTHITIS.

By balanitis is meant inflammation of the glans penis. By posthitis, inflammation of the inner or mucous surface of the prepuce. The two conditions generally coexist, and are therefore spoken of as *balano-posthitis.*

It occurs from want of cleanliness, and is predisposed to by phimosis, gonorrhœa, subpreputial chancres, and over-acidity of urine, as in the gouty and the diabetic. Different names expressive of different causes have been applied to balano-posthitis, such as venereal, catarrhal, gouty, diabetic, etc.; but such distinctions so far as regards symptoms and diagnosis are quite unnecessary, though in the treatment the exciting cause of the inflammation must be borne in mind.

Mr. Hutchinson has described a very chronic form of the disease in men past middle age, which goes on, if not treated, for years, and which he calls "balanitis perstans," a very threatening pre-cancerous condition.

Symptoms.—It gives rise to a sense of burning and itching, and the glans penis and inner aspect of the frænum are red, glazed, and covered by an offensive yellow secretion consisting of decomposed smegma, epithelium, and pus. The epithelium may become detached, and the surface of the glans and inner aspect of the prepuce then look superficially excoriated.

Diagnosis.—With a very phimotic prepuce there may be some difficulty in forming an opinion as to whether the discharge comes from the urethra or from a chancroid sore, or is due to balano-posthitis. The peculiar and disgusting odour of balano-posthitis, and the absence of heat and pain along the urethra during micturition, will exclude urethritis. When a chancre is present, it can, as a rule, be detected as a tender and perhaps indurated spot by squeezing the several parts of the foreskin between the finger and thumb, and there will in all probability be some inflamed glands in one or both groins. The inguinal glands may, however, be inflamed in balano-posthitis, but much less frequently. The division of the prepuce will at once make clear any case which cannot otherwise be diagnosed.

Treatment. — This consists in cleanliness, frequent syringing with a lotion of bicarbonate of soda, or a warm boracic or weak mercuric lotion, and if this does not effect a cure the surface should be rubbed over with a stick of nitrate of silver. Other remedies failing, the prepuce should be slit up and the inflamed surface lightly touched with nitric acid.

It should be remembered that prolonged balanitis, in elderly men, may run on into epithelioma, and this is, therefore, all the stronger reason for efficient treatment.

When due to diabetes, the diet and medicinal treatment suitable to this disease, aided by cleanliness and the local application of dry boracic powder, will generally suffice to cure the inflammation. Circumcision and slitting up the prepuce should be avoided in such patients if possible. All diabetic patients bear operations, even the slightest, badly. When due to gouty causes, the remedies suitable to gouty patients should be employed.

HERPES PROGENITALIS OR PREPUTIALIS.

Herpes zoster affecting the area of the ilio-inguinal nerve may attack the penis; but the more common form of herpes is of an erythematous order and of a more local character, and as it affects the glans penis as well as the prepuce, it is better named H. progenitalis than H. preputialis.

Symptoms.—It commences with itching and a sense of heat upon an erythematous patch of prepuce or glans penis, and soon afterwards one or several papules, changing into vesicles and then into pustules, appear on this patch. As the pustules shrivel, small excoriations are left, which heal in five or six days from the appearance of the papules. As a rule, to which, however, marked exceptions now and then occur, there is not much if any pain, and the patient usually seeks advice, fearing the eruption may be of a venereal character.

There is a great disposition for herpes to recur at intervals of a few weeks, and to go on doing so for a long time, until the disease wears itself out by degrees, and then ceases for several years, and until some venereal attack starts it afresh.

Mr. Berkeley Hill remarks:—"In a person who has once suffered, very slight causes, such as excessive eating or drinking, fatigue, or sexual intercourse, are sufficient to bring on an attack."

Men of a gouty tendency, and liable to psoriasis, eczema, lumbago, lithæmia, are the most subject to it.

Several French authors speak of H. progenitalis as being generally, if not always, preceded by some venereal affection—gonorrhœa or a soft chancre; but Berkeley Hill and Hutchinson do not speak so dogmatically on this point. The latter states that "herpetic vesicles may occur on the genitals of either sex quite independently of any venereal cause, and if they have occurred once, they are prone to occur again"; and he further says, "those who have never suffered from syphilis are liable to recurrent herpes, yet it is certain that those who have so suffered are infinitely more prone to it. In syphilitic subjects, too, herpes is often much more severe than in others." My own experience accords with these views.

Diagnosis.—There is not any difficulty in correctly diagnosing an uncomplicated case. Soft chancres will be distinguished from herpes by the larger size, greater depth, and more scattered distribution of the ulcers. A herpetic sore may become the seat of inoculation, or a herpetic vesicle may appear upon the spot at which the syphilitic virus has previously gained entrance, so that in either case the herpes may take on the specific characters.

Treatment.—A purge, some cooling saline mixture, and restricted, or, at any rate, properly regulated diet, together with the local application of a little Goulard lotion or boracic powder, are the simple remedies required for most cases. Where there is a disposition to recurrence, any gouty or other constitutional tendency should be attended to, the bowels and liver should be kept regularly in action, and some astringent wash daily used for the glans and prepuce.

Mr. Hutchinson speaks of the remarkable therapeutical value of arsenic in such cases. As the glans shares with the prepuce in H. progenitalis, circumcision, as recommended by Kauffmann, does not seem applicable; and Mr. B. Hill tried it without success in some intractable recurrent cases.

LUPUS AND LEPROSY

do, but very rarely, affect the penis.

Mr. Hutchinson records ("Arch. of Surg.," vol. ii. p. 17) a case of non-ulcerating lupus of the prepuce in a boy, associated with lupus of the face, limbs, and trunk. Circumcision was performed, and the parts healed and remained well. He also gives cases of syphilitic lupoid disease of the glans, and says that this disease is more difficult to cure there than on the skin.

Mr. Jacobson, and Dr. Rake, of Trinidad, have performed circumcision in cases of phimosis due to leprosy. The bacillus leprosæ was found in the nodules on the prepuce which was removed. The wounds healed rapidly.

LYMPHANGITIS

occurs in two forms, either as a single inflamed lymphatic, or as an inflamed network of small lymphatics.

When one trunk only is involved, it presents as a hard cord along the dorsum of the penis, extending often into the prepuce. It arises generally from balano-posthitis or acute phimosis, and occurs in young healthy men. It is to be distinguished from phlebitis by the cord-like feeling it causes on one side, and not in the middle line of, the dorsum, which feeling is directed towards the inguinal glands, and not beneath the pubes as is an inflamed dorsal vein.

The net-like or diffuse form may give rise to small, red and painful nodules, which suppurate and leave obstinate fistulæ.

Treatment.—Saline purges, lead lotion, and the horizontal posture are indicated. Demarquay recommends excision of the affected area of skin as the only efficient treatment for the superficial fistulæ left after the diffuse lymphangitis.

Another abnormal condition of the lymphatics of the penis is dilatation of one or more, or even a network, of these vessels from various causes, such as obstruction to the lymph current by an enlarged inguinal gland, or injury during coitus. The dull-white contents may be seen through the dilated vessel walls, or there may be an escape of chylous fluid from one or more places.

ERYSIPELAS, CELLULITIS, AND GANGRENE.

These diseases may attack the penis *de novo* or may spread to it from neighbouring parts. When they occur after circumcision, especially in weakly or dirty children, they may run on to gangrene and, even without doing so, may spread and prove fatal.

Both the dry and the moist forms of gangrene occur in the penis, the moist being much commoner. The gangrene may affect the prepuce only, or it may involve the whole organ, or extend along the skin of the penis to the abdomen or scrotum. It occurs, after the continued fevers, from thrombosis of the dorsal vein of the penis, or of the pelvic or prostatic veins; or it may be started by erysipelas, by the sloughing and inflammation of an acute phimosis, by paraphimosis, injuries of various kinds, long-continued priapism; by extravasation of putrid urine, the ulceration of a fragment of calculus in the navicular fossa, or by inflammation in the erectile tissues of the penis. Reclus observed gangrene of the penis in an old man with atheroma of the dorsal arteries. It has occurred in the young and apparently healthy without any ascertainable cause.

The course, prognosis and treatment of these affections when they affect the penis are much the same as when they attack an extremity.

NEURALGIA OF THE PENIS,

probably of gouty origin, occurs with and without neuralgia
of the testicle, or it may be induced by irritation of the trunk
or branches of the small sciatic nerve at a distance from the
penis, as in Hilton's case of pain on one side of the penis, caused
by fibrous thickening of the tissues near the tuber ischii, producing pressure on the perinæal branch of the small sciatic.

ACUTE GOUT OF THE PENIS.

Sir J. Paget has recorded a case of recurring attacks of great
swelling and inflammation, with pain and redness of the body
of the penis, and attended with urethral discharge and swelling,
in an elderly and gouty man. These attacks were always associated with other symptoms of typical and acute gout, yielded
to calomel, colchicum and liquor potassæ, and passed off with
the other symptoms, under this treatment.

AFFECTIONS OF THE BLOOD-VESSELS.

Small cutaneous nævi occur on the penis. They rarely, if
ever, involve the glans. They should be cured early by galvano-
puncture or ethylate of sodium, as they are apt to spread
and cause irritation, and thus lead to infantile masturbation.
Mr. Jacobson refers to a case under his care, of priapism caused
by nævus of the skin and glans of the penis. Varicose veins are
not very unfrequent, and as a rule cause no inconvenience and
need no treatment. Subcutaneous rupture of the fibrous capsule
of the corpus cavernosum may lead to a soft swelling, which
becomes hard and larger during erection, but feels like an
abscess at other times. Albinus and Boyer record such cases.
They should be left alone, not opened, on account of the
hæmorrhage which will follow.

Tuberculosis of the Penis.—Mention has been made of
the inoculation of circumcision wounds by the tubercular
bacillus by the saliva of the operator, just as a tattooed surface
may be affected when done by a syphilitic or tuberculous
person. The disease has also been known to commence *de
novo* in the glans penis; the tuberculous material extending
far into the substance of the glans and appearing on its
surface merely as irregular, cheesy-looking ulcers. In such

case the channel of infection is probably the circulation. Tuberculous lupus of the penis has also been described.

ELEPHANTIASIS

may affect the prepuce and the skin of the penis either separately or together with the scrotum. Negroes with long prepuce are said to be prone to elephantiasis of the prepuce. Out of

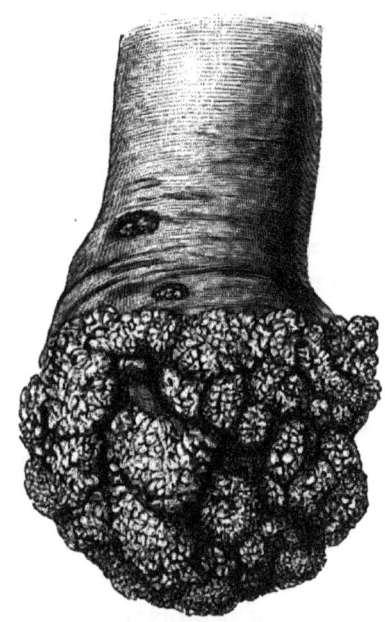

113 cases of elephantiasis in the Calcutta Hospital three affected the prepuce and one the penis. The proper treatment is removal of the diseased tissues. As in the case of the affection of the scrotum, it may occur either in association with the filaria sanguinis hominis; or in Europeans who have never been in the tropics independently of the presence of this parasite.

SEBACEOUS CYSTS

are occasionally met with in the prepuce, for which circumcision is the best treatment. Cysts connected with the glands behind the corona have been met with,

Fig. 52.—Papilloma of Penis.
(Hunterian Museum.)

sometimes single and as large as a hen's egg; sometimes multiple, and varying in size from a shot to a horse-bean. They should be excised in the usual manner for sebaceous cysts.

PAPILLOMATA

may be either moist or dry; they have often a venereal origin, and are produced by the irritation of dirt and discharges; but they may arise from the papillæ behind the corona, and from those of the glans and inner aspect of the prepuce without any venereal origin. They form red, vascular, sessile or slightly pedunculated, flabby, and foully-secreting masses or tufts (Fig. 52). The proper treatment is to remove them completely with scissors curved on the flat, taking care to remove also the skin or the mucous membrane from which they are growing. It is well to rub the raw surface with strong nitric or acetic acid.

This treatment should be carried out whilst the patient is anæsthetised. In the case of the drier variety of warts, or if the patient dreads an anæsthetic, an attempt may be made to wither and destroy them by calomel dusted over their surface, or by frequent application of glacial acetic acid or the acid nitrate of mercury. It is essential that they should all be thoroughly destroyed, otherwise a fresh crop will spring up from the portions left behind. It must be borne in mind that primary epithelioma or sarcoma may here as elsewhere, from the first, assume a papillomatous appearance. (*See* Mr. Lane's case referred to below.)

KERATOMATA, OR HORNS,

are occasionally met with on the prepuce or glans, and are developed from warts which grow on these parts or from a sebaceous cyst. They rarely attain to any considerable size ; they form flat plates or slightly curved projections ; are painless, striated, with a tendency to split, and yellowish or brownish in colour. They are often associated with phimosis, congenital or acquired. The proper *treatment* is excision, as they are prone to ulcerate around the base and to be followed by epithelioma.

PRIAPISM.

This is a condition of continued erection apart from any sexual desire. When complete it is very painful ; when incomplete not so. The corpora cavernosa are the parts affected. The corpus spongiosum generally is unaffected. It is produced by injury to the erectile parts of the penis, by excessive venereal indulgence, by leukæmia, in which disease it is caused rather by effusion of blood into the corpora cavernosa, or by the formation of thrombi owing to the great excess of white corpuscles ; and in children by phimosis, stone in the bladder, and worms. Injuries to the cervical and upper dorsal parts of the spinal cord cause only incomplete priapism—*i.e.* turgescence without rigidity.

The duration of priapism varies ; it often lasts from three to six weeks, and may continue for as many months.

Treatment is unsatisfactory. Tartar emetic, mercury, bromide of potassium, belladonna, leeches, and strapping have all proved useless. Camphor, belladonna, or morphia is needed to procure sleep. Incisions have been employed with some success, and deserve a further trial. When due to injury of the spinal cord no special treatment for the priapism is required.

DISEASES OF THE CORPORA CAVERNOSA AND CORPUS SPONGIOSUM.

There are several diseases of the erectile structures of the penis, all of which produce induration of the corpora cavernosa or corpus spongiosum, or both.

(1) **Inflammation of the Erectile Tissues** of a more or less acute or subacute kind is caused by injury, gonorrhœa, rapidly repeated and excessive sexual excesses, and by ulceration or sloughing of the glans. In these cases the skin of the penis becomes red and œdematous, and a portion of the erectile structures firm and hard; there are the constitutional symptoms of fever and perhaps also painful priapism. Later the hard masses may soften and suppurate, and pyæmia may carry off the patient unless active operative steps are taken to evacuate and antisepticise the diseased parts.

(2) **Chronic Induration in Gouty Subjects** takes the form of more or less flattened nodules due to fibrous or keloid-like thickening of the sheaths and trabeculæ of the corpora cavernosa or septum pectiniforme.

It occurs only in men as_t forty or forty-five, and is thought to be analogous in origin and character with Dupuytren's contraction of the palmar fascia. This thickening may be limited to a small area of the penile sheath, or extend all along the penis and involve the suspensory ligament. Similar indurations have been ascribed by Ricord to syphilis, and were regarded by him as analogous to the syphilitic thickening of the tunica albuginea testis.

Another form of gouty origin, and probably due to thrombosis of the venous spaces of the corpora cavernosa, presents itself as small nodules of the size of peas or horsebeans, circumscribed, hard and painless, which sometimes spontaneously disappear. Similar deposits have been observed in diabetic subjects, and have been also ascribed to injury and urethritis.

(3) **Calcification of the Septum and Sheath of the Corpora Cavernosa** analogous to atheroma of the middle coat of vessels is described. In some cases true bone has been found in the septum of the penis which had apparently been developed from cartilage.

No active treatment is required in forms 2 and 3. No local treatment is of any use, though the gouty thickenings sometimes disappear spontaneously. If syphilis, urethritis, or stricture coexist, the patient should be treated accordingly. The bony masses have been excised with benefit when they have gravely interfered with micturition and rendered coitus difficult or impossible.

(4) **Gummata** of the penis are very rare; they have, however, been described as occurring, not only in the glans and the other erectile portions of the penis, but in the prepuce and skin covering the body of the organ. They should be treated actively at first by potassium iodide, and if they do not yield under the drug, circumcision, excision or amputation should be performed. There is danger that the gumma or the scar of a gumma may pass into epithelioma.

I have reported a case in which both corpora cavernosa and corpus spongiosum were invaded with scattered hard masses which rapidly extended, and were very painful in spite of all kinds of treatment. Neither injury, syphilis, gonorrhœa, gout, rheumatism, nor tubercle appeared to be the cause. The man died insane, but unfortunately no examination was permitted after death (*Lancet*, 1895, vol. ii. p. 95). Where much pain and retention of urine are unrelieved by other remedies, amputation of the penis may be required.

MALIGNANT DISEASE OF THE PENIS.

Squamous-celled carcinoma, or epithelioma, is the usual form of malignant disease. A few cases of primary sarcoma of the penis originating in the erectile structures have been recorded.

In comparison with carcinoma of other organs, that of the penis is not very frequent. Out of 501 cases of cancer of various parts and organs of the body which came under my observation in the cancer out-patient department of the Middlesex Hospital during the ten years 1872-1881, there was only one instance of cancer of the penis. (*See* vol. vi. of the Transactions of the Medical Society of London.) In other statistics the penis is affected in from 1 to 3 per cent. of the cases.

A case has lately been reported by Mr. W. A. Lane of malignant disease commencing in the urethra, near the meatus, of a man aged 39. In the space of four months it

M

destroyed the floor of the spongy body and prepuce, and extended over the surface of the corpora cavernosa and spongiosum invading and destroying their capsules. The specimen was examined by the Morbid Growths Committee of the Pathological Society, and pronounced to be "an infiltrating epithelial growth" which originated in the urethra, closely resembled "duct carcinoma" of the breast, and which, like the latter, they considered should be included in the class of "villous carcinoma" (Trans. Path. Soc., Lond., vol. xliv. pp. 105-107). Other cases are recorded by Mr. W. H. Battle, E. H. Fenwick, Kauffmann and others.

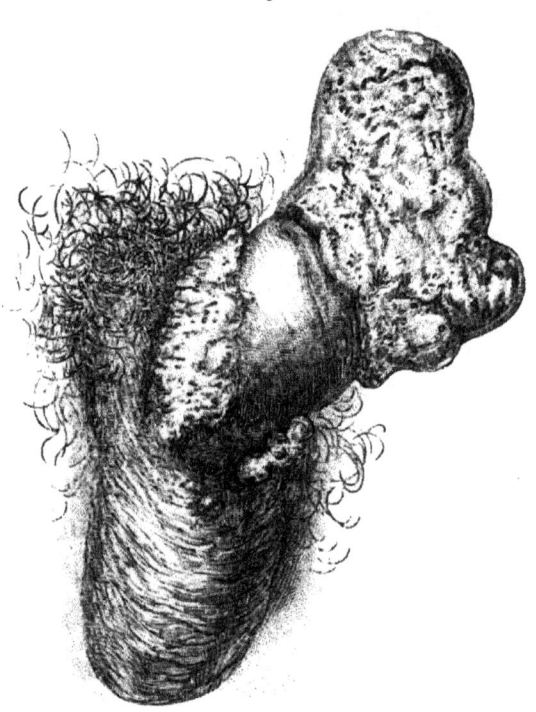

Fig. 53.—Anomalous Granuloma of Penis.
(*After Lunn.*)

A less malignant form of disease, described as "An Anomalous Granuloma" of 19 months' duration in a man 31 years of age, was brought before the Clinical Society by Mr. J. R. Lunn. (*See* Clin. Soc. Trans., vol. xxvii.)

In this case the glans penis and corona were covered with unhealthy granulations; a large, raw, granulating patch occupied the dorsum penis near its root, and several nodules were situated on the scrotum (Fig. 53). Some were commencing to break down, and there appeared to be some affection of the sebaceous follicles. The penis was removed by splitting the scrotum and detaching the crura penis from the pelvic arch.

Epithelioma of the Penis commences in a nearly equal number of cases on the prepuce and on the glans, the prepuce being perhaps more often than the glans the starting-point.

It may begin, like cancer of the tongue, in quite a variety of ways, as a wart upon the surface, or as a pea-like nodule beneath the surface; as a raw or excoriated patch, or as an ulcer; as a crack from injury or irritation, or as a leukæmic or ichthyotic patch such as often precedes epithelioma on the tongue, cheek, or lip. I have seen these ichthyotic patches on the vulva as well as on the prepuce. I have removed epitheliomata from such patches on the vulva, and the disease is described as occurring in a similar way on the prepuce.

The scars of wounds and the extension of the disease from the urethra and scrotum are other modes of onset of cancer of the penis.

Causes.—Epithelioma of the penis is a disease of late middle and advanced age, though it has fairly often been observed in men under thirty-five, and still more often under forty-five. Phimosis is a very pregnant cause, leading as it does to deformity, stunted growth, and irritation from retained secretions of the glans penis. Warts, chancres, the contracted scars of chancres, and every form of chronic irritation, such as gouty balanitis, sores, or cracks about a too short frænum, and the irritation of a urinary fistula, are other causes of epithelioma.

The manner in which the disease is propagated is by the lymphatics to the inguinal glands, or by infiltration, and dissemination of the malignant cells, in the corpora cavernosa.

Symptoms.—These differ in quite the early stage, according as the disease commences as a warty excrescence, or as a subcutaneous lump, or as a raw or blistered patch. But in whatever way the disease begins, its course soon becomes the same in all cases; an ulcer soon forms, and cauliflower-like excrescences arise here and there upon the epitheliomatous ulcer (Fig. 54). The ulcer varies in depth in different parts, its edges and base are very hard, the base being more or less fixed, and the edges more or less everted; the surface may be sloughy or ashy-grey, or nodular, or covered with exuberant granulations which bleed readily and scab over, forming a crust from beneath which a foul sanious discharge escapes.

The disease tends to spread locally, and though for a time resisted by the fibrous sheath of the corpora cavernosa, it does at length eat its way into the cavernous tissue, and there spread rapidly, entirely destroying the natural spongy character of the tissue. Separate isolated nodules of squamous epithelioma may be found in the corpora cavernosa at a considerable distance from the original mass of disease.

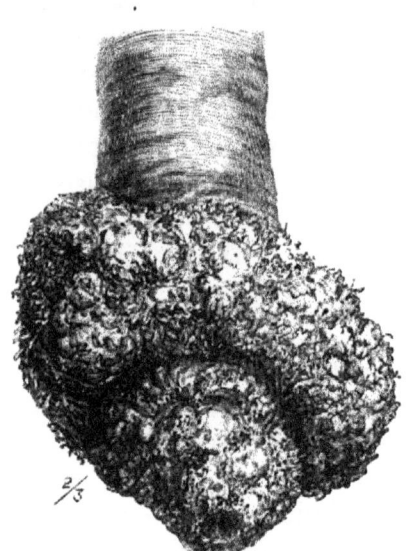

Fig. 54.—Cancer of Penis. (Royal College of Surgeons.)

As it is at the prepuce or glans that the disease generally begins, it is here that the chief mass of it is found, and sometimes the extremity of the penis is increased several inches in circumference. As a rule, the urethra escapes, and no obstruction to the outflow of the urine occurs. Occasionally, however, the urethra just behind or within the glans becomes perforated, and a urinary fistula is established in the floor of the urethra. One of the most severe attacks of urinary fever I have ever witnessed was started by the establishment of such a fistula during an act of micturition. Even when the end of the penis is converted into a huge warty mass of epithelioma, the urine will escape from the extremity of the urethra and make its way through the diseased tissues. Should obstruction in micturition occur, it is relieved later by sloughing of the disease.

There is but little if any pain as a rule till ulceration has extended (Fig. 55); pain then of a shooting and burning character occurs in the part, and radiates to the penis and perinæum. There is often a slight

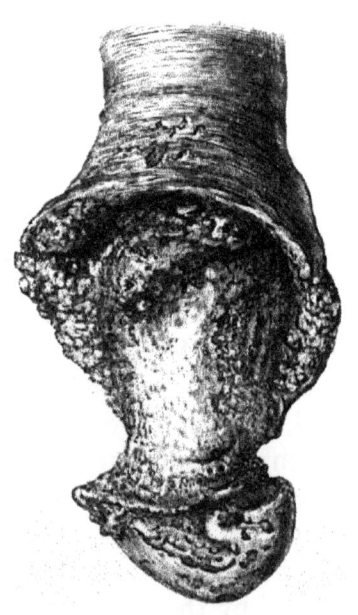

Fig. 55.—Cancer of Penis. (Royal College of Surgeons.)

amount of bleeding, but severe hæmorrhage is rare. One of the most marked features is the discharge of a foul, fetid, and abundant sanious fluid.

Too often when the patient first comes under the surgeon's notice the inguinal glands on one or both sides are obviously affected. Even if the glands are apparently unaffected, they may yet have been reached by the disease; it is this which frequently renders unavailing what appears to be the most complete removal of the primary disease. The abundant supply of lymphatic vessels on the penis, which run direct to the inguinal glands, and of deep lymphatics which run with the pudic vessels to join the glands along the internal iliac artery, explains the rapidity with which the disease is conveyed to these glands. This rapidity of invasion is the greater when the rate of ulceration is great, and when the disease commences on the under aspect of the prepuce. Warmth and moisture, and the rapid spread of the disease beneath a phimosed foreskin, are the conditions most favourable to an early infection of the lymphatics.

The position of the inguinal glands about the saphena and femoral veins, and their proneness to become inflamed as well as invaded by cancer elements, create difficulties in the complete removal of them, and explain the œdema of the lower limbs and groins, and the hæmorrhages which occur in the late stages of the disease. Another danger is that the glands soften, and ulcerate into one of the veins, and thus through the blood-stream distant parts and viscera are invaded.

Diagnosis.—An early recognition of the disease is of the utmost importance, so that its complete excision may be effected before the lymphatic vessels and glands are involved.

When the disease commences as a wart, by the time it becomes hard at the base and characteristically ulcerated on its surface, the disease has too often already invaded the lymphatics, and the most favourable time for operation has passed. Before the wart has become indurated and fixed at its base, the only reliable means of diagnosis are the microscopical appearances and the beneficial effect upon it of cleanliness and treatment or otherwise.

When the disease commences as a subcutaneous pea- or bean-sized nodule, it ought to be diagnosed as malignant at once.

Between cancer and primary chancres, or the sores of late syphilis the effect of a fortnight's treatment ought to settle the doubt. It should never be forgotten that an obstinate tertiary syphilitic sore on the penis, as on the tongue, leg, or elsewhere, is very prone to pass into an epitheliomatous growth. No time should be lost, therefore, in operating upon a doubtful ulcer which does not improve under specific treatment.

In all cases where an induration or a sore exists beneath a phimotic prepuce, the prepuce should be slit up and examined; or if the whole of the disease can be removed with the prepuce, circumcision should be performed.

Treatment.—In any case of doubtful wart or ulcer which has resisted the ordinary treatment of cleanliness and suitable local applications for a few days, and has persisted or returned after having been freely treated by acid nitrate of mercury, or fuming nitric acid, nothing remains to be done but the complete and wide removal of the diseased tissues.

When the disease is limited to the prepuce, circumcision will suffice. I have had most gratifying results in these circumstances from simple circumcision. It must, however, be borne in mind that there is a great tendency, when the disease commences on the under surface of the prepuce or on the glans penis, for both the apposed surfaces to become affected, and to form some amount of adhesion between them. When such is the case, amputation of part of the penis is requisite.

The amount of penis to be removed depends entirely on the extent to which it is invaded. In some cases amputation may be safe just behind the glans or through the organ half way between the pubes and the glans; or it may be required immediately in front of the pubes, or even still farther back, so that the whole of the erectile structures are taken away, including the crura penis, and the bulb of the urethra.

If the inguinal glands are enlarged, they must be freely removed. But when these operations are undertaken, the surgeon must be prepared for extensive and complicated dissections exposing the saphena vein and femoral vessels, and the anterior crural nerve.

CHAPTER IV.

CONGENITAL MALFORMATIONS OF THE URETHRA.

HYPOSPADIAS.

By hypospadias is understood an abnormal and congenital opening of the inferior wall of the urethra.

It is by no means a very rare malformation. Émile Forgue thinks it occurs once in every 1,200 to 1,900 males. It has been observed in several members of the same family through several generations. Lepelletier quotes the occurrence of scrotal hypospadias in each of three brothers.

It is the result of an arrest of development in early fœtal life. The urethra is developed in three portions: the prostatic and membranous urethra from the constricted, tubular, lower end of the urogenital sinus; the spongy portion, by the closing in below of the urogenital fissure posteriorly and of the groove beneath the genital tubercle anteriorly; and the *balanic* urethra (*i.e.* the urethra of the glans penis), which is hollowed out in the epithelial ridge on the inferior aspect of the glans, and subsequently joins the spongy portion of the urethra.

Any arrest in the evolution or union of these three component parts will result in one or other of the forms of hypospadias.

VARIETIES.—(1) **Hypospadias of the Glans Penis** (balanic hypospadias) appears most frequently as a longitudinal groove open below and formed by the superior wall of the navicular fossa. The urethral mucous membrane is continuous with the adjacent integument, and is often valve-like, so as to mask the entrance to the spongy urethra. This orifice is frequently contracted so as scarcely to admit a pin. There is a corresponding gap in the under part of the prepuce. There are several varieties of this form of hypospadias, which are shown in the accompanying diagram (Fig. 56). Torsion of the penis, and congenital adhesion of the penis to the front of the scrotum, sometimes complicate this form of hypospadias.

(2) **Penile and Peno-scrotal Hypospadias.**—The floor of the spongy part of the urethra between the bulb and glans

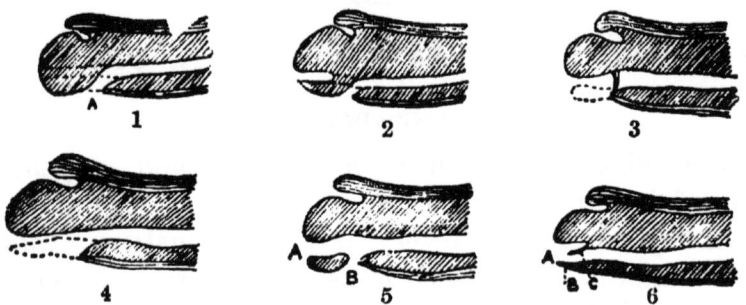

Fig. 56A.—Scheme of some Varieties of Balanic Hypospadias. (*After Kauffmann.*)

(1) Imperforate glans penis with opening of urethra at A ; (2) Canal through glans penis incomplete ; (3) A septum interposed between penile urethra and groove beneath glans penis ; (4) The common form of balanic hypospadias ; (5) Normal meatus A, with an opening behind glans B ; (6) A, Normal meatus, B, defective floor of urethra, C, penile urethra prolonged beneath glans.

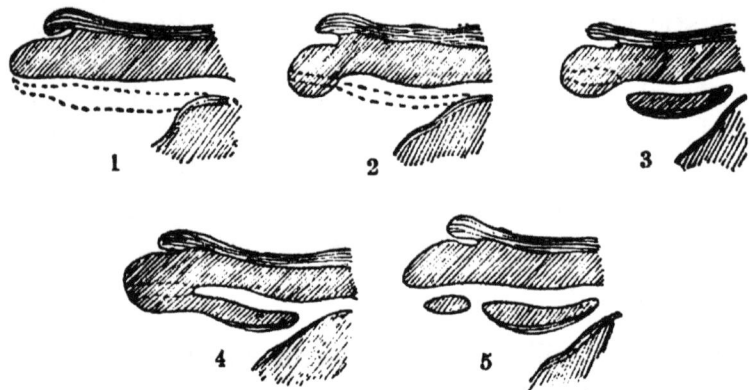

Fig. 56B.--Scheme of some Varieties of Peno-scrotal Hypospadias.
(*After Kauffmann.*)

(1) Absence of the whole length of the penile and balanic urethra ; (2) Peno-scrotal hypospadias with imperforate balanic portion of urethra ; (3) Imperforate balanic urethra with opening behind glans and another near front of scrotum, the intervening penile urethra being perfect ; (4) Imperforate balanic urethra, and penile urethra continued forwards in front of peno-scrotal opening and ending blindly at the back of the glans ; (5) Normal meatus with an opening just behind glans and another in front of scrotum, the floor of the intermediate part of urethra being present.

penis is wanting, and there is seen a moist vascular furrow, or more or less of a canal or a dense band of fibrous tissue, in place of the corpus spongiosum. With the latter condition, the penis is curved downwards and backwards to the scrotum.

In the penile hypospadias the urethra may open at any point between the peno-scrotal junction and the base of the glans. In the peno-scrotal form, the orifice of the urethra is immediately in front of the scrotum, but the scrotum is not bifid. There may be both the balanic and peno-scrotal forms of hypospadias present in the same subject.

The corpora cavernosa and glans penis are frequently well developed in this second form; but the prepuce, meatus,

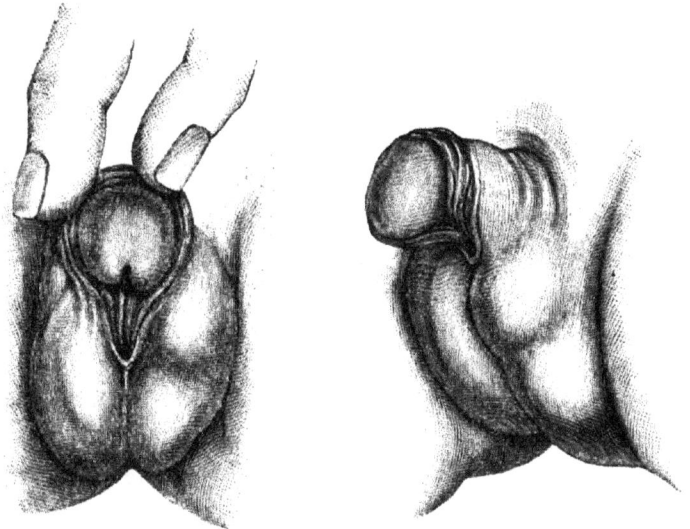

Fig. 57.—Peno-scrotal Hypospadias. (*After Duplay and Reclus.*)

glans and penis may be malformed; and the nearer to the scrotum the urethra terminates, the more likely are these malformations to be present.

(3) **The Third Degree of Hypospadias is the Scrotal and Perinæo-scrotal.**—In this form the arrest of development occurs earlier than in the other two, and the result is a near approach to the normal female formation, and the condition wrongly called hermaphrodism.

The penis is imperfectly developed and always curved downwards; the scrotum is cleft and the urethra opens in the perinæum; and the testicles may be small, ill-formed, ectopic, or retained; but if properly descended, each will occupy the separate scrotum of its own side (Fig. 57).

Symptoms.—Whatever troubles there may be in connection with the urinary and generative functions, incontinence is not one of them, because only the parts in front of the membranous urethra are involved in hypospadias. If the abnormal aperture is very small, the same symptoms may be produced as from stricture, and in many cases there has been retention of urine.

The nearer the aperture is to the scrotum, the more inconvenient is micturition. Persons with scrotal and perinæo-scrotal hypospadias must micturate in the squatting posture. An irritating erythema of the scrotum is caused by the frequent contact of urine in certain cases of the peno-scrotal group. Hypospadias of the glans penis, without much curving of the penis, does not materially interfere with erection, coitus, or fecundation. In the penile and peno-scrotal varieties, erection and coitus are difficult, or imperfect and painful, but frequently possible; fecundity is uncertain.

In scrotal and perinæal hypospadias, and in all cases where the incurvation of the penis is extreme, the sexual functions are imperfect, if not impossible.

Diagnosis and Prognosis.—As a rule there is no difficulty in the diagnosis. Should there be a fold or flap hiding the small aperture, it is only necessary to make the patient pass water to detect the abnormal opening. The history and general appearance will prevent a small hypospadias from being mistaken for a penile fistula. The sex of the subject in extreme cases of scrotal hypospadias will be settled by the detection of the testes in each lip of the vulviform slit, or in the inguinal canals; by the absence of a uterus interposed between a catheter in the bladder and the finger in the rectum; and by the absence of the catamenia, as well as by the outward appearances and the voice.

The unfavourable situation of the parts for plastic operation by the constant wetting with urine, and their variation in size from varying degrees of turgescence; as well as the thinness of the tissues out of which flaps have to be cut, are sources of uncertainty and failure in the operative treatment.

Treatment.—Hypospadias of the glans portion of the urethra rarely needs any operative treatment. Hypospadias of the penile or peno-scrotal needs operative treatment.

The details of the operation, as they have been laid down by Duplay, should be followed. As to the age at which operative measures should be employed, opinions differ. Bouisson prefers to wait till puberty. Duplay straightens the penis at the earliest age, and makes a new canal at the age of five or six years; but for the completion of the anastomosis of the different parts of the canal he waits till puberty, so as to obtain the advantage of the docile and intelligent co-operation of the patient. Probably the best rule to follow is that advocated by Bouisson and Émile Forgue—namely, to defer operating till puberty, except in those cases in which, owing to the narrowness of the abnormal aperture, or to the presence of a valvular fold, the emission of urine is interfered with: and in these cases an operation should be performed without delay.

The steps of the operation consist in first making an external meatus at the glans, then in covering in the penile portion of the passage from the glans to the abnormal orifice, and, thirdly, in freshening the ends of the old and new canal, and joining them together by horsehair sutures.

EPISPADIAS.

In epispadias, the urethra is exposed for more or less of its extent along the upper surface of the penis. It may or may not be associated with extroversion of the bladder.

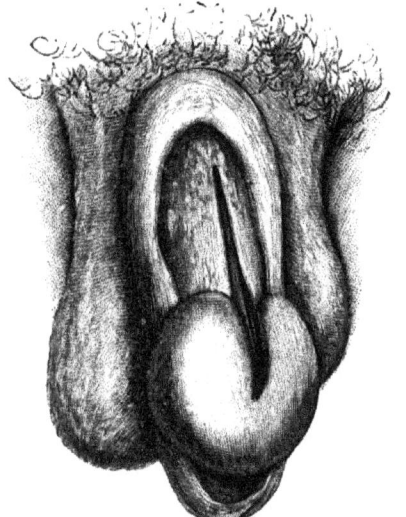

Fig. 58.—Epispadias. (*After Ammon.*)

Epispadias has been variously explained, but most of the theories are directly in conflict with embryological facts.

It is not, properly speaking, a division or deficiency in the upper wall of the urethra, but in the floor of the urethra, which has been transposed to the dorsal aspect, owing to torsion, of the penis. It is thus, in fact, a hypospadias reversed—*i.e.* upside down.

Torsion of the penis is probably explained by the outgrowth of one of the genital folds causing the genital tubercle (eminence) to deviate on one side and become twisted on its own axis. If such twisting or torsion takes place to the extent of half a circle, the corpus spongiosum and urethra will be on the upper surface of the penis. The corpus spongiosum rests on the groove of the united corpora cavernosa, these being situated on the inferior aspect of the penis, and the prepuce hangs from the inferior aspect of the glans.

Cases have been recorded by Gay, Follin, Dolbeau, and others, of epispadias associated with torsion of the penis.

Compared with hypospadias it is very rare. The proportion of the two sets of cases is 1 to 150.

There are three degrees of epispadias :—(1) That confined to the glans penis ; (2) that in which besides the glans portion a part of the spongy urethra is also defective ; and (3) that in which the epispadias is complete and extends the whole length of the penis.

In the first two degrees the penis is short but large, and the corpora cavernosa are complete. In the third degree, which is by far the most frequent, the penis is short and stunted and curved upwards and backwards, torsion is more or less manifest, the glans penis is normal, the corpora cavernosa are often defective or absent, and the prepuce is abundant, but often reduced to half its circumference. It is in this third degree that the several complications occur, such as extroversion and hernia of the bladder, separation of the pubes, and various abnormalities of the testes.

Symptoms depend upon the degree. Some epispadiacs urinate voluntarily, but with a misdirected stream ; some have great frequency of micturition, or even pass water involuntarily under physical and mental disturbances, such as coughing, laughing, etc. ; others have no control except when lying on their backs ; and in some there is continual dribbling of urine. Sexual functions are always difficult or impossible.

Treatment.—Several plastic operations have been practised with some measure of success. Wood's, Nélaton's, and Dolbeau's operations consist in covering the urethra with cutaneous flaps from the abdominal wall or scrotum. By Thiersch's method the canal is covered, but the curvature of the penis is not corrected. Duplay's operation is directed first to straightening the organ, and then to covering the canal by autoplastic flaps derived from the covering of the corpora cavernosa and prepuce. The operation is done in three stages :—1. Partial straightening of the penis by making one or more subcutaneous incisions into each cavernous body separately, and leaving the process of development to complete the rectification. 2. Covering the penile portion of the epispadias by quadrilateral flaps dissected from off the penis, and improving the shape of the organ by buttonholing the preputial skin. 3. Uniting the old with the new urethra.

Incontinence of urine was cured by an autoplastic operation in one of Dolbeau's cases.

IMPERFORATE URETHRA.

The urethra may be either incompletely or completely imperforate.

. **Incomplete Imperforations** are most frequently met with at the meatus, or a little way down the glans portion of the urethra, especially at the spot where this latter joins in the process of development with the spongy portion. The meatus may be simply very narrow or it may be contracted by valves. Another variety of incomplete imperforation is a cylindrical stenosis either of congenital origin or caused by irritation set up behind a congenitally narrow meatus. It takes the form of a ferrule or ring, and is most frequent just posterior to the navicular fossa.

A contracted meatus ought not to be ignored ; it causes in some cases cystitis, in others the symptoms of vesical calculus ; it also tends to prolong urethritis and gleet, and thereby to induce stricture and surgical ureters and kidneys. The only proper treatment is to divide the meatus with a blunt-pointed tenotome, and any sclerosed ring higher up the canal by the internal urethrotome.

Complete Imperforations occur either with or without an abnormal exit for the urine. They consist either (1) of a diaphragm or (2) of a transformation of part of the urethra into a fibrous cord.

(1) Diaphragms occur either in the lumen of the urethra or at the meatus. Sometimes two or more exist in the same

individual; or an imperforate meatus may coexist with a valve at the neck of the bladder, or with a diaphragm at some little distance from the external meatus.

(2) The part of the urethra most often replaced by a fibrous cord is the membranous. These cases are very rare.

Any complete occlusion without an abnormal exit for the urine, if it persists through the latter half of fœtal life, must result in dilatation of the bladder, ureters, and kidneys.

I have published a case of extreme congenital hydro-nephrosis, due to a diaphragm, easily broken down by a gum catheter, in the spongy part of the urethra. I have seen the same condition in a fœtus at full term caused by a small cyst in the floor of the spongy urethra, and quite obstructing its lumen, and another in which the bladder was hypertrophied and the ureters convoluted and dilated into pouches from torsion of the penis.

Complete imperforation of the urethra if there be an external communication with the bladder need not be attended with the disastrous changes in the bladder and higher urinary organs just alluded to. The abnormal opening through which the urine passes may be in the front wall of the rectum, in the perinæum, or on the under surface of the penis.

The proper *treatment* for complete simple occlusion is to break down the obstruction either with a tenotome or sound. Where the urethra is converted into a mere fibrous cord, a new urethra should be made, as in hypospadias.

PARTIAL OR TOTAL ABSENCE OF THE URETHRA.

Partial absence is less rare than complete. In the former case the penis may be represented by only an erectile warty appendix as in Goschler's case. The complete absence of the urethra, sometimes observed in the female, has been only twice recorded (so far as I know) in the male—namely, by Richardson and Revolat. In Richardson's case the bladder, as well as the urethra, was absent, and the ureters opened into the rectum. The patient lived seventeen years, passing water by the anus. In Revolat's case the anus and the penis were wanting, and both meconium and urine escaped at the umbilicus. The fœtus was born dead.

CONGENITAL DILATATION OF THE URETHRA.

Three or four cases are on record of a great dilatation into a flask-like sac of the floor of the urethra near the glans. They were not, apparently, dilatations behind a mechanical obstruction, but were due to the absence of the spongy tissue around,

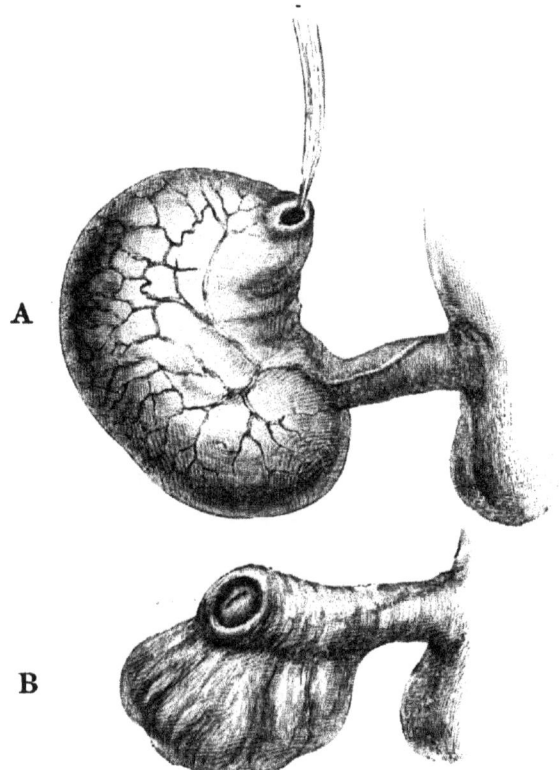

Fig. 59.—Congenital Urinary Pouch ; A, during micturition ; B, empty.
(*After Anger.*)

and the distension of, the mucous membrane of the affected part of the urethra.

The pouches became distended with urine at each act of micturition (in one case it held the whole of the urine discharged from the bladder), and were only emptied by pressing them between the two hands (Fig. 59).

The *treatment* is that practised by Hendriksz, of Amsterdam, who distended the pouch with tepid water and laid it open by two semicircular incisions, cut away a fold of urethral mucous membrane on each orifice of the pouch, and sutured separately the lips of the mucous membrane and the edges of the skin. (For Non-congenital Sacculation of the Urethra, *see* pages 268-9.)

ABNORMAL OPENINGS OF THE URETHRA, OR INTO THE URETHRA.

The urethra sometimes opens into the rectum, or externally, as stated under Complete Imperforation. Conversely the bowel may open into the urethra, as is described in all works on malformations of the anus and rectum.

DOUBLE URETHRA

is only met with in cases of double penis. Velpeau met with a case of double penis in a child in which each penis contained a urethra, and each urethra communicated with the bladder.

The glans penis may have several openings upon its surface, but only one of them will lead to the urethra, the others merely into a *cul de sac.* Cruveilhier records a case in which a canal ran from the corona along the dorsal aspect of the penis, under the pubic arch and between the corpora cavernosa, then bifurcated, and the branches passed round the sides of the prostate. He regarded it as an abnormal opening of the ejaculatory ducts.

Two other cases are referred to by É. Forgue : one in which the dorsal canal ended beneath the symphysis pubis, and another in which it seemed to have a connection with the prostate gland. (*See* Congenital Fistula of Penis.)

CHAPTER V.

WOUNDS OF THE URETHRA.

FROM its protected situation wounds of the urethra are rare, except when associated with wounds of the corpora cavernosa.

Punctured wounds are quite exceptional, and, like longitudinal incised wounds, as a rule heal quickly without interfering with the calibre of the canal.

Oblique and transverse wounds are situated almost always in the bulbous or penile portions, and are of more consequence. They are often attended with free hæmorrhage, derived, however, not so much from the wounded urethra as from the division of more or less of the cavernous bodies.

The most simple transverse wound, if not brought together soon by sutures, will heal, leaving a fibrous cicatricial stricture varying in extent according to the extent and mode of repair of the wound; whereas wounds involving even the whole circumference of the urethra, if accurately united by sutures and healed by first intention, have soft, lax cicatrices which encroach but little upon the lumen of the urethra.

RUPTURE OF THE URETHRA.

The urethra may be ruptured at any point from the prostatic portion to the meatus, but the most frequent seat of injury is the bulbous or membranous portion. Although in the flaccid state of the penis the penile portion of the urethra is well protected, yet in this state it has been ruptured by kicks from a horse (James Madden), and by compression, as in shutting a linen-drawer by pushing against it with the upper part of the thighs (Voillemier). During erection it is more exposed to injury, and in that state has been subcutaneously ruptured just in front of the scrotum by a pinch between the finger and thumb (Voillemier), by forcible bending of the penis upon its dorsum, and by forcible twists and undue violence during coitus. It has been said to rupture during strong erections in men suffering from inflammatory

N

deposits in the corpus spongiosum, owing to the inextensibility of the inflamed part preventing it from expanding *pari passu* with the cavernous bodies.

But the most frequent and most important forms of rupture of the urethra occur from violence to the perinæum; either by the individual falling astride of some resisting body, or from a kick or other blow inflicted upon the perinæum. Kauffmann gives the following statistics as to the mode of production of the rupture:—Out of 239 cases, 198, or 82 per cent., were caused by falls astride; 28, or 12 per cent., by blows on the perinæum; 9 by falls from a carriage; and 4 by injuries against the pommel of a saddle.

Pathological Anatomy.—Much discussion has been held as to the exact seat of injury in perinæal ruptures of the urethra; and many experiments and other observations have been made by surgeons, and especially by Cras and Terrillon, and, with certain reservations, their views may be accepted as correct.

When the rupture is caused by falls astride, it is situated at the bulbous portion of the urethra. If the contusing body is small, so that it can be driven up against the vault of the pubic arch, it rarely strikes the urethra in the middle line, but, inclined to the pubic ramus of one side, it twists the penis and forces the urethra against the opposite ramus of the pubis. If the contusing body is too large to be forced into the sub-pubic arch, the urethra is struck in the middle line and is crushed directly against the front of the pubes, or against the lower edge of the symphysis. Thus the spongy body itself, says Terrillon, or the anterior part of the bulb, is wounded, and the inferior wall of the urethra will be the first or the only part ruptured. The rupture will be jagged or flap-like.

Contusions of the perinæum caused by blows directed from before backwards cause lesions similar to the above, whereas direct blows on the posterior part of the perinæum directed from behind, damage the membranous part of the urethra immediately behind the bulb, but it is always the pubis which acts as the *point d'appui* for the rupture.

Iversen of Copenhagen agrees with Cras and Terrillon that the rupture is generally partial and involves the inferior and lateral, not the upper wall of the urethra. He also agrees with them that except in cases of fracture of the pelvis or disjunction of the symphysis, when the membranous urethra is apt to suffer, the rupture generally takes place just in front of the triangular ligament.

Poncet and Ollier attach much importance to the resistance offered by the triangular ligament, and assert that in rupture of the membranous urethra it is the upper wall which is injured against the edge of this ligament, and that in these cases a catheter can be passed by keeping along the lower instead of the upper part of the urethra.

Émile Forgue and Kauffmann consider the hypothesis of Ollier and Poncet erroneous, and their direction as to catheterism dangerous. With this view I am entirely in accord. Forgue found, by repeating the experiments of Poncet, that though the upper wall of the membranous urethra had been compressed, it was not lacerated. They agree with Terrillon as to the mechanism of ruptures involving the bulb—namely, that they are caused by crushing against the arch of the pubis.

It is the membranous urethra which is most commonly ruptured with fracture of the pelvic bones. The rupture is caused either by the penetration of the urethra by a broken fragment of bone, or by its being violently dragged upon and torn by the deep triangular ligament which is displaced with the broken bone.

In certain cases of falls astride upon the perinæum, the urethra may be ruptured at the bulb, and, the violence of the fall continuing, the pelvic bones are afterwards broken. In other cases, a simple dislocation of the symphysis pubis has caused rupture of the urethra by the temporary stretching apart of the sides of the pubic arch. The instances of so-called rupture of the urethra from muscular violence were probably ruptures from dislocation of the symphysis, or from an unrecognised fracture.

There are, according to Reybard and Terrillon, three degrees of rupture of the spongy urethra: (1) A trabecular rupture in which a hæmatoma is formed by extravasation of blood within the limits of the corpus spongiosum ; (2) a muco-trabecular or mucous membrane rupture in which the mucous membrane as well as the erectile tissue suffers; the damage to the mucous membrane may be either limited to the surface, or it may be torn in a ring-like manner with thin processes of the submucous tissue still connecting the two ends of the rent; (3) rupture of the fibrous sheath of the corpus spongiosum as well as of the erectile and mucous tissues.

The second and third degrees are anatomically and clinically justified ;. but, practically, the distinction is of little importance, because in each the urine can gain access to the injured tissues, and there are the same risks of inflammatory and septic changes. What is of more importance to the surgeon is whether the rupture implicates only part or the whole of the circumference of the urethra; because in the former case the undivided portion of the tube (nearly always the superior) forms a track for the catheter and a landmark in perinæal section ; whereas when the urethra is torn quite asunder, the mucous membrane wrinkles up, and the two ends retract, sometimes to the extent of an inch or more, making it extremely difficult to find the proximal opening. These differences of degree of injury do not, of course, apply to ruptures of the membranous urethra.

Dr. E. Deanesly, of Wolverhampton, in a succinct and instructive paper in the *Practitioner* (July, 1894), records a case in which a young man fell while running and struck his perinæum against the heel of his boot. At the operation, twenty-four hours after the accident, the sheath of the urethra was found intact, but a rupture of the inner wall could be easily felt on pinching the urethra between the finger and thumb, just in front of the bulb. On opening the urethra in this situation, a large V-shaped flap of mucous membrane and spongy tissue, the apex of which was directed backwards and embraced the lower two-thirds of the circumference of the urethra, was found detached from the floor.

Symptoms.—Bleeding from the urethra, difficulty in micturition amounting in some cases to actual retention, and swelling and ecchymosis in the perinæum are the leading symptoms ; but they are not invariably all present, nor are they always very prominent. *In penile rupture* of the urethra there will be a sudden pain at the moment, the trickling of a few drops of blood from the meatus, and a little ring-like thickening at the seat of injury, and that may be all at the time, but later a hard, intractable stricture follows. In other cases the symptoms are much severer; the hæmorrhage is very free, and recurring, there is complete retention of urine from blood-clot, and the pain at the moment of rupture may have been intense; though if the patient is the subject of chordee, there is an alleviation immediately afterwards of the pain of that condition. It has been said that " every rupture is a stricture in embryo."

The symptoms of *perinæal ruptures of the urethra* present the greatest variety in their degree of severity. In some few cases the pain is slight and soon passes off; there is but little difficulty or pain in micturition; there is slight ecchymosis of the penis and perinæum, and only slight, if any, swelling along the course of the urethra; the bleeding from the urethra is so slight as perhaps to have escaped the notice or the memory of the patient, and a catheter can be passed at once and with ease. But the subsequent effects may be most serious owing to infiltration of urine, inflammation and septicæmia; hence the necessity of carefully watching such cases for many days. In a far greater number of ruptures hæmorrhage from the urethra is free, continuous, or recurring, micturition is very difficult and painful, or there is partial or complete retention of urine; there is a swelling in the perinæum with ecchymosis extending more or less over the scrotum to the penis and thighs, and after a short time there may be a crepitant feeling over the swelling; it is possible the catheter can be passed if its beak follows the roof of the urethra, which may remain untorn.

In the most severe cases, and those in which the urethra is torn asunder, all the classical symptoms are pronounced—namely, free urethral hæmorrhage, total retention of urine, and a large perinæal swelling.

The introduction of a catheter is impossible, and attempts to introduce it can do nothing but harm; any effort on the part of the patient to pass urine, if successful, can but result in forcing urine into the torn tissues.

The whole condition favours infiltration, suppuration, gangrene, and infection, and these risks are, if possible, increased where the pelvic bones are fractured. Where the membranous urethra is the seat of rupture, infiltration of blood and urine spreads around the prostate and neck of the bladder, sets up pelvic cellulitis, and extends to the peritoneum.

If these, the earlier, ill consequences are escaped, or recovered from, a traumatic stricture of the most fibrous and inelastic kind is sure to follow later.

Diagnosis.—In rupture of the penile urethra, whether the patient is suffering from chordee or not, there is pain at the moment, followed by a few drops of blood from the urethra at least sufficient to stain the linen. The slight annular swelling around the urethra, and subsequently the development of a stricture, likewise point to the nature of the accident which has happened.

After a fall or a blow on the perinæum the discharge of blood by the urethra is sufficient to show what has happened, even without any of the other symptoms of rupture.

In the more severe cases of rupture of the bulb or membranous urethra, the symptoms are too marked to allow room for doubt.

The diagnosis as to the precise *situation* of the rupture will be made by careful inquiry as to the mechanism of the injury. As to the *degree* of injury, one is generally justified in concluding, where the symptoms are slight, that a part of the circumference of the tube is torn, and that, the inferior part or floor. Where the symptoms are very severe and well marked, we may fairly assume that the tube is torn across.

The doubtful cases are those in which there is no urethral hæmorrhage and where the patient can, at first, pass urine and there is no extravasation of urine. But in a day or two, or perhaps within a few hours, the diagnosis can be made from symptoms which become well developed.

Treatment.—In slight cases where there is no retention catheterism is needless, and may be dangerous, since it may excite bleeding which did not previously exist, and will tend to retard the healing of the wound.

In all cases, however, a close watch should be kept for infiltration of urine or inflammation of the injured parts.

In all cases in which partial or complete retention, urethral hæmorrhage, slight or much, and a swelling in the urethra, small or great, are present, external urethrotomy or perinæal section should be done, whether a catheter can be passed or not. There should be no temporising with a catheter retained in the bladder, hoping that hæmorrhage will be thus controlled and extravasation of urine and septic infection of the parts will be avoided.

An early perinæal section provides for the evacuation of blood and blood-clots from the wounded tissues; it enables the surgeon to control hæmorrhage completely, and also thoroughly to disinfect the wound. It enables a catheter to be introduced and retained, without inflicting unseen damage upon the lacerated parts, and it is the only means of preventing or minimising the subsequent stricture.

To wait is to increase the chances of sloughing, to allow extravasation and bacterial infection to be established, and to increase the difficulties of an operation, which will have to be performed later, by giving time for the retraction of the vesical end of the urethra in a mass of inflammatory tissue.

The steps of the operation of perinæal section for ruptured urethra cannot be given here in detail, but I desire to draw special attention to the importance of bringing the torn edges of the urethra together as soon as possible by means of sutures of catgut or fine silk. I practised this procedure for the first time in 1874, and I have taught and recommended it ever since.* In one of my cases I used silver wire sutures, in the others fine silk.

Suturing has been recently adopted in England by Mr. Wright of Manchester, Mr. Sheild, Mr. Woolcombe, Mr. Pearce Gould, Mr. Sutton, and by Dr. Edward Deanesly of Wolverhampton (*vide supra*); and on the Continent it has been performed by de Paoli, Vignard, Guyon, and Socin, and recommended by Kauffmann, Hägler and Émile Forgue.

Circular urethrorrhaphy consists in passing two, three, or four sutures of fine silk or catgut through the torn ends of the urethra, and thus tying them together around a catheter previously passed into the bladder. Buried sutures should hold together the torn fibrous sheath and the muscular layer, and a second set should bring together the edges of the wound in the integuments.

* Cavendish Lecture, *Lancet*, vol. i. pp. 1431-36, 1893.

Dr. Deanesly used horsehair and silkworm gut as sutures for the urethra, tied the ends together, and brought them out through the external wound, the rest of which was sutured. Primary union occurred except around the ends of the urethral sutures, and these were removed on the twelfth day, some little force being necessary to do this. A urinary fistula followed in the track of the sutures, but closed within a month from the accident. The calibre of the urethra since the operation has always allowed a full-sized instrument to be introduced, and twelve months afterwards there was no sign of stricture, nor was there any induration or thickening to be felt at the site of rupture.

There is much to be said in favour of non-absorbing sutures, as there is less risk of the wound becoming septic; but there is the drawback of having a suture track and a urinary fistula, even though of a temporary character, afterwards. Perhaps it will be found the best plan to use buried sutures of catgut or fine silk, and not to pass them through the free surface of the mucous membrane of the urethra.

If the torn ends are much bruised or lacerated, it will be advisable to cut a portion of them away before applying the sutures.

The catheter around which the urethra has been sutured should be retained from five to eight days, and afterwards a Jacques or gum-elastic catheter should be passed daily; or if the patient can pass it easily upon himself it would be well for him to use it for a week or two, every time he wishes to micturate.

CATHETERISM : FALSE PASSAGES AND HOW TO AVOID THEM.

Another class of wounds of the urethra are those which are caused by the ignorant, or careless, or too forcible use of catheters and sounds.

They are of the nature of contused and lacerated wounds.

In a normal urethra false passages ought never to be made. Strictures of the urethra, enlargements of the prostate, abnormally large lacunæ of Morgagni, the dilated orifices of mucous glands, and lacunar recesses in the prostatic urethra in which the point of an instrument can catch, are the conditions under which false passages are likely to be made.

Another predisposing cause is the flaccidity of the perinæum of old men, and the readiness with which the bulbous part of the urethra, owing to its feeble support in these subjects, becomes depressed by the point of an instrument carelessly or roughly handled. Guyon points out that in men with prostatic enlargement on whom the catheter has been frequently or constantly used there occurs such a degree of depression at the *cul de sac* of the bulb that it amounts to a "false direction"; in this the instrument may be suddenly arrested, and although there is not actually a "false passage," yet one will soon be made, if proper care is not exercised to avoid dipping the point of the catheter into this depression. The same risk exists after external urethrotomy or perinæal section.

In cases of enlarged middle lobe of the prostate a complete tunnel may be made through it, into the bladder, by the frequent thrusting of the point of an instrument against its base.

Sometimes the point of an instrument passes very readily and for some distance into the submucous tissue, and then re-enters the normal lumen of the urethra. This most likely is the explanation and mode of origin of those strictures which are called "bridle."

Symptoms.—As there is much less resistance to an instrument in passing it along the natural channel than in piercing the mucous membrane, the hand that makes the false passage probably realises at the moment an extra resistance, which it overcomes by the use of some amount of force. It should never be forgotten that *no force whatever* ought to be used in passing an instrument into the bladder. A sound or a lithotrite if properly handled will go along the urethra and enter the bladder by its own weight, and if a check occurs in its transit just as the handle of the instrument is about to be depressed between the thighs of the patient lying on his back, this will easily be overcome by raising the handle and withdrawing it a little, and then pressing with a slight downward drag over the hypogastrium with the other hand just as the handle of the instrument is again lowered.

I am constantly in the habit of showing the advantage of this little manœuvre, especially during lithotrity.

The lighter and gentler the manipulation of the instrument the easier will it pass into the bladder; and if an obstruction is felt, the catheter should be " coaxed," but not forced past it.

If the instrument is pushed out of the canal and to one side, it will no longer keep in a line with the linea alba, but the handle will be deflected to the side opposite to that on which the point has penetrated the urethra wall. This deflection need not occur, however, if the urethral floor and not the lateral wall is penetrated. So that the inexperienced surgeon must not be confident he is in the urethra merely because the handle of his instrument is in the median line.

The other symptoms are hæmorrhage, pain, abnormal resistance to the onward progress of the instrument, and the detection, by the index finger in the rectum, of the misplacement of the end of the instrument below or behind the prostate, and too near the bowel.

Rigors, fever, extravasation of urine, perinæal inflammation, and urinary abscess are the general and local complications which may arise. As a rule, in men in fair health, beyond slight hæmorrhage and the pain caused by the catheter, no inconvenience is felt by the patient if he is kept in bed and no further instrumentation allowed till the wound is healed.

Treatment.—To avoid making a false passage, the best course is to be very gentle and light of touch, and to keep the instrument towards the roof of the urethra. The advantage of hypogastric pressure has been alluded to above; its *modus operandi* consists, I believe, in diminishing the curve of the urethra and in putting it more upon the stretch—*i.e.* in making it " taut."

The object of catheters, coudée or bent up at the extremity, and of instruments with a strong curve, is to avoid the various irregularities, and especially those of the prostate, which occur along the floor of the urethra. They are particularly of use in enlargement of the prostate.

Another precaution is to keep the penis well drawn up over the instrument, especially whilst passing it through the membranous portion, and just before depressing its handle between the patient's thighs. In a case of false passage associated with stricture, in which a catheter is needed, the soft olive-headed instruments should be used; or a fine soft bougie should be passed, and then screwed to the end of a Holt's or Perrève dilator, and after the stricture has by this means been dilated, the urethra should be left uninterfered with by further instrumentation until the false passage has quite healed. If the patient can empty his bladder, no instrument whatever should be passed until the false passage has healed. Where there is retention, and catheterism is difficult or impossible, supra-pubic aspiration should be performed and repeated, if required, for three, four, or more days; by this means the urethra is placed at rest, the false passage is allowed to heal, congestion of the bladder and urethra cease, and in seventy-two hours, more or less, an instrument can probably be introduced without difficulty.

As a rule, there is no need of hæmostatics; but if hæmorrhage is severe, ice to the perinæum, the avoidance of instrument, the use of which will certainly cause fresh bleeding, and the internal administration of ergot or witch hazel, will suffice.

If pain and inflammation are present, warm fomentations should be applied to the perinæum, consisting of lead and carbolic or lead and opium lotion.

CHAPTER VI.

FOREIGN BODIES IN THE URETHRA.

VERY long would be the list of foreign bodies which have been pushed into the urethra by the insane, the lustful, the curious, and the foolish. Hairpins, slate pencil, pieces of stick, twigs of shrubs, seeds, pea pods, feathers, pins, needles, etc., are amongst the number.

The urethra of the inveterate masturbator becomes, by constant friction, sometimes very callous, its tonicity is lost, and incredibly large bodies are sometimes admitted.

Surgical instruments have been broken off in the urethra both during operations and whilst tied in, or when being passed. Renal calculi of small size are apt to be impacted either in the neck of the bladder or in the deep urethra. Foreign bodies may either remain in the urethra, or be driven out again by the urine, or travel back into the bladder.

It is probably very rare for them to be expelled through the meatus—at any rate, not in cases which come under the notice of the surgeon. A smooth, even, foreign body, such as a pea or bead, is likely to be expelled if the patient passes water very soon after its introduction. Chopart reported a case in which a piece of a bougie encrusted with phosphates was expelled after five weeks. When retained in the urethra, they may find a resting-place either in the penile or deep portions of the canal, becoming fixed either by partially piercing the urethra wall, or by catching in the orifice of a lacuna or gland duct.

In a considerable number of the cases (Émile Forgue says about one-third) the foreign body reaches the bladder. How this happens has been much discussed by Civiale, Ségalas, Mercier, Foucher, and others. Probably a foreign body to be thus drawn into the bladder must first be *entirely* introduced into the urethra. It then passes up the penile urethra to the bulb by the action of the longitudinal muscular fibres, aided by the frequent erections (and their after-subsidence) which are excited by the irritation of the foreign body. At the bulb it is temporarily, or may be permanently, arrested; but if it be of sufficient length to furnish a *point d'appui* for the longitudinal muscular fibres, it will·be carried on by them and by the muscles of the perinæum past the triangular ligament until it comes within the grip of the circular muscle fibres at the neck of the bladder.

Mercier says that the posterior part of the sphincter vesicæ, in contracting, rises higher than the front part, and that thus the foreign body is, so to speak, seesawed upwards towards the front of the bladder. The migration into the bladder may take place in twenty-four hours or less, according to the size, shape, and resistance of the object. Some patients feel the progressive movements, others are only aware of what has happened by the greater freedom with which they can urinate after the body has reached the interior of the bladder.

Symptoms.—Foreign bodies impacted in the urethra, as a rule, cause such serious inconvenience and trouble that surgical aid is soon obtained. When retained for weeks, months, or, as in some rare cases, for several years, they become encrusted with the salts of the urine, and cause dilatation of the urethra behind. That their residence for any length of time should be possible, urine must be able to escape by them. It is in the deep perinæal part of the urethra chiefly, in the prostatic occasionally, in the penile portion rarely, if ever, that the foreign bodies are thus lodged for a long time.

The first symptom excited after the introduction is a sharp pain in the urethra, radiating to the thighs, perinæum, and abdomen; this is much more severe as long as the body is in the penile portion than when it reaches the perinæum, where the sensation is more that of a weight.

Micturition is always more or less, and may be completely, obstructed. If, however, the body be such as a hairpin or a piece of tobacco-pipe, or catheter with its long axis in the axis of the urethra, the bladder can be readily emptied; even then micturition becomes more frequent, owing to reflex irritation of the neck of the bladder. Frequent erections may occur. After a very short time, it may be several hours, but generally about the second or third day, the mucous membrane becomes inflamed, giving rise to a sero-sanguinolent or purulent discharge from the meatus. The penis becomes swollen, tender, and œdematous, and the local inflammation may spread to the neighbouring parts, such as the scrotum and perinæum, and along the urethra to the bladder, or along the vasa deferentia to the testicles.

Unless the cause of offence is removed, the inflammatory conditions may become chronic. Abscesses may form outside and communicate with the urethra, and these may be followed by urinary fistulæ, or septic infection ; and suppurative pyelo-nephritis with dilatation of the renal pelves may slowly destroy the kidneys. It is rare, however, for cases to be so neglected as to give time for these more advanced changes to take place.

Diagnosis.—The history of the patient and digital examination of the penis, perinæum, and per rectum if necessary, will leave no doubt in most cases of the presence and the exact situation of a foreign body. If there should be any doubt, the passage of a metallic catheter or sound along the urethra, whilst the finger is in the rectum, will be sure to clear it up.

Treatment.—If the body be smooth and rounded or oblong, it may be expelled by gripping the end of the penis during micturition and then letting go, so that the rush of the urine shall carry the foreign body with it. If retained within the penile urethra, the attempt at extraction through the meatus with urethra-forceps, or a fine, blunt-ended probe sharply curved back near its end, may succeed If not, rather than continuing to make fruitless efforts at extraction, or running the risk of lacerating the urethra by forcing the body back into the bladder, or subjecting the patient to needless anxiety or danger by delay, the foreign body should be deliberately cut down upon and removed *in situ*, through a longitudinal incision, and the urethra should then be immediately and accurately sutured by buried catgut or fine silk sutures, as described in the treatment of ruptured urethra. A catheter should be retained for a few days.

The following case shows what excellent results are to be expected from this treatment :—George Williams, a grey-haired man aged fifty, but looking older, with a cleft meatus, when heavily intoxicated, introduced a hairpin, with the curve inwards, into his urethra. This he did on January 10th, 1893, and on January 13th, when he first came under notice, the ends of the pin could be felt through the wall of the spongy urethra, just in front of the scrotum. There was no blood or pus in his urine. On January 14th a small incision in the median line of the perinæuin, behind the hairpin, was made under chloroform by Mr. Andrew Clark, who, with a blunt hook passed forwards along the urethra, caught the pin by the curve and withdrew it. Two buried sutures of very fine silver wire were used to close the urethral incision, and the superficial wound was sutured with silk. A catheter was retained for a week. The superficial sutures were removed on the fifth day. No urine came through the wound from first to last, but the urine contained pus from the urethritis set up by the catheter. The patient was discharged well on the tenth day.

CALCULI IN THE URETHRA.

These are of two kinds: (1) those which are formed on the spot; and (2) those which are conveyed into the urethra by the urine stream, and are retained there for a longer or shorter time.

1. Those which are formed in, or in one of the recesses of, the urethra are composed of phosphate of lime; they are found occasionally in the recess on the floor of the urethra left after the healing of a perinæal section, or external urethrotomy; or in a urethral fistula, or an enlarged or dilated lacuna or pouch.

In some calculous subjects the mucous membrane has been lined, as the bladder sometimes is, with a gritty, mortar-like material, largely composed of phosphatic salts.

It is not always possible to say, until sections are made, whether these calculi and concretions are or are not encrustations upon renal calculi, or around minute fragments of a vesical calculus.

2. Calculi which have passed into the urethra from the

kidney or bladder, and have been retained there for a time, differ from those formed entirely in the urethra by having a nucleus and stratified layers. The renal calculi are generally small, round, flattened, or elongated and smooth composed of uric acid, and of a grey or greyish-red or buff colour. But I possess several which are very rough and uneven, and composed of an aggregation of coarse crystals and little lumps of crystals of uric acid. Sometimes they are passed as flat flakes, like shale of a dark slate colour; and in one instance I have met with the distoma hæmatobium (bilharzia hæmatobia) embedded in a mass of pus cells, epithelial débris, and uric-acid crystals. This was in a gentleman who had spent three or four months for three winters in succession on the Nile.

Portions which are detached from a vesical calculus are usually rough and irregular, and show fractured surfaces.

A small calculus or fragment of one not exceeding a few grains in weight, and not very angular, can traverse the urethra and cause but a few superficial scratches, or no injury at all. But a calculus or fragment of larger size, or of considerable roughness of surface, is forced tightly against or into the urethral wall and is there retained, and becomes the centre for further deposition of urinary salts. The bulbo-membranous portion of the urethra, and the canal just behind the meatus, are the usual seats of impaction. All ages are subject to it, but it most frequently occurs in infancy. Thus Kauffmann, out of 112 cases, gives 28·6 per cent. as having occurred between one and ten years of age; 15 to 16 per cent. between eleven and thirty years of age; the rest being distributed over all ages up to the eightieth year.

When a stone is impacted in the penile portion of the urethra, and goes on increasing, its nucleus of oxalate of lime or uric acid is eccentric, and nearer the anterior extremity; and if the calculous deposit is considerable and segmented, only the anterior segment will contain a nucleus, unless the several apparent segments are really individual calculi formed round as many separate small renal nuclei.

Penile calculi have, in several instances, ulcerated through the urethral wall, and then, either in the scrotum or within the prepuce, have gone on increasing to a great size. (*See* Scrotum and Prepuce.)

When a stone is impacted in the dilated membrano-prostatic urethra, and goes on growing, it may reach back into the bladder and there increase mushroom fashion. Such a stone will present the appearance shown in the specimen illustrated by Voillemier (Fig. 60); the nucleus then will be eccentric, and near to the inferior and anterior extremity.

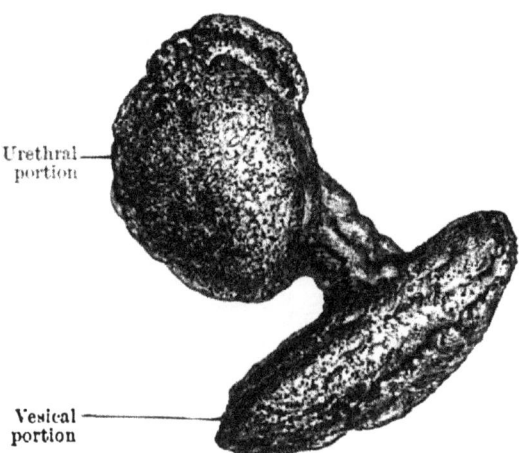

Fig. 60.—Urethro-vesical Calculus.
(*After Voillemier.*)

Several small calculi, or two or more calculi of much larger size, may be contained within an enlarged prostatic urethra. In 1889 I removed, by median urethrotomy, from an elderly man, the four facetted calculi shown in Fig. 61. The prostatic urethra was much dilated, but on making the attempt to use the lithotrite, I could not separate the blades until the beak of the instrument was pushed beyond the calculi, when it at once entered the bladder. The patient had had three previous operations for stone performed — lithotrity by Sir Henry Thompson, in 1870; lateral lithotomy in 1885 by the late Mr. Bellamy; and supra-pubic cystotomy in 1888

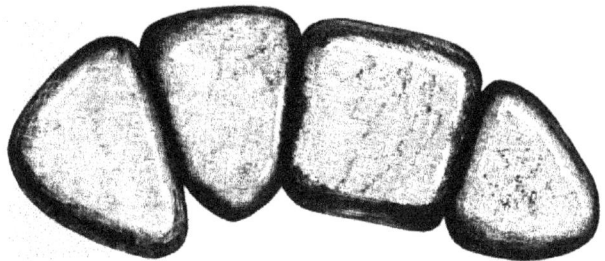

Fig. 61.—Calculi in Prostatic Urethra. (Middlesex Hospital Museum.)

also by Mr. Bellamy. In 1890, just eighteen months after my first (patient's fourth) operation, I again performed median urethrotomy upon him and removed another calculus from the dilated prostatic urethra.

An interesting and somewhat similar case occurred in the practice of Voillemier.

Occasionally, large urinary pouches are formed in the floor of the urethra, in which calculi are lodged (Fig. 62).

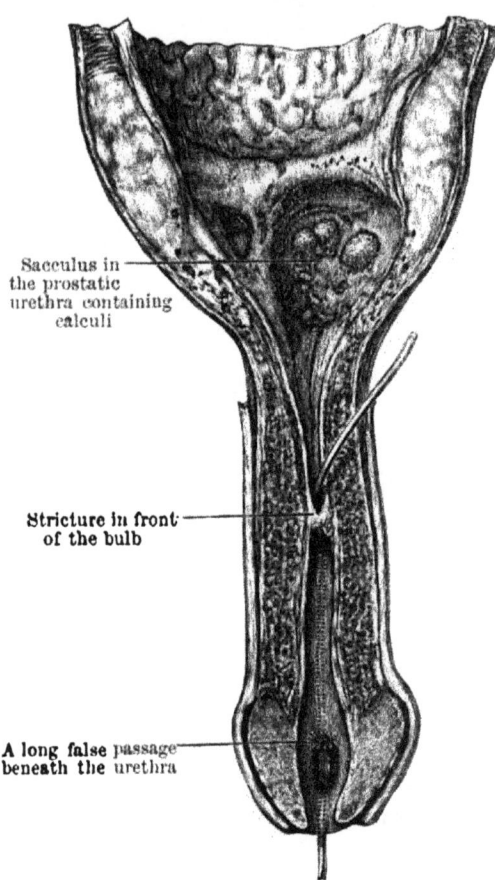

Sacculus in the prostatic urethra containing calculi

Stricture in front of the bulb

A long false passage beneath the urethra

Fig. 62.—Calculi in Prostatic Urethra.   (Middlesex Hospital Museum)

J. L. Petit records a case of a boy with retention of urine who had a large tumour, the size of a fist, between the rectum and scrotum, which had existed for seven or eight months. On pressing the swelling, a large quantity of urine escaped from the urethra, so that it gave the impression of being a hernia of the bladder. The calculus moved from place to place, and gave rise at times to retention, which the patient was able to overcome by lying on his back, when, presumably, the stone receded into the perinæal pouch.

In some cases, the calculus, having ulcerated through the urethra, comes to occupy a recess which may subsequently communicate with the urethra only by means of a very narrow orifice, so that little or no evidence of its presence can be detected by a sound in the urethra. Such has .been the case in some scrotal and preputial calculi of urinary origin. In other instances the calculi rest in an ulcerated cavity in the prostatic floor, as is shown in Fig. 63.

Urinary infiltration of the perinæum occurs, Kauffmann states, in one-fifth of the cases in which this ulceration takes place. In other cases the inflammation is circumscribed and ends in a urinary abscess, which, opening on the surface, gives exit to the calculus. In another case quoted by Petit, gangrene opened the abscess towards the perinæum whilst the patient was at stool, and the calculus, as well as the slough, fell into the bed-pan. " The gangrene," as Petit remarks, " performed the duty of the surgeon."

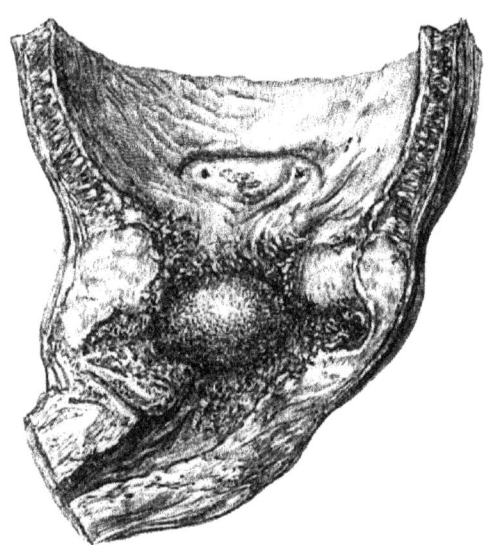

Fig. 63.—Calculus in Prostatic Urethra. There is an oval calculus one inch in diameter lying in an ulcerated cavity in the prostate. From a man aged 70, who had symptoms of vesical calculus for three years and a urinary fistula for a year. (Middlesex Hospital Museum.)

Symptoms.—An impacted urethral calculus suddenly causes stoppage in micturition. The patient, during the act of passing water, feels something enter and travel along the urethra till the stream stops, or nearly stops. In children this is generally the first symptom; in adults there have, as a rule, been previous renal and general symptoms suggestive of renal or vesical calculus, lithiasis, or lithæmia. Besides retention, or sudden stopping of the stream, there may be no other symptom. Pressure along the course of the urethra will reveal the presence of a hard body; the introduction of a bougie, catheter, or sound will detect it. Palpation per rectum will assist in deciding whether the calculus is in the bladder or in the prostatic or the membranous urethra.

Prognosis.—This depends upon the previous state of the higher urinary organs; and upon the presence and severity of any local complications such as have been mentioned above, and in connection with foreign bodies in the urethra (page 206).

If a stricture of the urethra of long standing has caused impairment of the bladder and kidneys, the prognosis is not favourable.

A calculus may block the narrow lumen of a stricture, and death may follow from sudden and complete retention and urinary infiltration, as in one of Verneuil's cases.

Treatment should be the same as for foreign bodies in the urethra. (*See* page 206.) A smooth-surfaced stone in the deep urethra should, if possible, be pushed back into the bladder, and there crushed and removed by litholapaxy.

But urethrotomy, followed by urethrorrhaphy, is so safe and successful that it is to be preferred to any forcible efforts to return the stone, especially one with a rough surface, to the bladder for the purpose of lithotrity.

When a calculus is impacted behind a stricture, external urethrotomy is indicated as the means of removing the calculus and dividing the stricture at the same time.

By urethrotomy and the use of immediate sutures, impacted calculi may be removed from the penile as well as from the perinæal urethra, with confidence that, with well-applied buried sutures and due observance of aseptic precautions, the results will be perfectly satisfactory. Should non-absorbing sutures be used for the urethra and left hanging from the wound till they are cut out, a urinary fistula will probably be formed; and as penile fistulæ are very troublesome to heal, such sutures should not, in my opinion, be used on this part, at any rate, of the urethra.

CHAPTER VII.

NON-SPECIFIC URETHRITIS—FOLLICULITIS—COWPERITIS.

NON-SPECIFIC URETHRITIS.

URETHRITIS is an inflammation of the mucous membrane of the urethra, and may be either of a specific or non-specific nature.

The specific, by far the most frequent form, is due to infection with the gonococcus microbe; and this infection may take place through the unbroken mucous membrane of the urethra. It is commonly known as gonorrhœa or acute blenorrhagic urethritis, and as such is not included within the scope of this work.

The non-specific form has many points of resemblance to gonorrhœa, and is caused by various micro-organisms other than the gonococcus. In the healthy urethra numerous saprophytic bacteria, and pyogenic micro-organisms have been discovered. Amongst those which have been seen by different observers in cases of simple urethritis are the chain cocci, the micrococcus pyogenes aureus, a diplococcus identical with the micrococcus albicans amplus of Bumm, and a micrococcus like the bacillus Zopfii—namely, the orange-coloured micrococcus of the urethra.

If there should occur some breach of surface from injury, or some perverted state of the mucous membrane or of its secretion, owing to disturbed vaso-motor influence or a morbid constitutional state, then the urethral mucous membrane may become affected by these non-specific micro-organisms, and suppuration with urethral discharge will supervene.

Causes.—This affection may be excited by excessive sexual indulgence and by the irritating effect of ordinary leucorrhœal or menstrual discharges; by exposure to cold; by the use of strong aromatic substances and drugs such as turpentine, balsams, iodide of potassium; or by abnormal conditions of the urine such as an excess of lithic acid or oxalate of lime.

The crystals of uric acid or oxalate of lime mechanically and chemically irritate the mucous membrane of the whole urinary tract. Foreign bodies impacted in the urethra excite urethritis by direct irritation; and a catheter retained in the passage is apt to do so also, as is often witnessed when a free purulent discharge escapes by the side of a catheter *en demeure*.

The reflex irritation excited by hæmorrhoids, fissures, and stone in the bladder is sometimes responsible for simple urethritis.

Symptoms and Diagnosis.—The symptoms are somewhat the same as those of gonorrhœa, but much less intense. A sense of heat, of fulness and tenderness along the urethra, with a cutting or scalding sensation during micturition and a muco-purulent discharge, sufficiently characterise the disease.

It is of importance to bear in mind that one who leads the purest of lives may be the subject of an acute urethritis, and that, for the peace of mind of others as well as of the patient himself, the surgeon should be able to diagnose the non-specific from the specific form.

In simple urethritis all the symptoms are much less acute than in gonorrhœa. There are never the itching, pain, and gaping of the external meatus, in the beginning; nor the chordee during the course of the attack, as in gonorrhœa. Simple urethritis usually ceases spontaneously in a few days after the removal of its cause, and never leaves behind a persistent gleet as gonorrhœa so frequently does.

Treatment.—This resolves itself into ascertaining the cause and removing it by appropriate means.

When the inflammation arises from digestive disturbances and an over-acid state of the urine, a carefully regulated diet, avoiding fats, sugar, and alcohol, and the administration of alterative and tonic medicines such as soda and gentian, or the mineral acids and preparations of iron, are required.

FOLLICULITIS AND PERIFOLLICULITIS.

The French surgeons have given a good deal of attention to the glandular apparatus of the urethra and glans penis which no doubt plays an important part in inflammation of this mucous tract. In the following description of Folliculitis and

Cowperitis, free use has been made of the article by M. Émile Forgue in the work edited by Duplay and Reclus.

Symptoms.—Small tender nodules giving the sensation of shot can be felt in the wall of the urethra ; they vary from the size of a pin's head to that of a pea. They are spherical or ovoid, smooth, fixed to the urethra, and the skin is movable over them. They are produced by engorgement of the mouth of the follicles, are temporary, and disappear often under examination. When the follicle is chronically inflamed, and obliterated, a retention cyst may form. Sometimes the follicle persists as a little indolent mass beside the urethra ; more often it inflames and suppurates, involving the cellular tissue and opening through the skin.

Hypersecretion of Littré's glands often follows urethritis. These acini afford nests for the gonococci, in which chronic discharge is maintained, and where materials are generated which lead to recrudescence of the disease.

Gonorrhœa does not attack a clear surface. It is rather " a sieve in the holes of which," following the comparison of Diday, " the malady extends, and into the holes of which remedies must penetrate."

In examining very close to the meatus, says Diday, one frequently comes across an interesting lesion. A narrow opening is seen upon one of the edges of the meatus, out of which may be pressed a small drop of liquid corresponding to that in the urethra. The canal extends 3 to 5 or 6 millimetres in a direction parallel to the urethra. On inquiry it is ascertained that this lesion occurred about the same time as the urethritis. The appearances at the edge of the canal are exactly like those at the edge of the meatus, both being red, swollen, painful, and glistening, or pale and indolent, according as the urethritis is acute or chronic. Urine does not pass by this small orifice. When the patient has had several attacks of gonorrhœa the same accompaniment is found in each attack and in the same form. It is a mucous folliculitis which has become gonorrhœal by primary or secondary contagion.

This lesion affords an example of what, in those suffering from gonorrhœa, occurs in the rest of the urethra. Lagneau, noticing in two of his patients small, spherical, hard, movable swellings situated on the side of the frænum, which opened and allowed a drop of pus to escape by a small whitish orifice alongside the frænum, asked himself if these tiny collections situated under the preputial fold, like a ranula under the frænum of the tongue, had not for their seat some one of the little glands described by Tyson in the coronal furrow.

This view is confirmed by Jadassohn and by Fabry, who have seen the glands enclosed between the two folds of the prepuce so affected, as well as the canals which, running parallel to the urethra, open in the neighbourhood of its orifice.

Fabry cites the case of a *confrère* who, being attacked fifteen years before by gonorrhœa, had recovered in the course of a few weeks without relapse. There was undeniably between the two folds of the prepuce a small tumour the size of a lentil, easily movable. On pressing upon it there escaped from a minute orifice close to the frænum a drop or two of liquid which contained gonococci. The urethra was dry and appeared healthy. The small tumour was excised. The histological examination furnished proof that a veritable gland existed there, constituted by an excretory duct lined by several layers of flat epithelial cells, which gland extended into smaller ducts furnished with a single layer of cylindrical epithelium. The flat cells and some of the interposed lymph corpuscles lodged the gonococci.

Gonorrhœa persists in the glands long after the urethra is dry, and therein lies a continuing danger of contagion.

The follicular discharge is trifling in quantity, intermittent, and escapes by a minute orifice which sometimes opens into the interior of the meatus. Both patients and surgeons ignore the existence of this follicular gonorrhœa, which maintains a latent form.

Diday quotes a case of repeated relapses, in which the follicular inflammation was more painful than the urethral. So long as the follicle is diseased the urethra is menaced with relapses. The bead of pus is small, and scarcely visible, and therein lies the peril. The ex-gonorrhœic disregards this inoffensive-looking oozing, which does not inconvenience him in the performance of any of his functions; but it is the cause of many an unexplained contamination.

Peri-urethral Abscess.—The majority of cases of peri-urethral abscess result from suppurating perifolliculitis; and the chronic nodules on the dorsum, from angeioleucitis, which is sometimes also acute and diffuse, or even complicated with phlebitis and gangrene.

Astruc recognised these venereal abscesses of the perinæum in gonorrhœics. They occur anywhere in the penile urethra, and are especially frequent at the frænum, beneath the fossa navicularis, and in the region of the bulb. It is in the course of a follicular blenorrhagia or chordee that they appear. Localised pain and tenderness, induration and œdema, mark the spot; in a few days suppuration occurs, and it is of the first importance not to retard the escape of the pus. In my own experience the abscess forms most frequently about the fourth or fifth week of gonorrhœa. A fistula may follow an abscess and burrow around the sides to the dorsum of the penis, beneath the skin.

In the spongy portion these collections are larger and more diffused, but situate in the median line; about the bulb they are racquet-shaped.

COWPERITIS AND PERICOWPERITIS.

The glands of Méry, described in 1684, have not failed to attract the attention of pathologists and surgeons. About 1702 Cowper said : " The glairy translucent liquid which appears at the end of an attack of gonorrhœa, and which in England is known under the familiar denomination of ' gleet,' has its source in these glands."

J. L. Petit recognised in certain perinæal abscesses an origin in these glands—a fact which Morgagni confirmed by several autopsies; and this teaching was renewed by Ricord in the present century. Suppuration of these glands as a complication of gonorrhœa is rare, for Ricord, in his immense practice, only met with about six cases in a year. Inflammatory engorgement probably is much more common. Inflammation commences in the third or fourth week of gonorrhœa; it may be caused also from traumatism, vigorous coitus, the passage of a bougie, or a too energetic use of the syringe. Tarnowski records an acute attack in a gonorrhœa of two years' standing brought on by riding.

When, towards the third or fourth week of an acute gonorrhœa, the bulbar region becomes painful, the pain being fixed, and the part very tender to the touch or the pressure of the trousers, cowperitis becomes probable.

Local examination reveals (Gubler) slight swelling, without alteration in the colour of the skin, which is perfectly free; and a clearly-limited rounded or oval tumour about the size of a haricot bean, the broader end being toward the anus, while the narrower is continuous with the bulb.

The cellular tissue is involved, but extension backwards is strictly limited by the transversus perinæi muscle. It is only when both glands are affected that any very noticeable swelling occurs; then the localisation is much less exact, and suppuration occurs within seven days.

J. L. Petit has insisted strongly that retention of urine is associated with swelling due to inflammation of the glands. According to Gubler, this is exceptional, but in 1884 Tuffier published a case in which the autopsy showed that the lumen of the urethra was narrowed and retention produced by a cowperitic abscess projecting towards the canal. A young man with gonorrhœa of three weeks' duration came under my care on account of increasing pain and difficulty in passing water of a week's standing. There was a slight convexity of the perinæum and extreme tenderness and pain on the left side of the raphé just over and posterior to the region of the bulb. A deep longitudinal incision into this slight swelling was made half an inch to the left of the median line, and about half an ounce of pus was evacuated. Immediate relief followed. I have no doubt this was an abscess in the left Cowper's gland, and it was the pain and increasing difficulty in micturition necessitating at last the use of the catheter that brought him into hospital.

Cowperitis may run a chronic course. It is probable, but has not been demonstrated clearly, that its secretion contributes to some urethral discharges.

Symptoms.—At its commencement cowperitis is characterised distinctly by tumour of the size of a haricot bean, its vicinity to the bulb corresponding to the seat of the gland. But the clinician rarely sees it at this period. The inflammation is generally phlegmonous, and a mass of diffuse cellulitis marks the central glandular focus. The condition is easily then confounded with a urinary abscess, especially as, in some cases, delay in opening a cowperian abscess gives time for perforation of the urethra and the complication of urinary fistula. The inguinal glands are apt to become inflamed.

Diagnosis.—The history may decide. Cowperitis follows a recent acute gonorrhœa, a urinary abscess, a contusion, wound, internal injury to the urethra, or old gonorrhœa. Distinction is difficult between cellulo-adenitis of Cowper's gland and a simple peri-urethral abscess following folliculitis occurring near the bulb; this latter forms a sort of expansion round the urethra, and when opened the probe has a wide range of movement in the cavity.

Englisch calls attention to a diffuse subacute inflammation in the bulbo-urethral triangle, associated with a thin urethral discharge in tubercular subjects, which extends towards the scrotum, emits thin pus when opened, and leaves a granulating sinus. It commences in Cowper's gland.

Treatment.—Incision should be early (lithotomy position) in cases of suppuration, otherwise perforation of urethra may occur, or follow later. Tubercular cases should be curetted.

CHAPTER VIII.

STRICTURES OF THE URETHRA.

By stricture of the urethra is understood a persisting diminution of its calibre by sclerosis, or by a cicatrix in its walls.

The so-called "inflammatory" and "spasmodic" strictures of older writers are falsely called "strictures." Inflammation and spasm are, indeed, causes of temporary obstruction and retention—in the one case owing to the congestive tumefaction of the mucous membrane; in the other, to spasm of the muscular parietes of the canal, or of the muscles surrounding the canal—but these conditions are not "strictures." The "carnosities," or "caruncles," and "excrescences" within the urethra, which were described by the old authors as causes of retention, and included as one of the classes of strictures, are now known to be extremely rare, except as little granulation masses behind organic strictures. "Bridle strictures" are in all probability nothing more than the effects of false passâges.

There is, perhaps, more warrant for retaining as a distinct class what Hunter called the "mixed strictures—composed that is, of a permanent stricture and spasm"; but, as he remarked, "there are very few strictures that are not more or less attended with spasms"; and as the spasms do but aggravate the degree of obstruction caused by the organic change in the urethral wall, and are—in part, at any rate, if not entirely—caused by the irritation excited by this organic narrowing, they have no right to the dignity of giving a name to a class by themselves.

Another group of cases has been spoken of by some under the title of Stricture. In a very few instances on record, obstruction of the urethra has been caused by "false membranes," varying in length from an inch upwards, and more or less adherent to the mucous membrane. Rokitansky speaks of "primary croup occurring on the urethral mucous membranes; it induces a circumscribed or a tubular exudation, according to the intensity of the process, and occurs chiefly in children." Sir Henry Thompson has examined several of the extant museum specimens, and reported cases of this kind, and considers some of the former doubtful, and having more the appearance of a dilated lacuna than of a flap of false membrane. He recognises as not unfrequent, the deposits upon the surface of the urethra, the result of inflammation, which Sir Charles Bell described "as a consequence of stricture," and as being deposited "like a crust of coagulable lymph" behind the stricture. But a croupal exudation from the urethra he believes to be extremely rare; and in this opinion he is supported by M. Guérin, who states that in not one out of a hundred cases which he examined had he found *any false membrane* on the free surface of the mucous membrane; "the plastic process," he remarks, "has acted either immediately beneath the mucous membrane or in the spongy tissue of the canal."

In two out of three cases recorded by Mr. Hancock, the false membrane, about an inch in length, was loose and raised at its posterior part, and formed a semilunar valve with its free border to the bladder, causing a very possible obstacle to the discharge of urine.

Mr. W. H. Battle, in a paper on Membranous Desquamative Urethritis (*Lancet*, 1893, vol. ii. p. 302), describes a case in which large casts of the urethra were passed off with the urine every morning for several months by a man aged forty-four. These casts were composed of a membrane of columnar epithelium, one or two layers in thickness, and numerous white blood-corpuscles. There were none of the usual evidences of inflammation, and no retention resulted.

Pitha speaks of croupous exudations formed in thick plates completely obstructing the lumen of the urethra.

None of these cases, however, properly come under the denomination of "stricture."

I follow entirely Sir Henry Thompson, who says:—" I recognise but one morbid condition of 'stricture'—namely, that organic or permanent change in the walls of the urethra which narrows them, or prevents their opening or dilating to the natural calibre."

Sir H. Thompson groups the several forms of stricture under the following heads—namely, linear, annular, indurated annular, and irregular or tortuous strictures; but I prefer to classify them, not according to the form of the stricture, but according to their mode of origin.

Etiology.—The two common causes are inflammation and injury. Thus we have "simple organic strictures," due to sclerosis following inflammation; and "cicatricial strictures," following rupture or injury. The frequency of the former is to the latter as fourteen or fifteen to one.

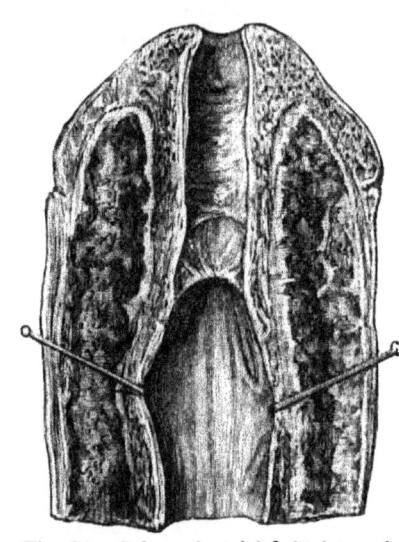

Fig. 64.—Sclero-cicatricial Stricture in the fore part of the Urethra. (*After Voillemier.*)

CITRATRICIAL OR TRAUMATIC STRICTURES

may follow any of the forms of injuries described in previous sections. Gross, writing on the connection between masturbation, which is one of the causes of slight traumatisms, and stricture of the urethra (*Med. News*, September 20th, 1888), says he found stricture generally near the meatus in 291 out of 331 habitual masturbators. The bulbous and membranous parts of the urethra are the commonest situations of cicatricial strictures from other kinds of injury. Their extent depends on the extent of the injury which causes them. They are nearly always single, generally crescentic, and occupy the floor and sides of the urethra: occasionally they are completely annular. They are frequently irregular or tortuous, generally very hard and cartilaginous, offer great resistance to instruments, and rapidly contract after dilatation. In some very severe cases the urethra is completely obliterated immediately in front of the rupture. They are often complicated with abscess, with obstinate fistulæ, and secondary changes in the kidney, ureters, and bladder, resulting in what are called "surgical kidneys." They are developed with great rapidity. Thus, Dr. Deanesly (*op. cit.*), in a case in which he had not used previous sutures on the urethra, but had retained a catheter for thirteen days, was unable, on the second day after removing the catheter, to introduce the smallest instrument. Twenty-three days after the accident the urine stream was no larger than a No. 2 English catheter, and a hard, spindle-shaped stricture could be felt in the perinæum just behind the scrotum, which, later, necessitated external urethrotomy. Guyon has seen a stricture developed by the fourteenth day; Lefort, by the twenty-fourth day.

SCLERO-CICATRICIAL STRICTURES.

If a man with gonorrhœa or gleet gets, from any cause, a crack or fissure in the urethral mucous membrane, the cicatrix which forms in the membrane is likely to be thickened by an inflammatory process which precedes the healing, and there is formed what M. Forgue calls a sclero-cicatricial stricture—that is, a fibrous stricture of hybrid origin, and due in part to the small wound and in part to the inflammation. They are formed rapidly, and are very resistant to dilatation.

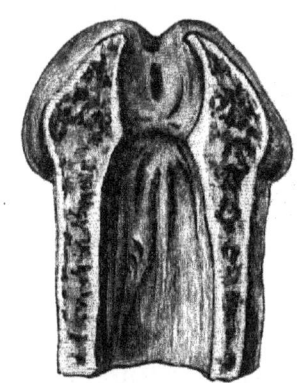

Fig. 65.—Cicatricial Stricture following Chancre. (*After Duplay and Reclus.*)

Two varieties of cicatricial stricture occur without the intervention of any injury—viz. those due to the cicatrices of small ulcerations which arise in the course of acute urethritis, and those caused by simple chancroids. The first occur along the middle line of the roof or floor of the urethra within an inch or two of the meatus (Fig. 64); the second affect the meatus and navicular fossa, only exceptionally being situated farther up the passage. The true or hard chancre rarely produces a stricture, and when it does so, it is not a narrow stricture, does not occur farther inwards than the navicular fossa (Fig. 65), and generally disappears in part—*i.e.* in so far as the thickening is due to syphilitic and not to cicatricial elements—under specific treatment. Tédenat speaks of very narrow cicatricial strictures of the meatus and navicular fossa in three instances in diabetics, following the ulceration that sometimes affects the extremity of the penis of these subjects.

SIMPLE ORGANIC (OR INFLAMMATORY) STRICTURES.

These are by far the commonest, and form what some authors speak of as the "simple organic strictures." They are not to be mistaken for the cases of retention of urine due to a swollen or œdematous condition of the mucous membrane during the height of an acute urethritis or gonorrhœa, which the old writers used to describe as inflammatory strictures. These simple "organic" (inflammatory) strictures are the result of a repetition of attacks of inflammation, gonorrhœal or otherwise, and they occur at a considerable time after the attacks have subsided. Whilst traumatic strictures follow quickly their cause, the inflammatory are tardily produced, and often delayed for years. Guyon collected 142, with the view of ascertaining the length of time which elapsed between the appearance of the stricture and the first attack of urethritis. He found that in

4 cases it occurred within			1 year.
10 ,,	,,	,,	2 years.
36 ,,	,,	between	2nd and 4th years.
19 ,,	,,	,,	4th and 6th years.
24 ,,	,,	,,	6th and 8th years.
49 ,,	,,	,,	10 to 15 years or later.

If a stricture occurs shortly after a gonorrhœa, it is because some slight rent or crack in the mucous membrane has occurred from one of the several causes that have been mentioned (p. 193), and the stricture is of the sclero-cicatricial kind. For the production of a simple organic stricture there must have been one or more attacks of inflammation of old date.

The conditions favourable to the production of these simple organic (inflammatory) strictures are profuse or prolonged suppurations, vascular changes favourable to arterio-capillary sclerosis, and any irritation within the canal. Astringent injections have been indiscriminately blamed. Whilst there was probably much truth in the accusations brought against the former use of solid caustics, there is little, if any, in those made against the mild astringent solutions which it is now the custom to use. Anything that tends to prolong a urethral inflammation predisposes to stricture. Hence a narrow meatus, as Valette, of Lyons, pointed out in 1875, is a very pregnant cause.

Pathological Anatomy.—**Traumatic strictures** consist of typical fibrous tissue, the thickness, form, extent, and degree of irregularity of which depend on the nature and extent of the original injury. Multiple fistulæ and much callous tissue are seen and felt in the perinæum, and in connection with these callous masses of tissue there is sometimes set up active inflammation running on to suppuration.

The **sclero-cicatricial strictures** present little islands of fibrous tissue, small sclerosed bands or nodules, which vary in shape and size according to the character of the cause of the injury. They are found in the anterior portion of the urethra.

The **(inflammatory) "simple organic" strictures** are frequently multiple. They are met with commonly in the fossa navicularis, in the anterior third of the urethra, in the subpubic portion, and in the scrotal and bulbous portions of the urethra. The bulbous is the most common seat. On laying open the urethra in the usual manner in the cadaver, the slender, fibrous, submucous ring which alone constitutes some strictures actually disappears. Very narrow strictures in the penile portion, whether single or multiple, are sclero-cicatricial, and caused by small traumatisms. In some extreme cases, the greater part of the urethra is pretty uniformly indurated by this chronic inflammatory tissue. Guyon points out that the urethra in these cases gets narrower as the bulb is approached, so that, though No. 15, French size, goes along the penile portion, the scrotal portion may not take more than No. 8 or No. 6, and this will be completely arrested at the level of the bulb.

The length of the strictures varies much, and the stricture tissue does not end abruptly but gradually, so that it is not always possible to distinguish a line of limit between the healthy and abnormal tissues. The changes in the submucous tissue are generally more marked below a stricture than above it. The degree of stricture varies extremely. It is, however, quite exceptional for the urethra to become completely occluded. There is always a passage through these strictures, though it may be tortuous and of capillary fineness. Brodie and Voillemier state, and I have witnessed the same thing, that if fistulæ exist and allow a very free escape, the stricture may close entirely.

When annular, the anterior orifice of the stricture may be in the axis of the urethra or to one side of it. If not annular, the stricture may involve any side of the tube, but is most frequently on the floor. It may present a smooth and gradual eminence to the bougie or be obtuse and ledge-like.

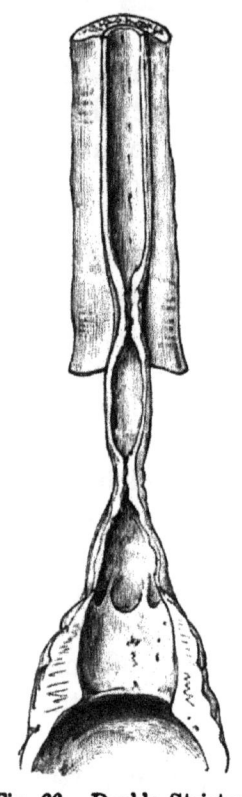

Fig. 66.—Double Stricture of the Urethra (in penile and bulbous portions) with Dilatation of the Prostatic Urethra. (Middlesex Hospital Museum.)

The urethra is, in old-standing cases, dilated behind the stricture, and may be enlarged into a pouch, the walls of which become trabecular from enlargement of the lacunæ of the mucous membrane (Fig. 66).

The fibrous tissue of which the stricture is formed is yellowish-white, with little hæmorrhagic spots towards its circumference. The changes in the tissues which constitute simple (inflammatory) organic stricture start from the mucous membrane and invade in turn every structure forming the urethral walls. So that in the beginning, and in slight cases only, the mucous membrane, or the mucous membrane and the submucous tissue, are involved, whereas in very advanced and long-standing strictures, the corpus spongiosum throughout, including its fibrous sheath and the tissues of the perinæum outside the sheath, are sclerosed.

Halle and Wassermann, in their memoir on the subject, have given a detailed account of the microscopic changes. The initial change is in the epithelium, which passes from the stratified cylindrical into the stratified pavement variety; first the surface cells, then the deeper layers, are flattened, and a horny condition is the result. Islets of hypertrophied, stratified pavement epithelium, with transparent tumefaction of the cells, and small projecting vascular papillæ, are formed. Later, the stratified pavement epithelium is quite dry, flattened, and horny. Pigmented granulations arise between the cells of the deep layer of the epithelium, the cells of which may contain a great deal of pigment.

The horny layer is not in any case produced in the changed epithelium of the posterior urethra, because of the different embryological origin of the two parts of the canal.

The subepithelial lesion does not progress *pari passu* with that of the epithelial; a great and extensive epithelial change can occur with but only a slight subepithelial one. The effects of the morbid agent, the gonococcus, are first produced on the epithelium only, and may be limited to it entirely.

The change in the basement layer of the mucous membrane consists in a sclerosis which may either surround the canal or be limited to one segment of it, especially the floor. Small papillary projections give a wavy line to the limit between the epithelial and subepithelial tissue. On these projections the change in the epithelium is the most marked; but being flattened by the epithelium, they do not stand out on the mucous surface.

In some cases, veritable vegetations, simple or branched, project into the canal and obstruct it, especially posterior to the stricture. These occur where the inflammation has been most intense.

The anatomical union which exists in the normal state between the constituent elements of the urethral wall is maintained in the condition of stricture. The lesion spreads from the subepithelial layer to the spongy body. The invasion may be complete and like a ferrule, extending as far as the fibrous sheath, including the trabeculæ, the arteries of which may be reduced to mere fissures devoid of blood. The lesion of the spongy tissue as well as that of the submucous tissue is most intense at the level of the stricture. The thickened trabeculæ show an increased amount of muscle bundles, which later undergo hyaline degeneration. The ring of elastic tissue which strengthens the mucous membrane of the urethra, especially in the posterior part of the penile region, may disappear in part or entirely.

Thus, besides the epithelial changes, inflammatory strictures often consist in a sclerosis of the mucous and

submucous tissues and the spongy body, and, in fact, of all
the layers constituting the urethral wall.

Symptoms.—A stricture in the first place causes symptoms
which have reference to the stream of urine and the manner
of micturition; it is thus a urethral affection. The stream is
altered in form, in its manner of leaving, and in the distance
to which it can be projected from, the meatus; and if the
obstruction is sufficient, it will be entirely arrested. In order
to overcome the obstruction, the bladder has to make com-
pensatory efforts, and may be worn out by over-exertion or
prove too feeble to respond; it is also exposed to the risks
of inoculation either by extension of urethritis or through
catheterism. Vesical symptoms then appear, and are superadded to the urethral. Finally, the ureters and kidneys
exposed to the effects of the urethral obstruction, namely,
to the forcible and frequent vesical contractions and to the
decomposition of urine, are dilated and suppurate, and add
to the gravity of the condition, and unfavourably determine
the prognosis.

Symptoms referable to the Urethra.—Too much attention has been given in the descriptions of the symptoms
of stricture to the "forked," "twisted," "corkscrew-like,"
and other variations in the form of the stream of urine; but
these changes are generally due to a narrow meatus, or to the
agglutination by mucus or muco-pus of the lips of the meatus,
and not to the stricture. A narrow stricture may be present
without any such change in the stream; or the changes in the
form of the stream may occur independently of stricture. A
stricture quite near the meatus might have the same effect as
a narrow meatus, but not so a stricture at the bulb with the
anterior part of the canal and the meatus of normal size.
With regard to the powers of projecting the stream, it must
be borne in mind that the bladder is more concerned than the
stricture. As Guyon has said, " One pisses with the bladder,
not with the urethra"; so that in this respect young men
and old men with strictures cannot be compared. If the
bladder is feeble the stream will not be projected far, whether
there be a slight stricture or no stricture at all. On the other
hand, if the muscular tissue of the bladder is good, and has
become hypertrophied owing to the obstruction, the projection

of the stream will be powerful, though the lumen of the stricture may be small. Old men with prostatic enlargement much more than men with old-standing stricture are the most likely "to water their boots and their trouser-flaps." Undoubtedly, in neglected stricture there comes a time when the bladder gets the worst of the competition; it can make no further efforts to compensate for the obstruction; or it no longer has the contractile power of earlier years. If the patient is feeble to start with, from age or disease, then we may expect loss of power in the bladder in quite the early stage of stricture; otherwise not.

But often other conditions, such as a congenitally narrow meatus (a common enough condition); an inflammatory œdema, excited perhaps by a gleet or a catheter; and spasms of the muscular wall of the urethra, add to the obstruction caused by the stricture. We prove this often in the case of spasms by passing a No. 8 or 9 instrument easily on a man with a very small stream. The farther forwards the stricture is situated, the greater the obstruction it causes.

Pain during micturition of urethral origin is caused by urethritis, but not by stricture.

Symptoms referable to the Bladder.—Frequent and painful micturition are the first symptoms complained of in some cases. They are of vesical origin and due to congestion or inflammation about the neck of the bladder. Many patients who have never noticed any change in the form or the force of their stream suffer from frequency of micturition, especially during the day, and the calls to micturition are more and more imperious. Later the same troubles occur during the night as well as the day. The patient may complain of no pain, but perhaps of a sense of weight only in the perinæum; but he may have severe pain at the end of micturition at the neck of the bladder. These symptoms are the result of inflammation about the neck of the bladder, and are delayed for a longer or a shorter time according as the bladder has time and power to become accustomed to, and to overcome, the obstruction of the stricture, or not. If not, the stagnation and the decomposition of the urine in the bladder will very soon set up cystitis and its attendant symptoms.

Dittel says that difficult and painful ejaculation of semen

is often an early symptom of stricture, and is complained of before there has been any difficulty in micturition. Personally I have not met with this symptom.

At variable periods, men with stricture are apt to get attacks of acute retention. A sudden chill, sexual indulgence or excess, indiscretions in eating and drinking, or going an undue length of time without passing water, may be the cause of this. Retention may occur in a young man with only a commencing or large-sized stricture, upon whom it is quite easy to pass an 8, 9, or 10 catheter. In these circumstances it is very likely that an inattentive or inexperienced hand will not detect the stricture. But acute retention happens much more frequently in cases of long-standing stricture. These acute attacks, which may last sometimes for twenty-four or more hours, are due to spasm or to hyperæmia (congestive tumefaction) of the urethra, and when they have passed off the patient makes water as before their onset. Whilst the occurrence of spasm is undeniable, these attacks are sometimes due to congestion rather than to spasm. This view, as pointed out by M. É. Forgue, is favoured by the following facts :—(1) The chief situation of the spasm is the membranous part of the urethra; but in these cases the catheter is frequently arrested at a spot much anterior; (2) the sudden onset accords well with the rapidity of vascular congestion in the spongy urethra; (3) the free bleeding sometimes caused by introducing an instrument; (4) the improvement which follows antiphlogistic medicines.

A very common cause of retention of urine of which sufficient notice is not taken is the impaction in the lumen of a stricture of a mass, or plug, of stringy muco-pus. This substance, which often obstructs the large eyes of a catheter, can very readily block the lumen of a stricture, as a cork does the neck of a bottle. Warm water, syringed or irrigated down the urethra, will sometimes dislodge this plug and drive it into the dilated recess behind the stricture, and then the patient can again pass urine.

Incontinence is a symptom of stricture, and occasionally a little dribbling of urine is the first thing complained of. It is brought about in the following manner :—Some dilatation of the urethra occurs behind the stricture, and a little urine remains there after the bladder has ceased contracting, but is forced through the stricture and out of the meatus drop by drop by the contraction of the urethra. It is the escape of what Dittel calls the "urethral residuum" of the urine, the discharge of which some patients are accustomed to hasten by pressing forwards with their finger along the perinæum.

This incontinence occurs at first only when the man is up and about; it does not trouble him at night; but as the condition gets worse the urine escapes at night also, and at length is incessantly dribbling just as water at a lock is incessantly dripping from the cracks and crevices of the lock gates.

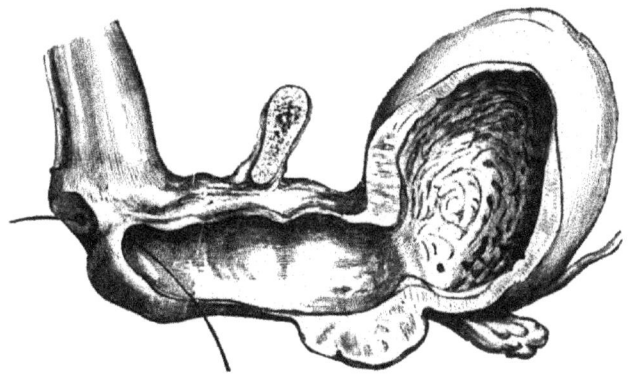

Fig. 67.—Great Hypertrophy of the Bladder Walls. Dilatation of membranous and prostatic urethra behind a stricture at the bulb. The stricture is indicated by the bristle. (Middlesex Hospital Museum.)

The dilatation of the urethra behind the stricture goes on extending backwards till the neck of the bladder is itself dilated and no longer serves as a sphincter (Fig. 67); but the stricture acts, as Reybard expresses it, like a sluice-gate (sert d'écluse), and the urine involuntarily escapes, especially in the standing or sitting position. If added to this condition the urine becomes ammoniacal, the bladder is so irritated by its presence that its expulsive efforts become more and more frequent and violent, and the inclination to urinate more and more imperious. How irritating such urine must be can be imagined by the effect of smelling salts upon the nose and eyes. This is the condition in which, as É. Forgue describes it, "the patient's life is one of pissing and suffering." The abdominal muscles are called upon to aid the efforts of the bladder; the patient assumes the squatting or such other position as will enable his bladder to act most favourably; he pulls at the end of the penis to relieve pain; gets prolapse of the rectal mucous membrane and congestion of the face, eyes, and brain from straining; and during a period of temporary retention may get an attack of cerebral hæmorrhage.

It must be borne in mind that *incontinence* and *retention* may occur at the same time. The bladder and urethra behind the stricture are full of urine, and cannot be discharged except by the process above described, corresponding to the leakings at the lock gates. This was called the "incontinence of retention" by the elder Gross.

Another fact which should be remembered is that the bladder becomes slowly thickened from hypertrophy of its muscular coats (Fig. 67), and its capacity is greatly diminished, so that it may be quite hidden behind the symphysis, and give no evidence of its distension by percussion or palpation. It is interstitially inflamed, and the inflammatory material invades the muscular fibres throughout, and impairs or destroys their contractile power.

Renal Symptoms.—From the time the bladder ceases to perform its functions naturally the kidneys are threatened in a double manner: (1) by mechanical distension; (2) by ascending inflammation and suppuration. At this stage the general system rapidly suffers. What has been called "the urinary cachexia" sets in. The digestive organs are disturbed, the mouth gets dry and furred, the tongue is reddened at its tip and edges, and its dorsum is dry and coated; thirst is great, the appetite is lost, vomiting and diarrhœa occur; there are attacks of feverishness alternating with periods when the temperature goes below normal in the morning and is little above normal at night; the face becomes sallow, pains in the loins are troublesome, the urine becomes purulent, and the patient dies of urinary poisoning.

Diagnosis.—There is the clinical history. In traumatic (cicatricial) cases a previous blow or fall upon the perinæum. In sclero-cicatricial there has been some slight injury during erection or coitus, or caused by erection with chordee. In simple organic strictures there is probably the history of repeated urethritis, gonorrhœa, or gleet; or of a long-standing gleet which from time to time has been aggravated into a more active condition by bad treatment, indiscretion in diet or hygiene, or reinoculations.

If the patient complains of a broken, forked, or twisted stream, of slowness of the stream, or of deficient force, the first thing to do is to eliminate any question as to a contracted or swollen meatus or a tight prepuce.

The first symptom noticed by many patients with recent stricture is either undue frequency of, or too imperious a necessity for, micturition; or a slight degree of incontinence; or the symptoms of inflammation at the neck of the bladder; or an attack of

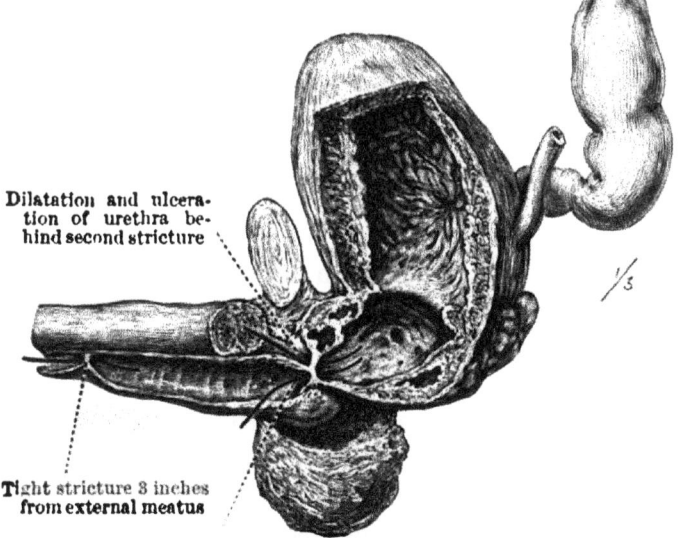

Dilatation and ulceration of urethra behind second stricture

Tight stricture 3 inches from external meatus

A second stricture near the bulb

Fig. 68.—Dilatation Effects of Stricture on Ureter and Kidney, with absorption of kidney substance. From a young man who died from extravasation of urine and gangrene of the scrotum. (Middlesex Hospital Museum.)

retention. The man with stricture strains throughout the act of micturition; he with prostatic enlargement at the beginning;

whilst one with vesical calculus does so at the end. There is often a very striking disproportion between the effort to micturate and the calibre of the stricture, and conditions other than the size of the lumen of the stricture (namely, congestion and spasm) cause obstruction and even retention.

When called to a case of retention, we must not be influenced too much by the age of the patient. As a rule, young and middle-aged men will be subjects of stricture, old men of enlarged prostate. The young man may, however, have a prostatic abscess; the old man may have a stricture, or inflammatory œdema from acute gonorrhœa.

The exploration of the urethra with an olive-headed bougie will remove any doubt. Instruments of this shape are to be preferred because, as Guyon says, the surgeon with them gets the resistance by the part of the instrument which fills the canal, not by the point, which may catch in any fold or recess which is not a stricture.

In passing the instrument, begin with a full size and gradually work down to the size which passes easily through the obstruction, so as in this way to avoid the error of overlooking a stricture of "large calibre."

To distinguish between stricture and spasmodic contraction, use a metal instrument instead of a flexible one. This instrument will be obstructed at the membranous part of the urethra by spasm, and *a slight gentle* pressure will often cause it to pass on through the spasmodically contracted part of the canal. On withdrawing the instrument there will be no gripping of it as there is when a stricture is present.

Prognosis.—This chiefly depends upon the promptitude with which proper treatment is commenced, and the regularity with which it is continued. If the stricture is dilated early, and the proper patency of the urethra subsequently maintained by the occasional introduction of a bougie, all will continue well. If, on the other hand, the stricture is left to take its own course untreated, sooner or later vesical and renal complications will arise.

A traumatic (cicatricial) stricture is severer and more rapid in its effect than a simple organic (non-traumatic) one. All the consequences of stricture are, as a matter of course, more rapidly progressive in old men with arterial sclerosis, or enlarged prostate, or chronic renal disease, than in young men with healthy organs.

Treatment.—This is (*a*) mechanical, and consists in dilatation, divulsion, internal or external urethrotomy, or perinæal section; and (*b*) constitutional, consisting in an unirritating diet, good hygienic conditions, and aseptic precautions.

The different mechanical means above mentioned for re-establishing the natural calibre of the canal meet with different degrees of favour from different surgeons; but though, in many cases, it is open to them to choose between one mode of treatment and another, still there are many others in which one method cannot, or cannot wisely, be substituted for another.

Dilatation.—All agree that for a large number of cases dilatation is sufficient, and that when it is so, no other operation should be substituted for it; moreover, it is nearly always requisite, as a complementary measure in maintaining subsequently the good effect of the other modes of treatment.

The most favourable cases for dilatation are recent strictures in young men. The most unfavourable are traumatic strictures, and strictures with long and tortuous, but not necessarily very narrow, lumen.

It is not the degree to which a stricture has been allowed to contract so much as the toughness in some cases, and the resiliency in others, of the material constituting the stricture, which make simple dilatation unfavourable.

There are conditions of the urethra, or of the patient, which militate against the treatment by dilatation. Such are an extremely irritable urethral mucous membrane, or one which bleeds readily; men highly neurotic who feel acutely; men without the courage to submit to any instrumentation without an anæsthetic; and men who, from having lived in the tropics or from other causes, are subject to attacks of urinary fever after every introduction of an instrument.

For such cases internal urethrotomy, or the rapid dilatation under an anæsthetic is the best treatment, unless the conditions which indicate external urethrotomy or perinæal section are present.

There are two different ways of employing dilatation not always suitable for the same case: (1) Dilatation without detention; and (2) dilatation with detention. It may be here premised that in all cases of stricture, if there is a narrow meatus it ought at once to be enlarged.

(1) *Dilatation without detention* (or interrupted dilatation as it is sometimes called) does not confine the patient to bed, because a catheter is not retained in the bladder. It is suitable for men who cannot or will not give up their time wholly to their treatment, who are not restricted to a limited time within which to be treated, and upon whom, even though the stricture may be very narrow at the commencement of treatment, there is no uncertainty or difficulty in introducing instruments; whose urethræ are fairly tolerant, and whose strictures are neither cartilaginous nor resilient, and who are not prone to urethral rigors.

To carry out this treatment let the patient first pass water. This relieves him of the anxiety that he is going to micturate over the hands of the surgeon all the time the bougies are being introduced, and it also flushes the urethra clean of any muco-purulent discharge. Next take care that the glans and meatus are quite clean. Then enlarge the meatus if contracted, anæsthetising the part with a 10 per cent. solution of cocain; after this, with a glass syringe, distend the urethra by injecting a drachm or two of simple olive oil or weakly carbolised oil (1 in 40), the penis being well drawn up, and the urethra compressed near the glans by the finger and thumb of the left hand of the surgeon. Then while the urethra is still distended with the oil, pass in an olive-headed bougie of such a size as is found by trial to pass readily through the stricture.

Supposing this to be No. 2 or 3, leave it in the stricture for a few minutes, then withdraw it and pass at once No. 4, and after another few minutes' detention of No. 4, pass No. 5, and so on until two or three stages of dilatation have thus been gained. On the second or third day afterwards, or even on the following day, if the patient can give the time, the same thing should be repeated, always commencing the procedure by passing the one or two largest-sized instruments which were passed at the previous interview.

In this way a week or ten days may suffice to dilate the urethra to the fullest size; or, on the other hand, three or four weeks may be required.

(2) *Dilatation with detention* (or continuous dilatation as it is sometimes called). By this plan the patient is confined to bed, or, at any rate, to his room and his couch. A catheter is passed, with the precautions just given, and is tied in the bladder, and allowed to remain twenty-four or forty-eight hours, when it is removed and another catheter one or two or more sizes larger is tied in. The rule should be that the catheter to be detained should glide easily within the strictured area. A catheter which nearly or quite fills the lumen irritates the diseased part, and, if there is any breach of surface, tends to increase the risks of absorption or extravasation of urine whereas a catheter which passes loosely through does neither; but in a rapid manner, which is often surprising, promotes the absorption and relaxation of the stricture tissue. A week or less is very often quite sufficient for full dilatation. During the retention of a catheter, the front part of the urethra should be frequently syringed out with Condy's fluid, or a weak solution of boric acid.

This mode of treatment is suitable for the same class of stricture as "dilatation without detention," when the patient can give up the time for it, or when it is requisite his treatment should be compressed within a few days. It is the best, therefore, for the in-patients of a hospital.

Some surgeons recommend a combination of these two methods of dilatation, employing dilatation with retention till No. 8 or 9, French size, can be passed, and then dilatation without detention at intervals of forty-eight hours, or longer, if the canal becomes inflamed.

There are cases of stricture in which no catheter or bougie can be passed, and yet the patients have no considerable difficulty in relieving their bladder, though from the small size and slowness of the stream the process takes a long time.

Such patients are liable to occasional attacks of retention, and it is frequently one of these which brings them under treatment. In such circumstances, a full dose of opium and a warm bath, or an attempt at catheterism in the hot bath, may be tried, if the retention is not very urgent and the patient is in fairly good health and strength; and it may succeed. But if the patient is old and feeble, it must be employed with caution if at all, as serious syncope has been induced by the hot bath. If it does not succeed, or cannot be tried, and in any case if the retention is extreme, the bladder should be punctured above the pubis with the aspirator needle, or trochar and cannula.

The effect of thus emptying the bladder is to relieve the congestion of the mucous membrane, and the spasms, and the patient may be able to pass water, or the surgeon to introduce a catheter within a few hours afterwards.

When retention does not occur, the patient should be kept in bed on a light farinaceous diet, with a moderate amount of barley-water to drink ; and, if the urine is acid, a mixture should be taken of bicarbonate of potash (grs. x) and tincture of hyoscyamus (ɱ xxx) three times a day. The patient after a . few days of this *régime* often experiences an improvement in passing urine, and by the end of a week or ten days the surgeon may slip in easily a No. 2, 3, or 4, though before the treatment commenced the stricture may not have admitted a filiform bougie. This point gained, dilatation with detention—*i.e.* the continuous dilatation treatment—should be employed.

It does sometimes happen, however, that though the patient passes a dribbling stream very frequently, and thereby gets sufficient relief for his immediate comfort, no catheter can be introduced after a prolonged trial of the rest, diet, and medicinal treatment just mentioned. Something must be done, however, otherwise the secondary changes in urine, bladder, and kidneys previously described will soon occur.

And, again, if the patient will not submit to this expectant treatment, and yet wishes to be put into a better condition, something must be done. He should be anæsthetised, and, remembering the advisability of enlarging a contracted meatus, and the necessity for the antiseptic precautions described above, a small catheter should be passed, if possible. If the surgeon, however, does not succeed, he should introduce Teevan's filiform bougie adapted to a modernised Perrève's or Holt's dilator, or to a Maisonneuve's urethrotome, and when this has been passed through the stricture into the bladder, one or other of these instruments should be attached to the bougie guide and passed on through the stricture or strictures, which will thus be dilated or divided.

When the penile urethra is the seat of stricture the internal urethrotome is the instrument of choice. The urethrotome I prefer is Sir Henry Thompson's. I dislike any instrument that necessarily cuts the roof of the urethra.

For strictures in the bulbo-membranous part which do not require external urethrotomy or perinæal section, Perrève's or Holt's dilator is an excellent instrument when properly used. As this instrument is made nowadays, the guide for the tubes to run upon is also a stiletted catheter, so that the surgeon can make sure by the escape of a few drops of urine that he is in the bladder and not in a false passage. Then the tubes, eight in number, should be passed, one after the other, in regular succession, from the smallest to the largest, and each should be allowed to rest in the urethra for several seconds. Each tube should be pushed quietly and steadily through the stricture so as to dilate it; not thrust in with a sudden jerk so as to divulse or split it. If there be as many as eight tubes of graduated size all of them may be introduced without causing a drop of blood to flow, the inference from which is that the instrument so employed *effects rapid dilatation without lacerating* the stricture. I am not in a position to state positively that this is so, because I am happy to say that, though I often use the instrument, I have never had the opportunity of proving the point.

At the present time the majority, I believe, of English surgeons prefer internal urethrotomy to this dilator. In an excellent clinical lecture on "Stricture of the Urethra" (*Clinical Journal*, July 25th, 1894), Sir William MacCormac, speaking of Perrève's instrument, says:—"It has been claimed for this method that it stretches the part without lacerating the mucous membrane, but I am very sure that in the majority of cases the mucous membrane is lacerated. . . . I do not know that at the present time this instrument is ever used. . . . I think the conditions for its use do not obtain. . . . Of course, these instruments had the advantage in the public eye that their use did not entail a cutting operation, though that really is not an advantage. . . . The objection urged against cutting operations, which certainly formerly entailed some degree of greater risk than we now incur, was that septic elements gained entrance ; but the antiseptic precautions we now take minimise the risk that formerly obtained." Sir William speaks of the method as "forcible dilatation," and of the graduated tubes as "divulsors," and when used in the manner these terms imply I have little doubt that breaches are made in the strictured tissue and adjacent mucous membrane. But in some cases this is even better than cutting healthy mucous membrane along the roof of the urethra and leaving the stricture tissue in the floor untouched.

Used as I have described above, the method is, *in principle*, the same as the "divulsion" method of Le Fort, which is advocated by Tédenat and É. Forgue, with this difference, that these surgeons do in two or three sittings, and without an anæsthetic, what can be done in one, either with or without the aid of anæsthesia.

É. Forgue remarks that "this method of Le Fort is not divulsion, but simply dilatation accelerated, and it renders good service when ordinary dilatation threatens to be prolonged, when one loses to-day the advance made yesterday, and when, also, the condition of the urethra and the higher urinary organs does not demand a more rapid result by the methods of urethrotomy." By rapid dilatation at a single sitting, this object also is accomplished, as well as by internal urethrotomy.

I entirely agree, and my practice is completely in accord with the teaching of Mr. Reginald Harrison, who advocates *the rapid method of dilating* a stricture, especially when cystitis, and offensive and muco-purulent urine, increase the sufferings and the danger of the patient. As he rightly points out, to tie in a small- or medium-sized catheter in such cases is a hazardous proceeding, as it merely draws off the more fluid and less harmful of the contents of the bladder, leaving the more poisonous and tenacious parts to cause trouble by frequent blockage of the instrument, and to become a source of infection to bladder, ureters, kidneys, and general system of the patient. I agree likewise with Mr.

Teale in his advocacy of rapid dilatation by the use of Lister's sounds, when he says, "It is my belief that full dilatation at the first sitting is safer than the older method of partial and gradual dilatation; and for this reason, that even in partial dilatation there is frequently some laceration or bruising of the surface at the strictured point. If the stricture be only partially dilated, there remains a narrowing at this sore point sufficient materially to arrest the flow of urine, and therefore there is urinary pressure on the raw surface, whereas in full dilatation the urine flows along the urethra equally and without undue pressure at any point, and puts no stress upon the tender and perhaps lacerated surface of the stricture." When Lister's No. 1 cannot be passed, Teevan's filiform guide is introduced and screwed on to the tip of a conical sound like Lister's without the bulb; this secures dilatation up to 4 or 5, and then the rest of Lister's sounds can be introduced in succession up to 12 or 14. Mr. Teale adds that "Rigors are extremely rare after the use of Lister's sounds. This rarity of rigor I am inclined to attribute to the fact that in nearly every instance dilatation has been carried *at the first sitting to 10, 11, or 12.*" The italics are mine, and I use them to emphasise what I believe to be the principle involved. My opinion is that it does not matter much by what means —Lister's sounds, Perrève's dilator, or the internal urethrotome—the complete dilatation is effected so long as it is accomplished at a single sitting.

Penile strictures are much more intractable than those of inflammatory origin near the bulb; they are all, or almost all, of the sclero-cicatricial kind, and partake largely of the characters of traumatic strictures. They are best treated by internal urethrotomy.

Internal urethrotomy is to be recommended for strictures in which dilatation of any form is insufficient or harmful, such as (*a*) cartilaginous stricture, (*b*) resilient strictures, (*c*) irritable strictures which bleed, or become readily inflamed, (*d*) which are frequently complicated by retention, cystitis, or orchitis, (*e*) when incontinence shows that there is considerable *dilatation* behind the stricture, (*f*) when instrumentation causes urethral fever, and when the kidneys are threatened.

Q

A disposition to urethral fever, and the presence of vesical and renal complications, are not reasons against, but in favour of, the operation; because fever may be prevented or checked, a free passage provided, and the kidneys and bladder relieved from over-distension by the operation.

The treatment by *electrolysis*, the technique of which was so improved by Le Fort, and which Mr. Bruce Clark and the late Mr. W. Stevenson in England have employed, does not seem to afford any advantages over antiseptic internal urethrotomy, either in regard to its simplicity, safety, or the greater stability of its results.

External Urethrotomy.—This consists in cutting through the stricture upon a staff passed into the bladder. It is the operation for choice (a) in traumatic strictures, (b) in strictures complicated by extravasation of urine, (c) in cases where there are perinæal fistulæ, especially when the fistulæ are old, hardened, and tuberculated, (d) in strictures that have returned after internal urethrotomy has been performed, and (e) in cases in which the patients, being careless, intemperate, or poor, will not or cannot attend to the regular periodic introduction of an instrument, requisite after dilatation or internal urethrotomy.

Perinæal Section consists in opening the urethra behind the stricture without a staff to cut upon. This, or Sedillot's or Wheelhouse's operation, is indicated (a) for strictures which are practically impassable—*i.e.* when no instrument of any kind can be passed after careful, prolonged, and repeated trials, aided by rest and dietetic treatment, and by anæsthesia; (b) in cases of retention where no instrument can be introduced under anæsthesia, and where the urine is known to be thick and purulent, and the bladder inflamed; (c) also, where no instrument can be passed, in cases of extravasation of urine, or urinary abscess due to perforation of the urethra behind the stricture. Sedillot's is most in favour in France, Wheelhouse's, a modification of Sedillot's, most employed in England; but perinæal section, provided it is followed up by the division of the stricture from behind forwards, is a most effective and satisfactory operation.

In most cases it will not be difficult (when the dilated urethra behind the stricture has been incised and the bladder emptied) to pass a bougie forwards from the wound through the stricture; but whether this can be done or not, the strictured tissues should be incised from behind forwards, taking pains to keep the bistoury in the middle line. A full-sized catheter can then be passed from the external meatus into the wound, and thence conducted upon a slender gorget into the bladder, after which the urethra behind the stricture, if in a healthy state, should be brought together by sutures.

In no single instance out of the many in which, during the last twenty-five years, I have performed Cock's operation have I contented myself with simply giving relief to retention, but in every case I have, either at the time or within some days subsequently (generally at the time), cut a way through the cicatricial tissue, and passed a catheter *en demeure* through the penis into the bladder, and thus induced the reconstruction of the floor of the canal out of the granulation tissue formed during the healing of the perinæal wound.

In Wheelhouse's operation, the search for the anterior orifice of the stricture is often very prolonged, and, from what I have seen, not unfrequently unsuccessful, so that Cock's operation, or supra-pubic cystotomy, has after all to be performed. The supra-pubic operation, either for the purpose of passing an instrument through the stricture from behind forwards (retrograde catheterism), or to relieve the retention, is unnecessarily severe, unsurgical, and unsatisfactory. The stricture cannot be treated without making a second incision, and all that can be gained by it can be better obtained by perinæal section, performed in the manner I have just described. The cases which require perinæal section and division of the stricture from behind forwards are rare; still they occur with sufficient frequency to make it necessary for the hospital surgeon to be always prepared to meet with them. At one time an impassable stricture with acute retention, or with foul, thick urine; at another time, such a stricture with numerous old fistulæ, or a perinæal abscess; and again, at another time, extravasation of urine, from rupture of the urethra behind an impermeable stricture, will require to be promptly treated by this operation of perinæal section (Simon's or Cock's operation, as it is called by St. Thomas's and Guy's men respectively). I have had to deal with four such cases in a fortnight, with three on three successive days, and I know of no field of surgery in which severe and even alarming conditions yield so readily and so satisfactorily to treatment.

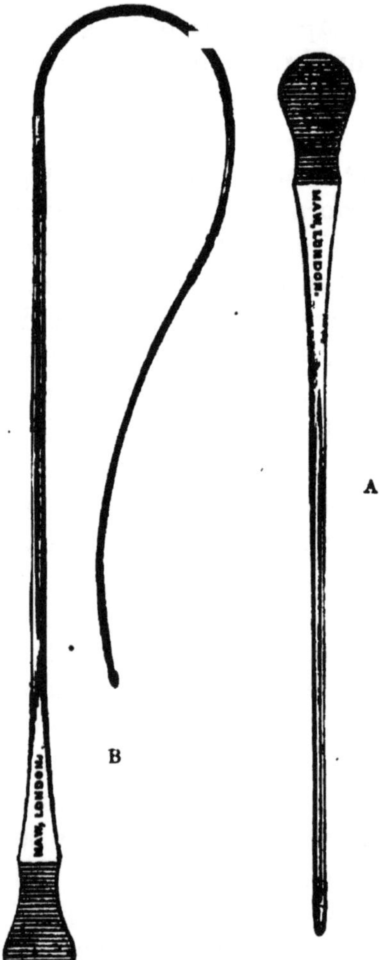

In many cases in which Wheelhouse's operation will prove difficult, tedious, or impossible, and in which Perrève's dilator, guided by the filiform bougie, cannot be passed, I have found the following plan answer admirably. Under chloroform I have passed the filiform guide bougie into the bladder, and have attached its outer end to a screw on a straight tapering staff made for me by Maw, Son & Thompson (Fig. 69). The staff, following the bougie guide, having been pushed as far into the stricture as it will go, is then cut down upon from the perinæum, and the front part of the stricture divided. Little by little the point of the staff is pushed inwards through the stricture and the knife run in its groove until at length the whole stricture is divided. I employed this instrument with great success in a case which had foiled Wheelhouse's method in another surgeon's hands. It is much simpler and easier than searching for the contracted anterior aperture of the stricture in a bleeding wound, especially in a deep perinæum. I strongly recommend the trial of the method to other surgeons.

Fig. 69.—A, Morris's Tapering Staff; B, with Filiform Guide-Bougie attached.

Puncture per rectum for retention from stricture has, I believe, no longer a place in modern surgery; it is certainly dirty and may be dangerous. If it is performed at all, it should be for retention from enlarged prostate. *Supra-pubic puncture* has quite taken the place of puncture per rectum. It is an excellent temporary expedient for the relief of retention where the general and local conditions are suitable for dilatation, as soon as the spasmodic and congestive stage has passed off. *Supra-pubic cystotomy* for the treatment of stricture ought not to be thought of, and will never, I imagine, be adopted by one who has sufficient confidence in his knowledge of anatomy, and in the steadiness of his hand and eye, to perform perinæal section without a guide after Simon's and Cock's method. If he declines to do perinæal section, let him adopt Sedillot's operation; or use the tapering staff.

There is no operation for stricture of the urethra which can compare with external urethrotomy, and perinæal section with division of the stricture from behind forwards, for the excellence and the permanence of the relief afforded.

I have, indeed, known a man go many years after the treatment of his stricture by Perrève dilator without the introduction of any instrument, and yet his stricture has shown no signs of return. But though this is the exception in cases which have been treated by dilatation or internal urethrotomy, the possibility of discarding catheterism or bougies is by no means very infrequent after cutting the stricture from without inwards; and if it is objected to these external operations that the convalescence from them is much more prolonged than from internal urethrotomy, the answer is that one can guarantee a large stream and a more lasting cure. There is no doubt that in some of the cases in which I have divided the callous " stricture " tissue from behind forwards, especially in two or three in which the stricture has been impassable for years, and all urine had been voided through perinæal fistulæ, I have made little more than a groove or inverted gutter in the tough cicatricial mass, and that the floor of the new urethra has been formed by connective tissue and integuments only, which have healed around a full-sized catheter detained from the time of the operation till convalescence. It is quite surprising how little tendency there is for the new-made channel to contract, the floor of which has a depressed pouch-like or sac-like condition.

The *excision of strictures* of the urethra dates from the beginning of this century at least, and though it has not been at any time extensively employed, it has of late come somewhat into vogue for old-standing cartilaginous-like, or tough fibrous, or very rebellious strictures, whether of traumatic or blennorrhagic origin.

Some surgeons, after resection, bring the cut edges together; others do not. Some have made good the deficiency by urethroplastic operations. Keyes utilised the mucous membrane of the foreskin for this purpose, and apparently with satisfactory result. When there would be much tension on sutures they should not, in my opinion, be used, because a good channel will result from granulation tissue built up around a retained catheter.

I have, in several cases, pared down the callous tissues about long-standing strictures, shaving it away without actually cutting out the stricture, and the results have given the patient and myself great satisfaction.

CHAPTER IX.

URINARY ABSCESS. EXTRAVASATION OF URINE.

WHEN a breach is made in the wall of the urethra, either by injury or disease, and is unaccompanied by a free external opening, urine escapes into the adjacent cellular tissue, and the result is either an abscess or extravasation.

If the urine issues slowly and in small quantity, and becomes circumscribed by inflammatory exudation, an abscess forms.

If the urine escapes suddenly or rapidly and in large quantity, it spreads far and wide in the tissues, unchecked by a barrier of inflammatory origin, and " extravasation of urine," properly so-called, is produced.

Traumatic Causes.—Extravasation may be caused by any of the kinds of wounds of the urethra described in previous sections. If the penile portion is ruptured during erection or coitus, or if the bulb is torn by a blow or fall on the perinæum, the urine will infiltrate the anterior and superficial part of the perinæum, and may spread thence to the scrotum, penis, and front wall of the abdomen.

If the membranous or prostatic portion is ruptured, the urine will escape behind the triangular ligament or between its layers, and, spreading thence to the anus and ischio-rectal fossæ, may ascend a long way into the pelvis. Thus it may infiltrate between the pubo-vesical ligaments into the pre-vesical space, and in severe and neglected cases may mount as high as the iliac fossæ, or even spread in the retro-peritoneal cellular tissue along the front of the vertebral column. It may also break through the anterior layer of the triangular ligament and become diffused also throughout the superficial part of the space.

The natural anatomical frontiers of the two perinæal spaces may be broken through, either at first by injury, as in fracture of the pelvis, or subsequently by suppuration, and in either way the extravasation may become general.

Pathological Causes.—The pathological ruptures occur spontaneously, and, as a rule, in the following manner:—The urethra behind a stricture, or other persistent cause of obstruction, is dilated, and the little urine constantly lodged here causes a degree of chronic inflammation, or even ulceration, with thinning of its walls. This effected, it only needs an attack of complete retention, or of increased difficulty in micturition, to be superadded to that which persistently exists, for the wall of the canal to give way under the more frequent and forcible muscular efforts of the bladder to expel its contents. Sometimes the rent in the urethral wall is large and the urine escapes rapidly, and then extravasation ensues; in other cases the breach is small and even minute, and the urine escapes *guttatim*, or nearly so, and then an abscess is the consequence.

Thus the predisposing cause is the thin, dilated, and friable condition of the wall of the urethra behind the obstruction; the immediate cause is the forcible propulsion of urine by the muscular contraction of the bladder.

In some cases in which this spontaneous pathological rupture occurs the degree of persistent obstruction is not great; indeed, it sometimes takes place behind what Otis has designated " strictures of large calibre."

URINARY ABSCESS.

If a few drops of urine leak into the peri-urethral cellular tissue through a small opening in the urethral wall, they set up a certain amount of inflammation which limits or circumscribes the extravasation. It does not matter how the urethra becomes damaged—whether by a false passage, or by the ulceration caused by the frequent hitching of the point of a catheter against the same spot, or by the fraying of the edges of a fissure or crack in the mucous membrane, or, as described above, by the giving way of the canal behind a stricture—the only conditions required are that the opening should be small and the leakage slow. In some cases the little opening cicatrises after the first leakage; in others, the leakage, by repetition, increases little by little. Hence the variations in the size of the abscesses, and in their rate of progress to a culminating point. The inflammation at the circumference of the involved area produces a plastic exudation of greater or less hardness; but sooner or later the tissues in direct contact with the extravasated and stagnant urine suppurate. If the patient is in bad health, if he is the subject of secondary kidney disease, if there is a frequent leakage of urine going on, or if the urine is not aseptic, suppuration will occur early —otherwise there may remain for a long time a quiescent, small hard fixed lump outside the canal, but without any active symptoms whatever.

Urinary abscess may thus be either acute, subacute, or chronic.

The *acute and subacute* are nearly always situated in the perinæum immediately beneath the urethra, but as they increase they approach both the scrotum and anus. They cause at first a small swelling, oblong or round in shape, hard to the touch, painless, and covered by healthy skin. In a few days they increase markedly and become painful, micturition

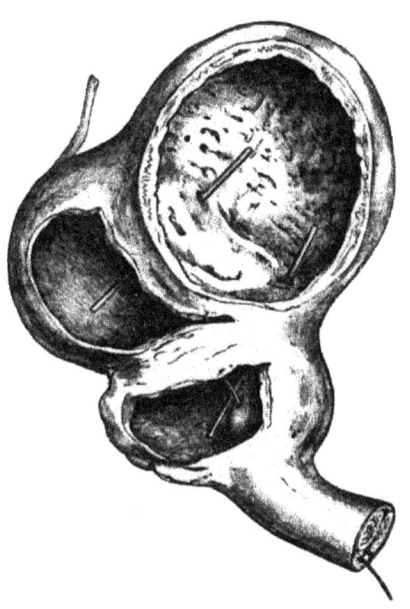

Fig. 70.—Abscesses resulting from Stricture; one abscess in the Prostate, the other behind the Bladder. Both communicate with the bladder cavity. (Middlesex Hospital Museum.)

is smarting or burning, the whole perinæum is tender, rigors occur, and the general symptoms indicative of local inflammation and suppuration are excited. At this stage the abscess (1) may burst into the urethra, when thick yellow pus is discharged with the urine, or drains away at the meatus independently of passing water, or can be squeezed along the passage; (2) or it may point towards the surface, and break, leaving a urinary fistula; or (3) without breaking through the skin, the abscess may burst into the bladder (Fig. 70), or into the surrounding tissues, when widespread extravasation may follow.

The *Chronic Abscess* is not so frequent as the acute and subacute. There is a small, hard swelling adherent to the under-surface of the urethra, scarcely recognised by the patient except for the slight occasional feeling of pain and burning in it when passing water. This swelling is hard and covered with healthy skin, and can be seen, felt, and perhaps slightly moved in the perinæum. It will remain quiescent for a long time, and then, after a long walk, a slight blow, or some increased difficulty in passing water, it will suppurate, soften, and increase in size, and burst through the skin or into the urethra. As in the case of the more acute forms of abscess, if it opens into the urethra it may, after some days, quite close, leaving an indurated lump beneath the urethra which may persist for months or years; if it opens on the cutaneous surface, fistulæ or widespread extravasation may follow.

There is a variety of urinary swelling, ill-defined, very chronic, and of almost stony hardness. It is generally situated in the middle line, intimately connected with the wall of the urethra, and well-nigh immovable. I have known them mistaken for fibromata or gummata; and Tillaux states that he has many times seen them mistaken by students for enchondromata or osteomata of the pelvis. I do not remember to have ever met with them except in the perinæum or penis, or at the peno-scrotal angle; but Forgue states that he has seen them in the neighbourhood of the symphysis and in the iliac fossa. They are caused by a drop or two of pure or aseptic urine, and consist of inflammatory fibrous tissue. Under provocation they may suppurate and become chronic, subacute, or acute abscesses, and then follow any of the courses just described. Before suppurating, they may cause a mechanical obstacle to micturition, and if so they should be excised like a tumour.

Diagnosis.—This will, in most cases, be made without difficulty by attending to the clinical history and the symptoms just described. When the abscess is connected with the penile urethra it is more difficult to diagnose than when in the perinæum. If the scrotum is swollen and œdematous, and less mobile than normal, and if there is a good deal of thickening of the tissues, through the midst of which the urethra seems to pass, a urinary abscess may be safely diagnosed when the history of the case is considered.

Treatment.—Although the urethra is not always clearly connected with the abscess, and urine does not invariably flow out through the incision when the abscess is opened, the urethra is, nevertheless, invariably involved by the abscess, and urine will, in almost every instance, trickle through in a day or two, if not at the time of opening the abscess. It is right, therefore, before making even a superficial incision into one of these abscesses, to inform the patient of its connection with the canal, and of the possibility of a urinary fistula following; otherwise, the surgeon may be blamed for want of skill in treating the case.

To prevent the abscess from bursting into the urethra, or from leaving a tortuous fistula, or from causing urinary extravasation, it ought always to be opened in good time.

Softening and fluctuation are not to be waited for, nor should the swelling be allowed time to enlarge, either towards the anus or scrotum. The method of operating when the abscess is in the perinæum is to pass a small staff, well smeared with carbolised oil, gently along the urethra beyond the swelling or into the bladder. The patient being in the lithotomy position, the surgeon cuts into the abscess and evacuates it completely with the finger or a scoop, and afterwards irrigates it well with carbolic solution (1 in 20). Then, taking a long, slender bistoury in hand, he passes its point through the abscess and into the groove of the staff through the median line of the urethra; depressing his hand, he pushes the point of the knife forwards and upwards along the staff until he has divided the whole of the stricture which is in front of the abscess. I have, in some cases, cut forwards through the floor of the urethra for an inch, or an inch and a half, and in some cases I have cut away a large portion of fibrous or cartilaginous-like strictured urethra. Other strictures, if existing, should be dealt with at the same time either with the internal urethrotome or by rapid dilatation. If a guide such as a filiform bougie and my tapering staff cannot be passed, I open the abscess by cutting the thick and œdematous tissue which lies between the skin and the pus; and then, if I can find the opening from the abscess into the urethra,

I pass a probe-pointed director forwards along the urethra through the stricture, which I divide as just described. If I cannot do this, I open the urethra at the base of the abscess (*i.e.* through the floor of the abscess) and deal with the stricture later; but this is seldom the case.

When the abscess is in the penile urethra, I open the abscess externally, and dilate, or internally divide the stricture or strictures in front of it at the same time.

In every case the contents of the abscess should be well cleared out, the abscess wall scraped and well rubbed with iodoform.

If the abscess has burrowed, as it very likely will have done, in a forward direction above the scrotum and towards the roof of the urethra, or laterally by the side of one of the cavernous bodies, the sinus should be cleared out in the same way as the abscess, and, if necessary, a counter-opening should be made in the integuments and a drainage tube introduced.

No catheter should be left in the urethra, but as soon as healing begins the urethra should be kept dilated by passing every few days a full-sized instrument.

M. Guyon teaches that it is best to open the abscess and leave the stricture to be treated by internal urethrotomy after the perinæal wound begins to granulate, the object of this being to avoid setting up, by way of the newly-made wound through the stricture, urethral fever or septic absorption— dangers which, I think, need not be feared if the abscess is thoroughly cleared out and antisepticised at the time of the operation.

Desnos and Forgue advise that the abscess should be opened and tamponed with iodoform gauze, and the stricture divided by internal urethrotomy at the same sitting, if the abscess is simple, does not burrow, and can be rendered aseptic at once, and if the urethra appears healthy. Otherwise, the internal urethrotomy should be postponed.

Horteloup practises the complete excision of the abscess. He censures the treatment by simple incision and drainage. He cites two cases in which the abscesses had been opened in the perinæum and the stricture treated by internal urethrotomy; and some years subsequently the patients presented themselves with a return of the strictures, and with a large amount of dense fibrous thickening external to the urethra, which he thinks persisted from the time of the abscess.

Horteloup's treatment is the same in principle as that recommended by me, but in the case of chronic abscesses is more extensive. He introduces a catheter, and, with the patient in the lithotomy position, makes two incisions convex externally, and cuts out a portion of tissue, including the abscess, like a quarter of an orange; then, with his finger in the wound, he feels for any indurated bands, which he snips away with scissors or a knife. The urethra is thus cleared of all surrounding indurated tissue, and appears at the bottom of the wound like an injected artery.

In acute abscesses he detaches the tissues with his finger and removes them in shreds. Then he treats the stricture either by internal or external urethrotomy, or by complete or partial excision of the stricture.

EXTRAVASATION OF URINE.

Extravasation of urine differs essentially from urinary abscess, although it occurs from the same pathological and mechanical causes. The tissues are infiltrated with urine so suddenly and in such large quantity, that they have no time to become inflamed, and thus, by throwing out a barrier, to prevent further infiltration. The consequences are dependent upon the quantity, and the degree of septicity, of the urine extravasated. It is true that pure, healthy urine can be poured out into a large vascular cavity without doing harm, until by its stagnation, decomposition, and widespread absorption under pressure, inflammation, suppuration, gangrene, or septic absorption occurs.

The toxicity of urine, slight as it is in the case of fresh, healthy urine, is doubtless increased in persons with renal inadequacy and chronic diseases of the bladder and urethra.

The septicity of urine is now known to be due to micro-organisms, and though streptococci and staphylococci have been found in urinary suppurations, the researches of several observers seem to point to the presence also of a specific form of bacterium—the pyogenic bacillus of urine, which some describe as identical with the bacterium coli commune.

In the gangrenous forms of urinary extravasation the "vibrion septique" of Pasteur probably plays an important rôle.

Symptoms.—When extravasation occurs in front of the triangular ligament, as it most frequently does, the perinæum in its anterior· half becomes tense and swollen. The deep layer of the superficial fascia, attached as it is behind to the base of the triangular ligament and along the sides to the ischio-pubic rami, directs the urine forwards into the scrotum, penis, and front abdominal wall. All of these parts may become much enlarged by œdema if the extravasation is great enough. If the rupture is behind the front layer of the triangular ligament, the urine passes backwards and upwards into the pelvis in the manner previously described.

In traumatic cases the extravasation does not always occur immediately or rapidly. In these cases, too, the urine is often healthy and unirritating, so that it is slow to cause inflammation or fever—in fact, it does not do so until it has undergone secondary changes, and therefore some days may elapse without serious local or general symptoms, if a catheter has been retained in the bladder. Again, the urethra behind the rupture may retract, or be closed by the compressor urethræ, or be blocked by blood-clot, and, further, the shock of the accident checks the secretion of urine; so that in this way again the local symptoms may be postponed for many hours.

When the urethra gives way behind a stricture, it is generally during an effort of the patient to pass water whilst his bladder is pretty well distended. Perhaps he is unable to start the stream, or has the pain of retention, when suddenly he feels a sense of great relief in his bladder without voiding any urine through his meatus. The bladder has partly emptied its contents into the tissues of the perinæum. But, in little or no time, in less than an hour perhaps, there are external evidences in the perinæum and scrotum of what has happened. Sooner or later—sooner if the urine is septic or a large quantity of it is poured out at once—the perinæum suddenly becomes tumid and tender, then red and painful, and here and there showing bullæ or spots of gangrene; fever progresses and rigors occur, and septic intoxication, or septicæmia, may follow very rapidly if operative treatment is postponed. Sloughing may be extensive, and in the scrotum may leave the testicles exposed. I have seen a robust man of middle age, the subject of stricture and untreated extravasation, die within three days of septicæmia, his body covered with septicæmic petechiæ; and at the post-mortem examination his lungs, heart, and abdominal viscera were found studded with minute hæmorrhages.

Diagnosis is much less difficult when the extravasation involves the anterior part of the perinæum than when it is confined to the deeper. The history and course of the case ought to exclude diffuse suppurative cellulitis or erysipelas. On examining the patient in the lithotomy position, the general aspect of the swelling, its course and limitations, its rapid increase, its sudden onset, all point to the diagnosis. Perhaps the symptoms have followed a false passage, a blow on the perinæum, or a fracture of the pelvis, or the ischio-rectal fossæ or the iliac fossæ give signs of distension or inflammation. In this manner we may be assisted when the extravasation is limited to the deeper parts.

Prognosis.—In most cases of simple extravasation, when treated in good time, the patients are at once relieved of fever, rigors, and pain by the incisions, and in three or four days are rapidly convalescing. Feeble, intemperate, unhealthy people, and those whose higher urinary organs are disorganised, run great risks, and recovery with them is much slower. Extensive sloughing will be followed generally in fairly healthy persons by rapid granulation and cicatrisation, and though both testes may have been bared of their integuments, they will soon become covered in again by newly-formed tissue.

Treatment.—This consists in making immediate multiple and free incisions into the perinæum, scrotum, penis, abdominal walls, ischio-rectal fossæ, or wheresoever the urine has penetrated, so as to provide exits for it, and to prevent fresh infiltration. Never wait for fluctuation. In the perinæum the incisions should be made in a longitudinal direction, and on each side of the middle line; in the scrotum and prepuce transversely, obliquely or longitudinally. All bullæ or sloughing parts should be incised. The wounds bleed very slightly. In making these incisions the urine often spurts out with considerable force owing to the great tension it exercises on the fascia and skin. The surgeon should be on the look out for this. As the floor of the urethra near the rent, in cases of pathological origin, is commonly in an ulcerated or sloughy state, it is proper to perform, at the same time that the incisions are made, external urethrotomy, and thereby to divide the stricture as well as the damaged urethra. This should be done also for the purpose of giving a direct exit to the urine from the bladder, and thus preventing further infiltration of the tissues.

In cases of extravasation from injury, if seen early, the treatment should be that recommended for rupture of the urethra. (Pages 198 *et seqq.*) When several hours have elapsed and the tissues are inflamed or threatening to become gangrenous, it is useless to employ sutures for the urethra. The surgeon must be content to make free incisions into the damaged tissues and to establish a direct outlet for the urine, and then wait until repair commences before introducing the catheter *en demeure.*

In the gangrenous and septic forms of extravasation some surgeons prefer the thermocautery to the knife. If the knife is used in these cases, the incisions will not give exit to the same amount of fluid as in the simple forms of urinary extravasation.

In the septicæmic and gangrenous cases with a tendency to coma, and a temperature descending below normal, only a fatal ending can be looked for. Neither free incisions nor quinine, nor large quantities of stimulants and nourishment, are likely to prevent it.

THERE are three varieties ot urethral fistulæ, viz.:—(1) The penile; (2) the scrotal and perinæal; and (3) the rectal. They differ from each other in origin, in anatomical characters, and in treatment.

1. THE URETHRO-PENILE.

Etiology.—The fistulæ that follow urinary abscess are rare on the penis, but they are sometimes formed in very chronic gleet by the inflammation, followed by ulceration or suppuration spreading from a follicle of the mucous membrane to the cutaneous surface. Englisch asserts that this occurs especially in tubercular subjects. Another cause is the progressive and deep ulceration of some soft chancres. They have followed the application of a tight string or ring round the penis, and also from various wounds and contusions of the urethra. They occur in the course of epithelioma of the penis.

Pathological Anatomy.—They are direct and short and free of branches, and open into the urethra obliquely from behind, forwards, or sometimes perpendicularly to the canal. The external opening is slightly depressed, not surrounded by granulations, except when it is situated in the peno-scrotal fold.

The internal orifice is funnel-shaped, and Voillemier says that he has ascertained this in so many cases in the post-mortem room that he regards it as an established fact. É. Forgue states that the external opening of the fistula caused by a chancre is a veritable hollow "wash-hand-basin shape"; whilst, on the contrary, the fistula resulting from a peri-follicular abscess has a narrow channel and orifice. The corpus spongiosum in the neighbourhood of the fistula generally atrophies and becomes so thin that the mucous and cutaneous openings seem blended in some cases. Where there has been much loss of substance, the opening may be from two to five centimetres wide with thin and bloodless margins, and the roof of the urethra can be seen through it. When

R

caused by cancer, cauliflower-like excrescences surround and surmount the orifice in some cases, or the opening is lost in the midst of the warty ulcer or cancerous mass.

Symptoms.—A variable amount of urine or semen escapes at the fistula. If the opening is wide and free, as much urine may pass through the fistula as through the meatus. If, on the other hand, the orifices and the canal are narrow, and there is a valvular disposition of either external or internal orifice, there will be only a few drops oozing through the fistula. The urine is not projected, but dribbles through the fistula and trickles over the scrotum and penis, and thus is apt to give rise to excoriations or erythema, and, by wetting the clothes, careless and dirty patients carry about with them a strong urinous odour. Sometimes a little pus is mixed with the urine, or a bead of pus escapes now and again independently of micturition.

In some cases, the fistula closes for long intervals and breaks open again and again to discharge a little pus, or pus and urine, for a few days only. Severe febrile symptoms attend the reopenings in some cases; and rigors, often quite severe, are brought on by the passage of urine through the fistula. A sharp attack of urinary fever is sometimes set up at the first bursting open of a fistula. The atrophy of the erectile tissue of the corpus spongiosum may be sufficient to cause slight arching of the penis during erection.

Prognosis.—The prognosis is only serious from the point of view of the difficulty in getting these fistulæ to heal in spite of the most varied and most careful treatment. There is no fear of secondary disease in the bladder or higher urinary organs. The rigors and feverish attacks which attend in some cases the patent stages of these fistulæ are not dangerous to life, though trying to the strength, health, and convenience of the patients.

I have known in one case an acute synovitis of the knee-joint, like gonorrhœal rheumatism, attack the patient, an elderly man, during one of the open and suppurating periods of the fistula.

Treatment.—For the very narrow fistulæ, cauterisation with a fine wire heated to white heat, or the point of a thermo-cautery, may succeed, but it is quite uncertain.

In a case I saw, in consultation, of a very minute fistula opening on the glans penis near the meatus, in which this treatment failed, the fistula was laid open into the meatus with a small tenotome; it finally healed from the bottom, but only after a tedious illness. The man was a fat Italian, very difficult to manage, who would not keep himself aseptic. He got erysipelas of the penis, and suppurating glands in the left groin.

In the majority of fistulæ a plastic operation, whereby "freshened" surfaces are held together by sutures, is the best plan to adopt. The plan of Nélaton was to raise a flap of skin on each side of the fistula and unite the two raw surfaces. Voillemier's method is to widely "freshen" the parts all around to the extent of a half-centimetre, and to suture the raw surfaces together (Fig. 71).

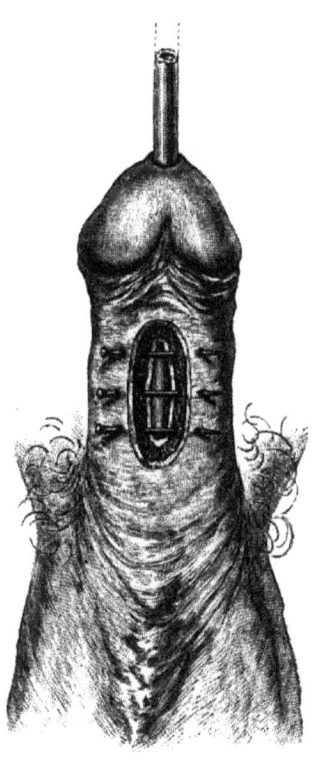

Fig. 71.—Voillemier's Method of Freshening and Suturing the Edges of the Fistula of the Urethra.

When the fistula is wide, various methods have been employed by Cooper, Delpeck, Duplay, and others, for closing it by flaps of skin transplanted from the neighbouring parts. They are described in works on "Operations."

After either of these operations, a catheter should be retained in the bladder so as to protect the sutures from contact with urine.

In very troublesome cases, where much urine escapes through the fistula, and other measures have failed, an opening should be made in the membranous urethra and the bladder drained through it, during the process of healing after an operation on the fistula.

2. URETHRO-SCROTAL AND URETHRO-PERINÆAL FISTULA.

These are nearly always the result of urinary abscesses formed in association with stricture. Traumatic ruptures sometimes terminate in fistulæ, as do surgical operations on the perinæal urethra or on the bladder. Immediate sutures to the urethral wound, when possible, should be used after external urethrotomy, or even after perinæal section, if the stricture has been divided, and a full-sized catheter passed into the bladder at the time of the operation. These means would be a security against fistula. Fistulæ after lithotomy are not very uncommon, and are due probably to contusion, to the septic state of the urine, and to the deposit of urine salts in the track of the wound. Other causes are peri-urethral abscesses which open both into the canal and through the skin. Suppuration of one of Cowper's glands, breaking down tuberculous and gummatous deposits in the perinæum, are illustrations of this class. Prostatic abscesses, opening externally, are also occasional causes.

Pathological Anatomy.—The internal orifice is commonly single, and if even the membranous or prostatic urethra is tunnelled by several tracts, they communicate with a single opening into the canal. But, as a rule, there are more than one, and very often there are several cutaneous openings, and these may be widely separated and far away from the perinæum. They may burrow through the pelvis and open on the buttocks, or near the trochanters, through the great sacro-sciatic foramen; or they may come to the surface near the anus, in the groins, loins, or hypogastrium. Cruveilhier has seen a case in which the fistulous track opened near the inferior angle of the scapula. In some, the openings are at the summit of a hard vascular wart, or in a *cul de sac*, whilst in others they are hidden behind a fold of skin. They may be either separated from one another by areas of healthy or cicatricial skin, or they may be grouped together amongst fungous granulations.

Though, in recent cases, they are sometimes single and direct in their course, yet in the great majority of cases they are irregular, tortuous, and branched in all directions; the branches ending blindly in the little recesses filled with pus, or pus and urine. The sinus tracts are lined by thick, soft, fleshy, pus-secreting granulations, if the fistulæ are not very chronic; or, if of long standing, they may be almost free of secretion, and covered with a layer of squamous epithelium. The surrounding walls are tough and hard, and give to the finger the sensation of firm cords; but in some cases the whole of the perinæum and the scrotum, and even the penis, are thickened, brawny and enlarged, and in a condition of false elephantiasis; in other cases, isolated fibrous masses of various sizes, formed of circumscribed sclerosed tissue, are studded about the scrotum and perinæum.

These sinuses are sometimes coated with a layer of the urinary salts, chiefly phosphates; they are sometimes the resting-places of calculi from the kidney, bladder or prostate, and increase *in situ* by the deposition of salts from the urine as it flows over them.

Symptoms and Diagnosis.—The history of urethral stricture, followed by that of urinary abscess in the scrotal or perinæal regions, and the escape of urine by the external openings, is sufficiently characteristic. The amount of urine which issues through the fistulæ varies; but even when it is very little, the skin of the surrounding parts is moist, and often excoriated or erythematous. If the internal orifice is large, and the stricture just in front of it is very narrow, the greater part of the urine may pass through the fistulæ, instead of by the normal meatus. If a metallic sound is passed along the urethra and a fine probe along the fistula, the two can generally be made to touch one another; but owing to the sinuous direction of the fistula, the probe may not get into the urethra, so that if the two instruments do not touch one another, it is not to be concluded that the fistula is not in communication with the urethra.

The fact that urine occasionally or constantly passes, or, by squeezing the glans penis during micturition, can be made to pass through the fistulous openings, will suffice to exclude from the diagnosis simple, or tuberculous peri-urethral abscess, or sinuses connected with necrosed pelvic bones. Some fistulæ in ano with only an external orifice if opening far forwards in the perinæum, and especially if a gleet and a stricture are also present, are very difficult to diagnose. I have recently had such a case under my care; and the diagnosis was not made until the orifice was enlarged, and then its rectal connection was established by finding that a probe passed readily upwards, just beneath the mucous membrane of the bowel.

In doubtful cases, assistance might be derived by injecting a coloured solution—a weak aqueous solution of fuchsin —into the meatus and finding it escape at the fistula. In some cases connected with suppuration in or around the prostate, a Y-shaped fistula exists, with a single arm towards the perinæum, and a branch to the urethra, and another to the rectum.

These cases cause much difficulty in diagnosis; but the history of an attack of inflammation or suppuration connected with the prostate clears the way.

In fistulous openings connected with diseased bone, the probe may detect the carious or necrosed surface.

The fistulæ formed by cancer of the bladder, prostate or deep urethra, will be readily diagnosed by their history and the enlarged inguinal glands, by the cauliflower-like outgrowths, and by the microscopic appearances of a fragment of one of the growths.

Prognosis and Treatment.—The treatment consists in dividing the stricture of the urethra by an external urethrotomy, following up and laying open the branches of the fistulæ; scraping their surfaces or cutting away their cord-like walls, and thoroughly asepticising the tissues by the liberal application of strong carbolic acid, or of iodoform, freely rubbed into the surfaces. Of course, any calculus should be extracted, and if the sinus tracts are lined by earthy salts, they should be well rubbed, or scraped with a blunt scoop.

The treatment by retention of a catheter in the bladder is disappointing, though in some cases successful. Boyer relates a case of a young man of Abbeville who had worn a catheter for eleven months, and whose fistula closed within a few days after the catheter was removed.

Injections are of little value, especially in chronic cases. The thermo-cautery is more likely to succeed. The plan recommended by É. Forgue, if the fistulæ are numerous, sinuous, and complicated with burrowing tracts and old indurations, is to open the urethra from the perinæum, lay open the sinuses, scrape away or excise the indurated tissues around the fistulæ, and resect any peri-urethral nodules.

3. URETHRO-RECTAL FISTULÆ.

They are sometimes traumatic, having been made at the time of, or following, lithotomy, or in the course of the operation of excision of the rectum. Rarely, they have resulted from the ulceration of foreign bodies, either from the urethra into the rectum, or *vice versâ*. Suppuration in or about the prostate is, in the great majority of cases, the cause of these fistulæ. The double opening of periprostatic abscesses into the rectum and into the urethra is very common. Segond found that in twenty-one out of forty-three cases of this sort, the abscesses opened into the urethra as well as into the rectum.

In some cases, the periprostatic abscess communicates with an intraprostatic pouch, and thus with the urethra; in others, the abscess takes a course behind the prostate gland and opens into the membranous urethra. Tuberculous disease of the prostate and cancer of the prostate are other causes of these fistulæ.

Pathological Anatomy.—There is usually a prostatic or retroprostatic cavity which is the meeting-place of the fistulous tracks opening respectively into urethra and bowel. In old cases, the walls of the space are thick and indurated, and the cavity itself is covered with a sort of false mucous membrane which renders it tolerant of its urinous and fæcal contents.

The urethral orifice is single, and generally in the prostatic urethra on one side of the veru montanum. It is rarely in the membranous urethra. As the urethral orifice is almost always situated on a higher level than the rectal, it is much easier for the urine to escape into the rectum than for fæces to get into the urethra. The course of the fistula is usually sinuous and branched, and its walls are indurated.

The rectal opening is above the sphincter; it is sometimes masked by a tongue of mucous membrane, and, though sometimes small, is in other cases wide and easily detected.

These fistulæ sometimes open by a branch sinus in the perinæum, or in the groin, or in the thigh. Sometimes, in old cases, a kind of stricture of the rectum is caused by the bridling effect of the tough and contracted connective tissue outside and around the bowel.

Symptoms and Diagnosis.—Urine escapes into the rectum and accumulates above the sphincter ani, and is discharged as the fæces are. The mucous membrane is not always well tolerant of urine; and if the latter be septic, an inflammation of the mucous membrane of the bowel of a dysenteric character may be excited.

In some cases there is a frequent and considerable escape of semen into the bowel, quite independent of erections, as well as by ejaculation at the time of coitus.

Fluid fæcal matter may get into the urethra and be discharged at the meatus, or into the bladder, and set up acute cystitis. A patient under my care some years ago with cancer of the rectum used to pass rectal gas when micturating, and bubbles of air emerged from the urethra with the urine, bursting as they dropped on to the ground or in the vessel. The poor fellow described them as being like to round clear "bladders" or berries.

The diagnosis is clear if rectal gas or fæcal matter passes per urethram; but if this is not the case, a small quantity of urine passed into the rectum is likely to be overlooked. An examination with the finger in the rectum and a sound in the bladder will often discover the cause of the fistula, as well as reveal the existence of the rectal orifice. If the orifice is obscured by a fold of mucous membrane, it may be detected at once by injecting coloured fluid down the urethra, or by getting the patient to micturate whilst the surgeon inspects the rectum by the aid of the speculum.

Treatment and Prognosis.—The treatment consists in endeavouring to keep the fistula dry of urine by drawing it off through a catheter retained in the bladder. Sir Henry Thompson cured a young man in six weeks by insisting on his passing urine whilst lying on his stomach, and never in any other position. In a very severe case under my care at the Middlesex Hospital in December, 1886, I drained the bladder by supra-pubic cystotomy, after fruitless trial of perinæal section and erasion of fistulæ at another hospital. This treatment, especially if followed by erasion or excision of the callous fistulous tracts, promises to give excellent results in very bad cases which have resisted other methods. Some cases in which the fistulæ arise from a prostatic abscess heal spontaneously after several weeks.

It should be an object to keep the rectum clean by daily washing it out with boracic or weak mercuric lotion. When the fistulous track is hard and callous, it should be slit open and scraped, or cauterised, and arfy bands of callous, fibrous tissue between the rectum and bladder, or prostate, should be divided. Various rather extensive operations with the object of completely detaching the rectum from the prostate, and closing each of the openings into the bowel have been recommended or performed by Astley Cooper, Tillaux, Quenu, and É. Forgue. Mr. T. Myles, of the Richmond Hospital, Dublin (*Med. Press*, Dec. 6, 1893), after establishing supra-pubic drainage, cut out the fistulous tracks and made a longitudinal incision in the roof of the urethra opposite the deficiency in its floor, and was thereby able to suture the cut edges of the floor together around a No. 8 catheter. The result was a complete success.

When the urethra is wounded, as it easily may be in some cases, during excision of the rectum, the fistula rapidly closes as the healing of the wound progresses.

URETHRAL FISTULÆ OPENING EXTERNALLY THROUGH THE WALLS OF THE ABDOMEN.

In extravasation of urine from stricture of, or injury to, the urethra, and also occasionally after lithotomy, the urine may find its way behind the triangular ligament into the pelvic cellular tissue, when, unless death quickly takes place, suppuration is excited, and matter may point above Poupart's ligament on one side or the other. Thus a urinary fistula is formed. I have seen this happen after lateral lithotomy; the pus burrowed up through the pelvis and along the spermatic cord, and was let out below the external abdominal ring. The patient, a man aged fifty-six, died fourteen days after the lithotomy, from a large abscess in the liver.

When the urine, after extravasation in front of the triangular ligament, finds its way beneath the skin of the abdomen, it may travel as high as the umbilicus, and a fistula may form in the groin or elsewhere upon the front or side of the abdomen.

In these cases, as in those of deeper-seated extravasation, suppuration is generally very free, but the fistulous opening will soon emit urine if the patient lives through the period of suppuration. Wilmot relates a case of extravasation of urine from a ruptured urethra, complicated with fracture of the left ramus of the pubis. Perinæal fistula formed, and others opened in the thighs, right groin, and above the pubes. All of them discharged urine, nearly the whole of which fluid escaped by the fistula for more than a year, until Mr. Cusack, under whose care the patient was, re-established the normal urethra by dividing a fold of false membrane which had been obstructing the canal opposite to the seat of fracture. Sir Benjamin Brodie found, after death, " a large abscess in front of the pubis, extending half-way towards the navel ; another among the muscles of the right thigh, as far outwards as the foramen ovale of the ischium, the periosteum having been destroyed and the bone itself rendered carious ; and all these abscesses could be traced into an abscess in the perinæum, communicating with the urethra, behind a stricture, by a small orifice." In an interesting inaugural dissertation on " Urinary Fistulæ," by J. Antonius Jagielski, a case is related of a farm-labourer, who, in June, 1819, was gored by a bull, the horn of which passed through the middle of the right thigh, towards the perinæum and scrotum, blood trickling from the urethra. A stricture of the urethra followed ; an immense urinary fistula resulted, and opened on the inner and posterior aspects of the upper part of the thigh, in the scrotum, and in the ischial regions ; urine had also burrowed amid the cellular tissue of the pelvis, and led to a large stinking abscess, as well as to contraction of the tissue around the rectum, with exposure of the three inferior sacral nerves.

Matter pent up behind the deep perinæal fascia is likely to burrow in the pelvic cellular tissue, and, dissecting its way by the side of the bladder, to open into the vagina, rectum, or some other part of the bowel ; and thus to establish a complete uretero-rectal, or uretero-vaginal, or vesico-rectal, or vesico-vaginal fistula. (*See* Chap. XII. Part III.)

Treatment.—No general rules can be laid down, but enough has been said to show that the cause of the fistula must be ascertained, and the treatment directed accordingly.

One thing will always be requisite, namely, to establish a free and, if possible, natural channel for the escape of urine. Thus, if stricture exists, it must be treated ; if a foreign body is in the bladder, it must be taken away. All causes of inflammation around the bladder must be removed, and, if extravasation has occurred, the prompt surgical treatment demanded for that emergency, and for the cause which has given rise to it, must be at once brought into effect.

In most cases the condition is very pitiable, and a cure is consequently all the more to be desired. Every act of micturition is attended with the escape of urine through the fistulous channel. When the channel is wide and direct, precaution can be taken to keep the clothes dry and clean ; but, when it is oblique or tortuous, the urine dribbles away long after the act of micturition is over, there is an ammoniacal odour always present, the clothes cannot be kept dry, nor the skin free from excoriation, and the state of the patient is one of loathing and disgust. If, in these circumstances, relief is not obtained, the health of the patient fails gradually and death ensues.

FISTULÆ CONNECTED WITH COWPER'S GLANDS.

Reliquet ("Fistules urétrales non-urinaires"—*Gazette des Hôpitaux*, 1885) has described a form of fistula opening near the orifice of the male urethra which is not in connection with the urethral canal. If the orifice is very small and close to the meatus, and the fistula is a source of a chronic purulent discharge, it may give rise to the diagnosis of gleet, and the patient may perhaps wrongly be suspected of having exposed himself to the contagion of gonorrhœa, of which the gleet is the result.

A fine bristle may be passed along such a fistula for two or three inches or more, running parallel with the urethra, but nowhere opening into it. Mr. R. Harrison states that he has seen the same kind of fistula on several occasions. Reliquet suggests that they arise from suppuration in connection with one of Cowper's glands, but this has not been actually proved to be their origin.

Treatment.—The occasional passage of a fine probe is in some cases enough to stimulate the fistula to heal soundly.

CHAPTER XI.

SACCIFORM DILATATIONS OF THE URETHRA.

POUCHES or sacciform cavities containing urine are occasionally formed by diverticula from the wall of the urethra.

They are sometimes congenital; sometimes the result of weakening of the wall by abscess or ulceration; and sometimes they follow injuries or operations. After a punctured wound of the urethra, the wound may heal, and then yield in the same way as an artery does in the formation of a traumatic aneurysm. After external urethrotomy, when urethral sutures have not been used, there is frequently developed a thin-walled pouch, in which urine collects in the situation of the cicatrix.

The largest of these pouches are formed behind a foreign body or a calculus long impacted; but most frequently they are sacciform dilatations of the floor of the urethra behind a stricture.

Their commonest situation is just·behind the scrotum. Much more rarely they occur in the spongy part of the urethra just in front of the scrotum, or just behind the glans penis.

When they dilate towards the perinæum they are oval or rounded swellings, sometimes of considerable size, covered with healthy integuments, which form with the stretched urethra thin, flaccid walls. When in connection with the spongy urethra they are oblong or sausage-shaped. They sometimes contain a calculus which may remain in the dilated sac, or which may shift out and in, as was the case in J. L. Petit's case. (*See* page 210, Urethral Calculi.)

Symptoms.—There may be a little leakage of urine continuing for a long time after micturition, and a little difficulty, as from stricture, in passing water. The urine may dribble away and wet the clothes for several minutes after the bladder seems to be emptied. If, then, an examination is made of the perinæum or under-surface of the penis during micturition there will be found a globular or sausage-shaped tumour below the urethra, and on pressing this between the fingers urine is discharged; but the sac may fill again as soon as pressure is relaxed. Generally, a little urine is left behind in the pouch or sac.

This swelling, which increases with each act of micturition, and can be made to disappear with the discharge of urine on compressing the swelling, is soft and painless, has no appearance of inflammation about it, and is covered by healthy integuments. These symptoms are characteristic and serve to exclude perinæal abscess, foreign bodies, or malignant disease. On passing a catheter its beak may be made to enter the pouch and to be felt in it by the fingers on the perinæum. If there be a stone either in the urethra or the sac, it will be felt, and might be removed by the lithotrite. If the extraction of the stone in this way is impossible, it must be removed by external urethrotomy, and then the pouch can be excised and the urethra closed by suture. So in cases of stricture, the stricture can be divided by external urethrotomy and the sac removed and the urethra sutured at the same time.

Treatment.—A catheter retained in the urethra may suffice to cause the contraction of small pouches communicating with the urethra by a narrow orifice, but for the larger sacs a perinæal incision and the partial excision of the walls of the sac, as well as the removal of the calculus or foreign body, or the division or dilatation of the stricture, will be needed.

CONGENITAL DILATATIONS.

Sacciform dilatations of congenital origin have been met with occasionally, and a few such have been recorded. (*See* Chap. IV. Part II.: On Congenital Malformations of the Urethra, pages 191—192.)

CHAPTER XII.

PAPILLOMA, POLYPI, AND CYSTS OF THE URETHRA.

PAPILLOMATA,

or vascular growths, excrescences or vegetations (as they are indifferently called), are often seen in the urethra of women, but are very rare in the male urethra.

Linhart, at a post-mortem examination on a male, found two small very vascular growths, consisting of a stroma of connective tissue covered with epithelium on the right wall of the urethra; and a little farther down near the bulb two similar very vascular and pedunculated growths were attached to the roof.

Similar tumours are to be seen in the Musée Dupuytren and in the Museum of Anatomy and Pathology at Vienna. They have been known to sprout from the cicatrix after division of a tight meatus.

A papilloma which grows but slowly in the navicular fossa, and which can be seen on separating the lips of the meatus, will increase rapidly as soon as it appears on the outside of the urethra.

When growing from the mucous membrane of the deeper parts of the urethra, they cannot often be diagnosed except with the aid of the endoscope. As a rule, they cause little, if any, obstruction to micturition, although sometimes the symptoms of stricture are present. They cannot be felt with a sound. Sometimes they cause considerable hæmaturia, or the feeling as of a foreign body in the urethra; there is often a slight chronic urethral discharge recurring, or aggravated by slight causes, and sometimes cystitis is excited, as in a case described by Sir Henry Thompson.

Their presence may be inferred if an instrument, passed easily and without pain, causes free bleeding, or if one, or a part of one, of these growths is caught in the eye of a catheter and removed.

MUCOUS POLYPI,

varying in size from a pin's head to a pea, were found, post-mortem, in a man who died of ischuria, by Roger. They were scattered in clusters over the urethra from the meatus to the bulb.

Small polypi, like nasal mucous polypi, have several times been accidentally caught and removed from the male urethra in the eye of a catheter. They may be pedunculated or sessile, and are met with in every part of the urethra, although the favourite site is near the meatus (Fig. 72). They vary in size from a hemp seed to a lentil or a pea, or larger, and are either single or multiple.

Treatment.—If one of these benign tumours should make its presence felt by feelings of discomfort in the urethra, by hæmorrhage, urethral discharge, or slight obstruction to micturition, it should be destro ed with the curette or nitrate of silver. If near the meatus, it can be seen and

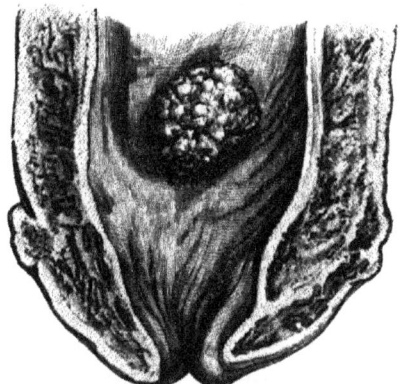

Fig. 72.—Polypus of Urethra. (*After Duplay and Reclus.*)

reached on separating the meatus. In many cases its exact location can be detected by the experienced surgeon by the slight catch or obstruction he meets with in searching the different parts of the urethral wall with a catheter or bougie.

If he does not thus succeed, the endoscope will often afford the necessary information on careful search being made with it. Gruenfeld, who has written upon Endoscopy, has described several different metallic snares, scissors, and forceps for extracting these growths under the light of the endoscope. But it is not so much as an adjunct to treatment as to diagnosis that this instrument is of service. When the exact situation of such a growth has been ascertained, the surgeon will be able to destroy it either by caustic, or the curette, or a catheter with a stylet which exactly fills but glides smoothly within it. When the last-mentioned instrument is employed, the growth, when caught in the large eye of the catheter, the stylet being slightly withdrawn, is crushed off by quickly pushing the stylet home again into the end of the catheter.

CYSTS OF THE URETHRA.

Retention cysts formed in connection with the glands of the urethral mucous membrane are rare. Gruenfeld relates one about the size of a hemp seed, which was causing a urethral discharge, and which he detected and punctured with the aid of the urethroscope.

I have referred to a case of double congenital hydronephrosis with dilatation of the ureters caused by a cyst the size of a pea, found in the urethra near the bulb of a still-born male infant. (*See* page 190, Congenital Malformations.)

CYSTIC TUMOURS

of Cowper's glands have been described, but the accuracy of the diagnosis in some of the cases is a matter of question. They have been found in adults as well as in the new-born; some of small size indenting the floor of the urethra, others large enough to be felt in the perinæum, and even to bulge the perinæum between the anus and scrotum. In a case quoted by Émile Forgue, a man fifty-one years old had a perinæal tumour extending as far back as the anus, growing for four years; after the second year it broke and discharged a large quantity of viscid, inodorous fluid. It would close and reopen again about every three weeks. When punctured, 150 grammes of thick, grey viscid fluid were withdrawn. The patient refused further operation.

CHAPTER XIII.

CARCINOMA OF THE URETHRA.

PRIMARY cancer of the urethra is exceedingly rare, very difficult of diagnosis in its earlier phases, and almost hopelessly unfavourable for removal in its later. As an extension from the penis, prostate, or bladder it is not so very infrequent. In Reclus and Duplay, reference is made to several cases of primary cancer. In three, the patients were the subjects of old strictures, and had suffered for a long time from troubles in connection with micturition; in two, the presence of the tumour and trouble in passing water were first noticed at the same time. In all, the situation of the tumour was the perinæum. In two others a perinæal abscess formed about the growth and was opened by the surgeon, and in one of them, after the incision had been made, large masses of florid malignant granulations bathed in urine and surrounded by active inflammation appeared at the opening. In two other cases the perinæum ulcerated and became more or less riddled with fistulæ, from which urine mixed with pus and blood escaped. In one of these cases (Mikulicz's) a large fistulous opening formed at the peno-scrotal angle, and the penis was much swollen and very œdematous.

The *diagnosis* may be made by the history of the case, by means of the endoscope, or by examination per rectum. In one case, Grüenfeld, by means of the endoscope, discovered the growth in a man fifty-nine years of age, who had suffered for eight months from hæmorrhage from the· urethra and difficult micturition, which necessitated the use of the catheter every six or eight hours. The disease was situated at the prostatic portion of the urethra, and was seen to be ulcerated.

As this tumour could be felt per rectum, the endoscope cannot be considered to have told any more than the finger; that it was ulcerated, on its urethral aspect, was only what was to be inferred from the long-standing urethral hæmorrhages.

When ulceration or an incision has led to an opening in the perineum, or fistulæ have formed, the ichorous discharge, and the budding outgrowths of the tumour from these

s

openings, and the enlarged inguinal glands sufficiently declare the nature of the disease. A microscopical examination of a piece of the exposed growth will clinch the diagnosis.

Mr. Marcus Beck reported a case of primary squamous carcinoma of the bulb of the urethra ("International Clinics," vol. ii., 2nd series, 1892), and collected ten other cases of primary cancer of the urethra, in five of which the diagnosis was confirmed by microscopic examination. Mr. Beck thought it possible that in some of these the cancer might have commenced in the skin around a perinæal fistula and not from the urethra.

The *symptoms* of primary cancer of the urethra are described by Mr. Beck as follows (*opus cit.*):—"It occurs in men over fifty who have most commonly suffered from some previous disease of the canal, usually gonorrhœal stricture. The most prominent symptom is the gradual formation of a hard lobulated mass round the urethra. Micturition becomes increasingly difficult, and is almost always very painful—far more so than in simple stricture. Hæmorrhage, especially before and after micturition. . . . The corpora cavernosa and their crura become implicated, and the disease advances past the scrotum into the penile portion of the urethra. The glands in the groin enlarge, and the patient looks cachectic. The passage of instruments is from the beginning difficult, and is always followed by bleeding. The next stage of the disease is the formation of a foul cavity containing blood-stained purulent fluid in connection with the urethra. The discharge from this may be recognised escaping from the urethra. As the cavity enlarges, a perinæal abscess forms, which reaches the surface, bursts, and leaves a fistula. The carcinomatous growth then extends to the skin and superficial structures along the line of the fistula."

Mr. R. Harrison is of opinion that instances are met with where urinary fistulæ become epitheliomatous. The openings usually, he says, present a worm-eaten appearance, are indurated and warty, and no kind of treatment does any permanent good. The object should be to prevent the supervention of cancer on chronic indolent fistulæ. Many a cancerous ulcer might be averted by timely surgical treatment or removal of any fistulous track which shows signs of being the seat of continuous irritation. ("Surgical Disorders of the Urinary Organs," 4th ed., p. 167.)

Treatment can be but palliative. Great comfort will be given by draining the bladder. Mikulicz, in his case, enlarged the fistulous channels, scraped away the masses of cancer, and amputated the penis; but the disease almost immediately returned. If, however, relief to suffering can be afforded by partial operations, they ought to be undertaken, just as they rightly are in the same disease of the tongue, face and elsewhere.

MALIGNANT DISEASE OF COWPER'S GLANDS.

This is very rare. One or two isolated cases—namely, those of Pacquet, Kocher, and Gussenbauer—have been reported. Gussenbauer's case was a soft carcinoma, the others cylindromata. Pacquet's case was an encapsuled tumour the size of a nut, hard, and adherent only with the bulb of the urethra. The patient was sixty-five years old.

The tumour operated upon by Kocher sent branches into the parts around, one of which was adherent to the right ischio-pubic ramus, and another projected over the dorsum of the penis beneath the symphysis; it was intimately connected with the urethra and the front wall of the rectum. The patient was fifty-seven. In Gussenbauer's case, which was one of cancer in a lad aged nineteen, the tumour had a narrow connection with the membranous urethra and involved the bulbo-cavernosus muscle and the wall of the rectum; the lymphatic glands were early and widely affected, and the growth of the tumour was very rapid, having fully developed in two months. A catheter was obstructed at the bulb before the tumour was removed, but not afterwards.

When not encapsuled and limited as in Pacquet's case, but large, branched, or widely spread, it must be impossible to be sure that the disease originated in either of Cowper's glands.

In Pacquet's and Kocher's cases there was no difficulty with the catheter, but there were early difficulties with micturition and defæcation, and pain in walking and sitting.

Treatment.—The early and complete removal would be the treatment, but the operation, if delayed, may be extensive and very complicated, or even impossible.

CHAPTER XIV.

INJURIES OF THE PROSTATE.

FROM the protected position of the prostate behind the arch of the pubis, injuries to it are very rare.

Wounds from without inwards are inflicted on the gland occasionally in the old operation of puncture per rectum for retention of urine, and in lateral or median lithotomy; others from within outwards, as in false passages. Surgical wounds are more frequent than accidental ones, although the prostate is liable to lacerations and contusions in fractures of the pelvis, and may be punctured or lacerated by a foreign body introduced through the rectum, or may be impaled on a spike entering from the perinæum. Gunshot wounds are very rare.

Infiltration of urine and hæmorrhage are the two risks.

Infective phlebitis is not unlikely in an organ so richly vascularised.

Bleeding may be free and even alarming, either by way of the urethra or through the wound; or blood may flow back into the bladder, especially if the neck of the bladder shares in the injury.

Extravasation to some extent must occur if the prostatic urethra is involved, and may spread either in the deep or superficial perinæum, according as the deep perinæal fascia is wounded as well as the prostate, or not.

Wounds inflicted from the perinæum or rectum may cause violent hæmorrhage without damage to the urethra; and in fractures of the pelvis the gland may be much contused or pulped without the urethra being entered.

Incontinence occurs if the neck of the bladder is divided..

The ejaculatory ducts may be divided or otherwise damaged as they traverse the prostate, and may in consequence become subsequently obstructed.

Treatment.—This will depend on the amount of hæmorrhage and the tendency, or otherwise, to extravasation of urine. A catheter retained in the bladder will allow of the wound, if in communication with the perinæum, being packed with iodoform gauze, or the lithotomy petticoat plug, or the expansion bag of Buckston Brown may answer better.

If hæmorrhage cannot be stopped by these means, or by the application of ice to the perinæum, rectum, and hypogastrium, or by the internal use of ergot of rye, a free incision made in a crescentic manner across the perinæum in front of the anus will probably enable the surgeon to directly control the bleeding vessels. If the wound is of the nature of an incised or incised punctured one, aseptic sutures should be introduced into the wounded parts; they may even be sufficient, when judiciously placed, to completely control bleeding. Sutures would be worse than useless in contused and contused lacerated wounds, as they might tend, by shutting in discharges, to promote sepsis.

CHAPTER XV.

ACUTE PROSTATITIS AND PERIPROSTATITIS.—ACUTE PROSTATIC AND PERIPROSTATIC ABSCESS.

Acute prostatitis arises from various causes, direct and indirect. Amongst the so-called direct causes are injuries, inflammation extending from neighbouring organs, various direct irritants such as caustics to the urethra, cantharides internally administered, irritation caused by the use of instruments or by calculi or foreign bodies in the prostate. Again, the congestive states induced by horse exercise, by sedentary habits, constipation, masturbation, and excessive coitus are included by Segond amongst the direct causes. The so-called indirect causes are cold, sitting on iron or stone seats, or on wet grass or damp cushions; and the infective diseases.

There are few if any observations to prove that cold or many of the above-named so-called direct causes, apart from urethritis, gonorrhœa, or gleet, have ever produced acute prostatitis or acute prostatic abscess. A few cases are on record of suppuration of the prostate occurring in the course of variola, suppurative phlebitis, and other infectious diseases; but it is very doubtful whether many of the other supposed causes ever do more than predispose to prostatitis.

Injuries, the presence of calculi in the prostate, the irritation which goes on behind an old narrow stricture of the urethra, are certainly occasional causes; but gonorrhœa and gleet are, beyond all question, the common causes of the disease. Segond found sixty-nine out of ninety-eight cases of prostatic abscess due to gonorrhœa. In most cases the acute inflammation of the gland commences about fourteen days or later after the onset of the gonorrhœa. In some cases no satisfactory cause can be assigned.

I have had under my care a case of very acute prostatic abscess in a young gentleman twenty-two years of age, which developed during convalescence from nephrolithotomy, and for which no satisfactory cause could be assigned. He had no urethral discharge, no anal trouble, and no instruments had been used in the urethra till the catheter was passed for the relief of the retention caused by the inflamed prostate.

Pathological Anatomy.—In the early and middle periods the prostate is much swollen, the prostatic venous plexus loaded with blood, and the urethral mucous membrane is somewhat congested. On section, a reddish, turbid fluid exudes, composed of a mixture of blood, serum, and the prostatic secretion. A little later this fluid contains pus, and the gland ducts, distended with pus, may be seen as minute whitish-yellow spots. Still later these pus spots increase in number and size and coalesce. Sometimes hæmorrhages or little masses of gangrenous tissue are found in the prostatic tissue.

The pus from a prostatic abscess is said to have a peculiar glutinous character; but I have seen very typical pus, as from any acute abscess elsewhere, passed per urethram, or let out by an incision from prostatic abscesses.

Recent histological researches show that the first lesion is of the epithelial elements, and that the interstitial changes, which may pass on rapidly into suppuration, are secondary.

The different parts of the prostate are affected in different degrees; some portions are intensely inflamed, whilst others remain healthy.

Lallemand first pointed out that the ejaculatory ducts became dilated and ulcerated and bathed in pus, and may be ultimately quite destroyed. Even the vesiculæ seminales may contain pus. Blood has been mixed with the semen when discharged during acute prostatitis. The testicles wasted in one case after prostatic abscess.

Periprostatitis and periprostatic abscess occur in the cellular tissue of the space between the rectum and prostate and the deep triangular ligament of the peritoneum; and though they may be secondary to inflammation of the rectum, bladder, or vesiculæ seminales, they are most frequently developed as extensions from acute prostatitis. The extension may take place by several routes, by the cellular tissue itself, or by the veins or lymphatics.

Segond and Guyon describe two forms of periprostatic abscesses, viz. those which occur by "diffusion"—*i.e.* when the intra-prostatic abscess breaks into the surrounding cellular tissue, and those which occur by "propagation" of the inflammation, whether along the lymphatics, veins, or the cellular tissue. Sometimes the inflammation or abscess is periprostatic at the outset, the prostate being but little inflamed; in other patients, on the contrary, the inflammation has throughout the disease affected the prostate and the surrounding cellular tissue equally. The periprostatic abscesses are always situated behind the prostate, and are in some cases quite limited and small, and in others large and diffused, dissecting out and bathing in pus, the rectum, vasa deferentia, and vesiculæ seminales. Tortuous and chronic fistulæ sometimes follow.

Symptoms.—The symptoms caused by these affections are very similar, and are at first a sensation of weight and fulness in the perinæum and some pain at the neck of the bladder. Micturition is more frequent, and is painful, especially towards the end of the act. There is rectal tenesmus. The pain increases and becomes throbbing, and is felt in an agonising degree when urine comes in contact with the urethra and the sphincter vesicæ is in action. The perinæum is tender and hot. Defæcation is very painful, and the anus is swollen and prominent, and large piles may form. At length there is retention, and the catheter has to be used, causing alarm and intense physical suffering. On introducing the finger into the rectum great pain is caused, and the bowel is felt to be tumid, soft, and very hot; large arteries are felt throbbing in the wall of the bowel, the outline of the prostate is very distinct, and the gland itself excessively tender and projecting against the bowel. In periprostatitis the outline of the gland is lost.

If suppuration has occurred the prostatic swelling as felt per rectum is soft, and, maybe, gives a sense of fluctuation, especially if the perinæum is at the same time pressed upon by the fingers of the other hand. If suppuration has not occurred, the gland feels tense and more or less hard. Pains in the loins, groins, and down the thighs are constantly experienced. Painful erections may occur. Fever, with its attendant constitutional symptoms, occurs at the outset of the local symptoms, and increases as the local changes heighten. Rigors most probably usher in the suppurative stage, which, as Desault says, is to be expected if the symptoms of inflammation continue to the eighth day, and if, having gone on increasing up to this time, they subside for a while, to increase again with a fresh rise of evening temperature.

As the abscess ripens, one of two or three things may happen, if it is left to take its own course. It may burst into the urethra spontaneously, or it may be ruptured by the introduction of a catheter to relieve retention, or it may burst into the rectum, either directly or after having caused a " diffusion " abscess in the periprostatic tissue.

Segond has recorded that fifty-five out of one hundred and fifteen intra-prostatic abscesses discharged per urethram either spontaneously or after having been ruptured by a catheter or sound. Abscesses which discharge in this direction generally get quickly well ; but if the exit for the pus is not free enough, troublesome and tortuous fistulæ may form in the neighbouring parts, and urinary infiltration or purulent infection may result, unless a free opening is provided by making an incision into the prostate from the perinæum.

Periprostatic abscesses may break either into the rectum or forwards in the front part of the perinæum, or at the side of the anus on the perinæum, or into the membranous urethra. Segond, analysing seventy-seven cases as to the course taken by the pus, divides them into three groups—the frequent, the rare, and the exceptional. The frequent are those which open into the rectum and urethra, perinæum and ischio-rectal fossæ. He found twenty-one out of sixty-seven cases opened both into the urethra and rectum. The rare cases are those which open in the inguinal and obturator regions; and the exceptional cases into the peritoneum, at the umbilicus, or at the great sacro-sciatic foramen.

Diagnosis.—The sense of weight in the perinæum, the pain and straining at stool, the still greater pain in micturition, the retention of urine, and the detection of a large, hot, pulsating swelling against the front wall of the lower part of the rectum, together with the fever, and perhaps the attendant rigors, form a group of symptoms which ought at once to lead the practitioner to diagnose acute inflammation or abscess of the prostate.

. There are, however, cases, rare though they be, in which the diagnosis cannot be made for certain, though the condition is suspected in spite of the absence of some of the most characteristic symptoms. I have witnessed this difficulty in the case of a short, thick-set, middle-aged gentleman whom I attended with Mr. S. Mills, and who a year previously had had a left lumbar swelling diagnosed as inflammatory and connected with the kidney. He had recovered from this illness without any operation, except that he had since always passed a little pus in his urine. He had not had any urethral discharge or bladder trouble, till one day (April 3rd, 1894) he complained of having to strain a good deal to pass water. This went on increasing till April 11th, when his bladder was sounded. On the following day (April 12th) complete retention set in, and he required frequent catheterisation till April 15th. There was no fever whatever, no pain or tenderness about the perinæum, no actual pain when a Jacques catheter was passed, no pain, or tenderness, or heat in the rectum, and no enlargement of the prostate detectable. He was able to get up, and walked daily from room to room, and, but for the retention and the feeling of irresistible and urgent straining to pass water, he felt quite well. At 9 a.m. on April 15th I passed a soft catheter to draw off his urine, and he remarked that it went in more easily than upon any previous occasion. I also at this time examined him per rectum, and again with negative result. In the evening of the same day he had an urgent desire to pass water, strained to do so, and whilst straining about two ounces of thick, laudable pus suddenly passed from his urethra, and immediately afterwards he relieved his bladder. The greater part of the urine voided on this occasion was passed into a separate vessel, and it was seen to be clear and normal-looking, and contained no more albumen or pus than it had done any time during the previous twelve months. From this time there was no relapse of the retention, and the patient made a satisfactory recovery.

The fever of simple acute prostatitis or of a small periprostatic abscess is not necessarily very great; there is generally a sudden elevation of one or two degrees for some few days, which subsides entirely at the period of defervescence. If the fever is prolonged, with evening elevations, the probability is there is pus pent up. When the temperature is very irregular, going up occasionally two or three degrees, phlebitic complications and purulent infection are to be feared. In traumatic cases the temperature may rise suddenly, and at once, to a very high point, and assume the character of the temperature of urinary fever. There is but little difference in the symptoms of acute prostatitis and acute periprostatitis; the dysuria is perhaps less, the sense of weight more diffused, and defæcation is perhaps more painful in periprostatitis than in prostatitis; and on examination per rectum, instead of feeling the prostate enlarged and tender, with its outline more distinct, as it is in prostatitis, the gland is masked by a doughy, ill-defined mass.

From inflammation of the neck of the bladder acute prostatitis and periprostatitis can generally be diagnosed by digital examination per rectum. From acute inflammation of Cowper's glands the diagnosis can be made in the same way and also by the fact that the greater tenderness and swelling are in the fore part of the perinæum in inflammation and abscess of Cowper's glands, and rectal symptoms are generally absent.

From stricture, hypertrophy of the prostate, and vesical calculus they are to be diagnosed by the sudden onset and acuteness of the symptoms, by the fever and other constitutional disturbances, and by the introduction of a sound.

Prognosis.—Recovery is the common termination when the abscess breaks into the urethra, or is opened in good time by the perinæum. So when they open into the rectum before the matter accumulates largely, or is widely spread, a rapid cure often follows. When both urethra and rectum are penetrated, troublesome fistulæ, with the discharge of more or less, or the whole, of the urine by the anus, may follow. Fistulæ also follow the spontaneous openings in the ischio-rectal fossæ; and, unless an early incision is made, the pus burrows forwards in the perinæum, and the corpora cavernosa may be dissected out, or the skin of the penis undermined, as in two cases under Guyon and Demarquay respectively.

The total destruction of the parenchyma of the prostate may leave a chasm incapable of being filled up, and which may be the meeting-place of several fistulæ; or, as is also the case when the prostate is destroyed by calculi, incontinence of urine may be the result, owing to the shrinking of the prostate and the consequent change at the neck of the bladder. Exhaustion, hectic, septicæmia, or pyæmia are the most common causes of death. Segond states that out of twenty-five fatal cases, death was caused by pyæmia in nine.

Treatment.—From the outset of the symptoms, hot fomentations to the perinæum, and the injection of hot water at frequent intervals into the rectum, should be employed, as they give much comfort by diminishing pain, mitigating the straining, and making micturition easier. Leeches to the perinæum, followed by a hot hip bath, relieve the congestion and swelling of the prostate and stop much of the pulsating pain. Morphia (gr. $\frac{1}{2}$) combined with belladonna (gr. $\frac{1}{4}$) in a suppository is useful as a palliative of pain and spasms. So also are suppositories of cocaine (gr. 1), but they need more frequent repetition.

To relieve retention a Jacques catheter, or a soft coudée if the Jacques will not pass, of No. 5 or No. 6 size, is the best instrument.

Frequent—*i.e.* every second day or so—digital examination of the prostate per rectum should be made, and as soon as pus is diagnosed, either by the softening of the prostate or the swelling of the cellular tissue, or by the occurrence of increased tension, and perhaps of rigors, a free deep incision into the prostate, or periprostatic tissue, as the case may be, should be made from the raphé of the perinæum. For the last twenty years I have employed this plan. The operation is easily done when the patient is in the lithotomy position. First make an incision in the raphé of the perinæum about an inch long, ending behind about half an inch in front of the anus, through the skin and subcutaneous tissues, avoiding the urethra in front and the rectum behind; then with the index finger of the left hand in the rectum, on the apex of the prostate, a long straight bistoury (I always prefer one with a double-cutting edge) should be introduced into the wound and pushed steadily upwards parallel with the finger in the rectum till the pus trickles down its surface; the knife should be kept *in situ* till with the left hand a grooved director has been passed along the blade into the abscess, then the knife should be withdrawn and a pair of dressing forceps introduced along the groove of the director and the blades separated so as to dilate the opening of the abscess; after this is done the forceps should be withdrawn and a drain tube introduced into the cavity of the abscess. The drain tube should be tied in, and hot antiseptic fomentations should be applied and continued for twenty-four hours. Subsequently, dry antiseptic dressings should be kept over the wound. The drain tube should be removed when the discharge has almost ceased, and the wound should then be allowed to heal.

It is only when an abscess has so far worked its way towards the rectum that it is almost through the rectal wall that it should be opened, or be allowed to open spontaneously in this direction. Even when far advanced towards the rectal wall, the pus may be successfully diverted by the perinæal incision. Very serious hæmorrhage will follow an incision through the rectal wall, unless care is taken to avoid the dilated and forcibly pulsating arteries in it.

In some cases which have spontaneously discharged into the urethra, no improvement follows until a free incision in the perinæum has provided a ready and direct exit for the pus. I have had to operate on a few such cases, and have found immediate benefit was experienced and a rapid cure effected by the perinæal incision.

CHAPTER XVI.

CHRONIC PROSTATITIS AND PROSTATORRHŒA.

Since the publication, in 1857, of a memoir on this subject by Hawkesworth Ledwich (*The Dublin Quarterly Journal of Med. Sciences*, t. xxiv. p. 30, August, 1857), text-books have generally devoted a chapter to chronic prostatitis. Swédiaur (1809) and Lagneau (1815), writers on syphilitic and venereal diseases, had referred to it as one of the complications or results of gonorrhœa. Gross, of Philadelphia, contributed to our knowledge of prostatorrhœa; Guyon has still more recently written on the chronic prostatitis in his admirable "Leçons Chirurgicales"; and E. Forgue has contributed an excellent summary of what is known of the affection ("Traité de Chirurgie" of Duplay and Reclus). Sir Henry Thompson has examined several cases and given an account of the morbid anatomy of the disease.

Etiology—Gonorrhœa is by some considered the only—it is certainly the chief—cause of chronic prostatitis. The gonococcus, by passing into the gland ducts and glands of the prostate from the deep urethra, sets up in these structures an inflammation very difficult to cure. Cold and damp, venereal excesses, old-standing stricture, chronic cystitis, and calculus are said by Sir Henry Thompson to be occasional causes. The patients who suffer chiefly are the neurotic and the weakly. It affects men of this sort between the twentieth and fortieth years, when gonorrhœa is most prevalent, when the sexual fires are at their height, and when the genital functions most engage their attention.

Pathological Anatomy.—The prostate may or may not be enlarged, but is a little less firm and somewhat more spongy than normal. On section, more fluid than usual issues from the tissue; it is of a dirty colour, and may be mixed with blood or pus. A few deposits of pus, from the size of pearl barley to that of a pea, are scattered in the tissue, or there may be a chronic abscess of some considerable size communicating with the urethra. The mucous membrane of the prostatic urethra may be more vascular and the duct orifices dilated, or the surface may be coated in places with organised lymph. There may be one or more chronic periprostatic abscesses behind the prostate.

Symptoms.—A little muco-purulent discharge from the urethra and a slight increase in the frequency of micturition are the early symptoms; then is experienced a sensation of weight, and perhaps a little dull pain, in the perinæum, increased by standing, walking, or horse exercise, and by sexual intercourse. Aching about the groins, loins, and thighs is experienced, and on digital examination per rectum there is some increased sensitiveness on pressing the prostate. On introducing a catheter or sound, increased sensitiveness, if not actual pain, is complained of, and the surgeon will often detect a creaking sensation like that of wet leather, if he is observant, just before the instrument enters the bladder. At the end of micturition there may be a little pain, and occasionally a drop or two of blood, and sometimes even more, so that vesical calculus will very likely be suspected. Sir Henry Thompson says :—" I know no other complaint in which the symptoms so strongly resemble those of stone in the bladder in a mild form." He also lays stress upon the diagnostic value of having the urine of the same micturition passed into two vessels, when it will be found that the first part contains shreds of tenacious muco-pus and epithelium, whilst the second and remainder part is clear, or nearly so.

· The patients may have diminished sexual desire and power, yet may be troubled with seminal emissions. They are nervous and debilitated men as a rule.

If a chronic abscess forms and bursts into the urethra, it may go on suppurating for a long time; urine gets into the abscess, keeps up irritation, and causes pain and decomposition, and in this manner the patient may be worn out or killed by septic infection or purulent phlebitis.

Diagnosis.—There is a form of chronic prostatitis which is the sequel of acute prostatitis. It is marked by induration and enlargement of the organ, due to the unabsorbed inflammatory products of the acute stage, and is sometimes mistaken for senile hypertrophy of the prostate. But chronic prostatitis ought not to be confused with hypertrophy. Inflammatory enlargement affects the young adult and middle periods of life; is almost always preceded by gonorrhœa, or a urethral discharge, or an acute prostatitis; is accompanied by some pain in micturition; and occurs in men in weakly, nervous condition.

Hypertrophy, on the contrary, occurs only in elderly men, and is not associated with any of the above symptoms.

The simple chronic prostatitis does not always, or perhaps often, cause enlargement of the organ, and is not preceded by acute prostatitis, so that it is easily distinguished from the chronic inflammatory affection which is the remnant of the acute attack. The latter does not require for its treatment counter-irritation and caustic applications, but the internal administration of iodides and bromides and saline aperients.

Treatment.—These cases require to be treated by counter-irritation with blistering fluid applied to the perinæum every five or six days. Care must be taken not to let the blistering fluid irritate the anus or the scrotum, and the blistered surface should be dressed daily by a little unguentum boracis. This treatment should be tried for six or seven weeks, and if there should still continue flocculent masses in the urine and pain at the neck of the bladder, with or without a little blood at the end of micturition, a solution of nitrate of silver (commencing with 5 grains to the ounce) or chloride of zinc (1 grain to the ounce) should be applied to the prostatic urethra by means of a perforated metal catheter carrying a piston and a sponge, so that the fluid can be squeezed out when the catheter reaches the prostatic part of the urethra. Rectal suppositories of iodoform (1 to $1\frac{1}{2}$ grain) and of ichthyol (4 to 5 grains) have been recommended. In certain chronic cases, when the prostate is enlarged but not painful, the cold douche to the perinæum may be tried daily.

The digestive organs should be attended to, the bowels kept open by a little compound extract of colocynth and nux vomica, and an unstimulating but simple and nutritious diet, and a mixture of iron and quinine should be taken. Cod-liver oil, pure air, and, if it can be obtained, a sea voyage are highly valuable.

If a chronic abscess forms and goes on discharging a quantity of pus per urethram for a length of time, an aseptic incision from the perinæum should be made into it.

PROSTATORRHŒA.

Causes.—This occurs occasionally in young men who have indulged in masturbation or undue sexual excitement, as well as in the habitually constipated, who have to strain a good deal to expel the contents of the rectum.

Symptoms.—It is characterised by the discharge of a ropy mucus of a greyish-white colour from the urethra at the end of micturition. The quantity varies from a few drops to a teaspoonful. It is sometimes attended with the presence in the urine of minute thread-like particles of inspissated mucus from the prostatic duct. It is due to a congestive state of the prostate gland, associated with dilatation of its follicles, but is not itself inflammatory, nor necessarily preceded by any inflammation of the prostate. It is attended by an extremely despondent state of mind, the patient often supposing that the discharge is seminal and that he is gradually becoming impotent.

Diagnosis.—It is to be distinguished from the discharge of chronic prostatitis or of folliculitis, as well as from ordinary gleet, by the discharge being entirely free of pus; from spermatorrhœa by the entire, or almost entire, absence of spermatozoa.

Prostatorrhœa is not necessarily preceded by gonorrhœa, being in fact most likely to affect those who have never had sexual connection.

Treatment.—The patient should be mentally reassured, and his fears should be removed by reasoning or ridicule. His mind should be healthily occupied. A nutritious but unstimulating diet should be taken. Tonics, especially quinine, strychnia, cod-liver oil, and perhaps iron, should be prescribed, and the bowels should be kept freely and regularly open. If he sleeps badly or is troubled by lascivious dreams, a draught of bromide of potassium and a little tincture of belladonna, or a pill of camphor and henbane, should be taken at night. The cold hip-bath night and morning, or the cold douche to the perinæum, is of much importance in remedying the dilated condition of the follicles and the general congestion of the gland to which the discharge is attributed. Dr. Hayes Agnew recommends that the sacrum, hips, and perinæum should be well whipped with a muscle-beater for ten minutes a day.

CHAPTER XVII.

CHRONIC ENLARGEMENTS OF THE PROSTATE.

THERE are several forms of chronic enlargement of the prostate, but it is necessary to draw a sharp distinction between two of them—namely, the inflammatory and the non-inflammatory. The inflammatory form is an affection of young and middle life, and has been already described, and the means of diagnosing it from the non-inflammatory have been mentioned on page 288.

We have now to consider the non-inflammatory forms, which are comprised under the ordinary name of Hypertrophy of the Prostate. These enlargements occur *only* in men past middle age; they are due to an excess of nutrition, yet are the result of senile changes which by no means invariably, or even usually, take place in elderly men. From a large number of observations Sir Henry Thompson's figures show that whilst it is probable that a slight tendency unrecognisable during life exists in one out of every three men over sixty, that only one out of every seven or eight at or over that age have any appreciable enlargement.

Etiology.—It would be quite useless to consider here the very numerous theories which have been advanced by most distinguished surgeons, from John Hunter to those of the present time, respecting the causation of enlarged prostate of elderly men. The reader who wishes to consider them must refer to the exhaustive chapter on this subject in Sir Henry Thompson's work on the Prostate.

This much should be stated, that inflammation is certainly not one of the causes. Nor are there good grounds for believing that either vesical calculus, urethral stricture, syphilis, gout and rheumatism, engorgement of hæmorrhoidal or prostatic veins, nor indulgence in sexual excesses in any way act as causes, beyond tending to an increased determination of blood to the part.

These enlargements never appear except in advanced years They do not exist during the period of greatest functional vigour of the gland, nor is their occurrence coincident with, or immediately subsequent to, the greatest and most prolonged sexual excesses. They are, therefore, not like hypertrophy in general, and have no analogy, for instânce, with hypertrophy of the kidney. Neither are they true hypertrophy of the gland in another sense, for in the great majority of instances the component tissues of the prostate are not all increased—certainly not all increased so as to preserve their relative proportions. Neither as a glandular nor as a muscular organ are they instances of hypertrophy, for it is neither the glandular nor the muscular tissue of the prostate that is commonly most developed.

The probable cause of these enlargements, as of the similar enlargements of the uterus—the only organ of the body like the prostate, both in the nature and arrangement of its component tissues—is a special proclivity or tendency of their structure, which may be, perhaps, brought into action by anything which induces an active determination of blood to these organs or their immediate locality.

Pathological Anatomy.—No new structures whatever are formed in any of these " chronic enlargements of elderly men." They consist simply of an augmentation of the normal elements of the gland, not necessarily, however, in the same relative proportions, nor arranged in the manner of the normal prostate.

Structurally regarded, Sir Henry Thompson groups them under four headings :—

A. True hypertrophy—*i.e.* over-development of the glandular and stromal tissues in normal proportions throughout the prostate. This is less frequent than the next and the fourth forms. The degree of enlargement is not very great.

B. Over-development of the white fibres, but not of the muscular fibres of the stroma, nor of the glandular elements. To this form the name of *Fibrous hyperplasia* is appropriately given. This is the most common form, and attains the largest size (Fig. 73). All the very large examples are of this nature. When the muscular as well as the white fibres are increased, it is a *Fibro-muscular hyperplasia.* But the muscular fibres are rarely, if ever, increased as much as the white fibres.

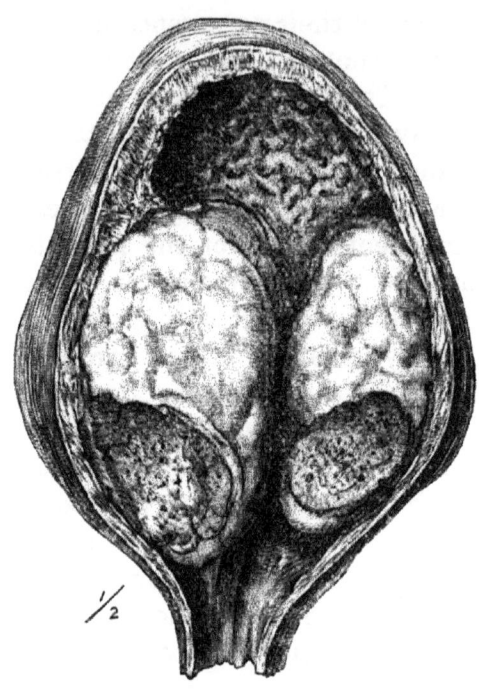

Fig. 73.—Lobulated Fibrous Hypertrophy of Prostate, forming a large Tumour half filling the Bladder. (Middlesex Hospital Museum.)

C. Excess of glandular tissue, not of the stroma, is the *Glandular hyperplasia.* It is very rare.

D. Simple tumour formations (Fig. 74). These are very frequently met with in prostates which are enlarged throughout, but occasionally they alone constitute the enlargement. They may consist either of glandular or stromal tissues, and may either be embedded in the substance of the prostate, or be more or less polypoid.

The embedded tumours are rounded masses distinct from the surrounding prostatic tissue, and are easily enucleated. They vary in size from one-tenth to five-eighths of an inch in diameter, and may be found in any part of the organ, in the lateral or median lobes, just under the capsule, or projecting the mucous membrane near the neck of the bladder.

In the polypoid outgrowths the glandular structure is generally more developed than in the embedded tumours. Like the latter, they may occur in any part of the gland, but the most frequent, and clinically the most important, are those from the median portion (Fig. 75). These form rounded swellings, varying in size from a

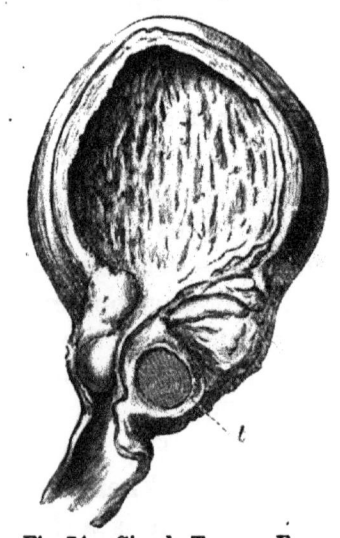

Fig. 74.—Simple Tumour Formation of the Prostate, *t.* (Middlesex Hospital Museum.) ("Manual of Surgery.")

pea to a small pear, standing up in front of the neck of the
bladder, or ultimately projecting into the cavity of the bladder.

They are always
continuous with
the rest of the
gland by means
of their own
ducts, which
open on the
floor of the
urethra.

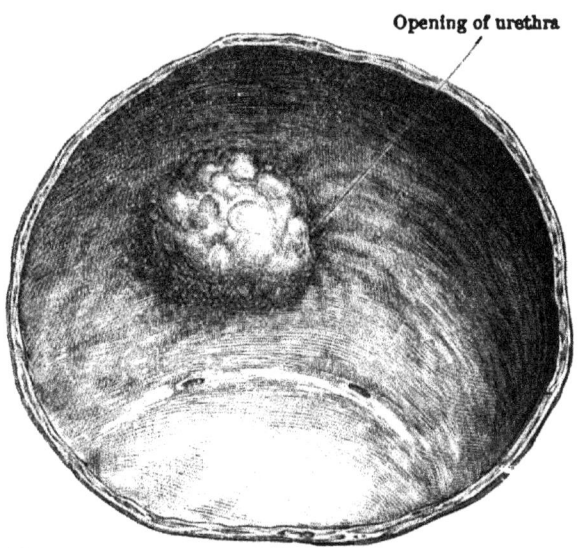

Opening of urethra

Fig. 75.—Median Prostatic Adenoma, sketched from
within the Bladder. From a Man sixty years of age.
(*After J. Bland Sutton.*)

The prostate
may be uni-
formly enlarged,
or the lateral
lobes may be
more enlarged
than the median
portion, or *vice
versâ*, or one
lobe may be much more enlarged than the opposite.

The most common form is for the whole gland to be
enlarged pretty equally throughout; and when one portion
predominates, it is more usually the central part.

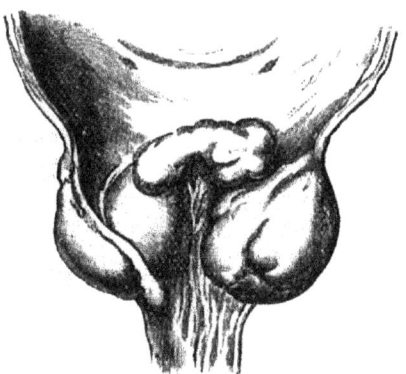

Fig. 76.—Hypertrophy in the Form of
Nodular Tumours of the Prostate.
(Middlesex Hospital Museum.)
("Manual of Surgery.")

The total amount of en-
largement varies much. It is
quite usual for it to amount
to double the natural weight,
which is six drachms, and in
exceptional cases great size
is attained, even that of a
cocoanut.

The enlarged prostate is
generally firmer and denser
than the normal, and on
section shows more variation
in colour. The cut surfaces
of the embedded isolated

mass stand prominently forth. There is more fluid than
normal oozing from the cut tissue of the glandular, and less

from that of the fibrous, hyperplasia than from the cut surface of the normal gland.

The anatomical changes wrought by the enlarged prostate on the prostatic urethra and the neck of the bladder are clinically of importance. Obstruction is the commonest effect, but incontinence is an occasional one. Obstruction, sometimes amounting to actual retention, is brought about by the chink-like narrowing of the urethra produced by the increase of the lateral lobes, or by an actual barrier caused either by the elevation of the middle portion or by a small tumour at the vesical orifice. Incontinence, which is very rare, exists when the urethro-vesical orifice is widened out in a crescentic manner by the increase of the posterior central portion, so that the urine escapes between the sides of the central eminence and the lateral lobes. The prostatic urethra is lengthened so as to measure, in some extreme cases, three inches instead of one inch and a quarter. It deviates to the right by enlargement of the left lobe alone, to the left by enlargement of the right lobe only, upwards by enlargement of the centre portion, or it may be tortuous by the unequal enlargement of different portions of the gland.

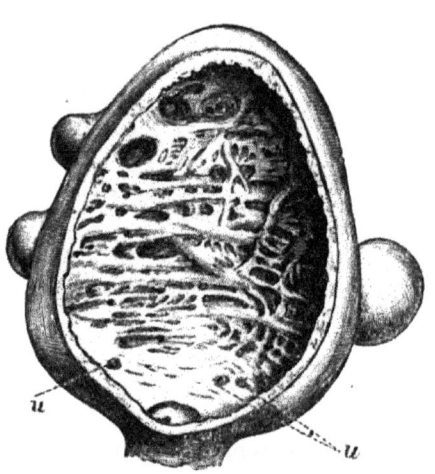

Fig. 77.—Hypertrophy with Sacculation of the Bladder. *u*, Orifices of the Ureter, double on the left side. (Middlesex Hospital Museum.) ("Manual of Surgery.")

The common effect upon the bladder is hypertrophy, with dilatation and sacculation (Fig. 77). The muscular trabeculæ are thickened and become very prominent, as seen from the interior of the viscus; strong interwoven bands project everywhere except at the trigone. The mucous and peritoneal walls are very thin, and sacculi are formed by the bulging outwards of the mucous layer between the muscular trabeculæ. Calculi and stagnant urine may lodge in the sacculi, or the wall of one of them may rupture. In some instances the bladder is found hypertrophied and contracted, more like the change which occurs from stricture; in other instances there is great dilatation, with little, if any, hypertrophy of muscular tissue. These differences depend partly on the suddenness and completeness of the obstruction caused by the enlarging prostate, and partly, perhaps chiefly, on the tone and physical strength of the individual. If the obstruction increases slowly, and the muscular power of the bladder is good, compensating efforts on the part of the bladder to overcome the obstruction will lead to hypertrophy, and only when this power is worn out will dilatation occur. If, on the other hand, the patient's powers are very enfeebled, dilatation will take place early, and there will be little or no hypertrophy of the vesical muscular tissue. Hence the differences observed in the post-mortem room.

Symptoms.—The onset of the symptoms is very insidious, and when the enlargement does not specially affect the central lobe, it may have advanced to a considerable degree before anything abnormal in connection with micturition is observed. Usually, the first symptom is an undue frequency of micturition with some difficulty in starting the stream, and with diminished power in projecting it. Increased effort to make the urine project clear of the trousers in some cases increases the difficulty, by bringing the bladder wall into closer contact with an enlarged middle lobe.

As the disease advances, the calls to micturate become more and more frequent, and micturition is not followed by the sense of complete relief. There is a feeling of fulness and weight in the perinæum and rectum not relieved by passing water. The patient often rises several times a night, and it is frequently owing to the disturbance of his night's rest —not to pain, which is rarely present, and not to the altered character of his stream, which he probably thinks natural to advancing age—that he is first induced to consult the surgeon

It is astonishing, not only that medical men sometimes do not appreciate the importance of these symptoms in their patients, but do not question their significance when occurring in themselves, and go on until they are brought face to face with their condition, which has been steadily increasing, by an attack of complete retention.

It thus occasionally happens that complete retention following a chill, an extra quantity to drink, or a slight prolongation of the interval from the last micturition, is the first announcement of the fact that the prostate is enlarged.

The patient will sometimes squat or lean forwards, so as to bring more force to bear on the bladder during micturition, and inguinal hernia is sometimes the result. The expulsive efforts of the bladder, aided by the action of the abdominal walls, lead to involuntary defæcation sometimes accompanying micturition. Hæmorrhoids and prolapsus ani are brought on ; and as the disease advances, soreness in the urethra, pain at the neck of the bladder, and radiating to the groins, thighs, and end of the penis, trouble the patient. Erections from simple turgescence, unaccompanied by sexual desire, annoy the patient, and dribbling of urine makes him uncomfortable and gives an offensive odour to his clothes.

This uncontrollable escape of urine occurs from different causes: (1) the last efforts of micturition may be powerless to empty his urethra, and thus a little urine escapes after the end of each act, just as occurs in some cases of stricture; (2) there is in rare cases actual incontinence from distortion by the middle lobe of the prostate of the urethro-vesical orifice ; (3) there is the incontinence of retention in cases where there is a very large quantity of residual urine left in the bladder after each act of micturition, and the catheter is not used ; (4) urine drains away during sleep, when voluntary control over the sphincter ceases ; but, later, during the daytime as well, from partial loss of voluntary control.

Hæmorrhage to a trifling degree sometimes occurs spontaneously after fatigue, exposure to cold, or excitement, and the blood may be either discharged externally or be retained in the bladder. Rough catheterism may cause very violent hæmorrhage ; and I have seen very considerable bleeding in cases of sudden acute retention of urine from congestion of the prostate, where due precaution and a soft catheter have been employed.

The alteration in the urine must be noted. At first a little residual urine, afterwards more and more, remains in the bladder; and though for a long time, owing to its constant admixture with the fresh secretion, its decomposition is prevented, yet at length changes occur. At first there is a slightly offensive odour and some turbidity, then the urine becomes ammoniacal and more and more offensive; a little muco-purulent discharge appears in the urethra, perhaps followed by some tenderness or swelling of the testicles, and a glairy, tenacious muco-pus, mixed with crystals of triple phosphates, may be deposited from the urine. The chemical reaction of the urine is neutral, then alkaline; it is generally of low specific gravity, rather increased in quantity, and deposits bladder epithelium, blood-corpuscles and pus cells, and triple phosphate crystals in abundance. Under these circumstances, vesical calculi are likely to form, and complicate and aggravate the prostatic symptoms, and set up cystitis. Acute cystitis may occur without the formation of calculus, in the later stages of the disease. The ureters and renal pelves become dilated, and secondary changes occur in them due to infection from the inflamed bladder. *Pari passu* with the renal changes, the general health suffers, rigors and attacks of fever occur, and uræmic poisoning, or septic infection and coma, bring about a fatal termination.

Diagnosis.—The increased frequency of micturition, the difficulty in starting the stream, the slow, narrow flow, which can only be projected a little way beyond the penis, and, perhaps, the dribbling of a few drops after the cessation of the expulsive efforts, when occurring in an elderly man, are sufficient to excite our suspicion; and if on examination per rectum an enlargement of the organ is discovered, we have sufficient evidence for making a diagnosis. Our next step should be to ask the patient to pass water. This he will do with the confident assurance at the end of the act that he has emptied his bladder. If now a soft catheter be at once passed, the surgeon will in all probability draw off an ounce or two or, it may be, several ounces of urine; and to the astonishment of the patient, and perhaps to his own also, this quantity of residual urine may amount to thirty or forty or even sixty ounces. Of course, if so much as this is retained, there will be a large dull tumour to be detected in the hypogastrium, and the acts of micturition will be very frequent, or there may be a constant overflow of urine going on. The hypogastric tumour may be in the median line or not. I have known it in some very aggravated cases take a direction distinctly to the right or to the left of the middle line, and cause some doubt as to whether so one-sided a swelling could possibly be a simply distended bladder.

Some indication will be given, on passing a sound or stiff catheter, whether the enlargement is due to the middle

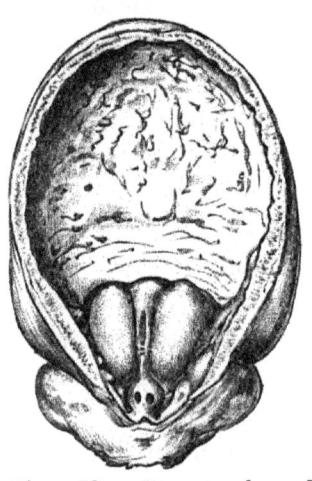

Fig. 78. — Hypertrophy of Prostate. (Mansell-Moullin, " Manual of Surgery.")

or to one of the lateral lobes. In any case, the prostatic urethra being lengthened, an instrument of ordinary length will pass in nearly its whole length before it reaches the cavity of the bladder. When the middle lobe forms the enlargement, the beak of the instrument will have to ascend over it, and the outer end must be depressed to a corresponding degree between the thighs. When one of the lateral lobes is unduly increased, the beak will pass to the opposite side, and the opposite end must be deflected towards the thigh of the same side as the enlargement.

From *stricture* of the urethra, enlarged prostate is distinguished by the obstruction to the sound being further down the urethra and not in the penile or bulbous portions, and by the fact that stricture makes its appearance before middle life, whereas enlarged prostate never occurs before fifty-five or thereabouts.

From *calculus*, by the pain at the neck of the bladder and at the end of the penis not being so severe, not being increased by exercise or any jolting movement, and by the absence of any sensation elicited by sounding the bladder with a short-beaked sound. Hæmorrhage is much more frequent with calculus than with enlarged prostate, especially after exercise. It must be borne in mind that calculus is often formed as the result of the changes in the urine induced by the retention caused by enlarged prostate.

From *vesical tumours* the absence of frequent, severe,

sudden, unprovoked, and intermittent hæmaturia, extending
often over many years, together with the changes in micturition above described, and the detection of an enlarged
prostate per rectum, will aid the diagnosis. Bleeding from
papilloma may be excited by the gentlest catheterism. Frequent microscopic examinations of the urine will probably
detect fragments of the tumour. Cancer of the prostate or of
the base of the bladder gives rise to irregular-shaped, hard
tumours as felt per rectum, not to enlargements of the smooth,
uniform, and typically-shaped outline of enlarged prostate;
moreover, the rate of growth of the swelling, and of the
development of the symptoms, the greater pain and more
abundant hæmaturia, the rapidly-failing health, and the emaciation of the patient, and, in all probability, the enlargement
of the inguinal lymphatic glands, will point to malignant new
growth in distinction to non-malignant simple hypertrophy
of the prostate.

Atony and paralysis of the bladder may give rise to many
of the symptoms of enlarged prostate, but the easy passage of
a catheter, the feeble flow of urine, and the absence of any
prostatic enlargement to be felt per rectum, will clear up the
question at once.

Treatment.—The most essential thing is the early recognition of the fact that a patient has an enlarged prostate
which prevents him from completely emptying his bladder,
and then inducing him at once to enter upon what is called
catheter life. If he acquiesces, he will certainly promote his
comfort, save himself from many distressing complications of
his disease, and, in all probability, retard the rate of increase in
the gland, and add considerably to his chances of prolonged
life. It is a fact that some men with enlarged prostate, the
enlargement being chiefly *eccentric*, as it is called—*i.e.* affecting the circumference and chiefly the posterior aspect of the
gland, and not the urethral aspect—can always empty their
bladders, and yet suffer much from the increased frequency of
micturition, from rectal tenesmus, from hæmorrhoids and prolapse, and from aching pains in the perinæum, groins, and thighs.
And these are the patients who get no relief from catheterism.
For such there is nothing but strict dietetic *régime*, much
rest in the horizontal position, regular moderate exercise two

or three times daily, attention to the regular evacuation of
the rectum, the use of large soap and warm water enemata
for this purpose, and soothing suppositories of cocain, belladonna, or conium, and anodyne ointments to the perinæum.

But in the great majority of patients the chief troubles, and
certainly the chief dangers, accrue from the urethral obstruction. For them, the regular use of the catheter is their sheet-
anchor. How often the catheter will be required will depend upon
the amount of residual urine. If there be only two or three
ounces, it will suffice to empty the bladder completely every
second or third day; if more, the catheter should be passed
every day. The best time to pass the instrument is at night
on going to bed, so that the bladder may be in repose, and the
patient too, for several hours. If complete retention first
brings the patient under surgical observation, and there are
many ounces (thirty or upwards) of urine in the bladder, it
is best not to draw off all the urine at once, but to remove
two-thirds of it and leave the rest to be removed in two, three,
or four hours. Do not let the urine flow away too quickly; never
compress the abdominal walls, or allow the patient to make
voluntary muscular efforts whilst the catheter is being used.
These precautions will tend to prevent sudden hyperæmia
and subsequent serious changes in the kidney and bladder,
as well as free capillary hæmorrhage from the mucous membrane of these organs—risks which are run by the too sudden
evacuation of a distended bladder.

A soft catheter, preferably Jacques or a coudée of medium
size, should be used. If a silver instrument is required, it
should have a very large curve.

Another precaution elderly men with enlarged prostates
should observe, is to take advantage of frequent opportunities
to pass urine—at least every two or three hours—with the
object of avoiding the risk of distension of the bladder.

Every man with enlarged prostate should avoid high-
feeding, excess in alcohol, and sexual excitement, chills, damp
and fatigue, or horse exercise. He should live not necessarily
abstemiously, but simply and regularly, and clothe himself
sufficiently warmly, wearing animal fabrics, not cotton, next
his skin. During catheter life there is always the chance
that inflammation of the bladder, or hæmorrhage from

congestion of the bladder and prostate, may occur from cold, fatigue, excitement, or some departure from rules of diet.

Should acute or chronic cystitis occur, it should be treated as described under these headings. To check hæmorrhage, it will usually be sufficient to keep the patient in bed, apply warm fomentations to the hypogastrium, and use the soft catheter as required.

If, in spite of this treatment, the prostate increases and catheterism becomes difficult or impossible, is there anything more which can be done?

For retention caused by sudden increase in the prostate from congestion of the blood-vessels, supra-pubic aspiration of the bladder is the immediate remedy. In some cases the relief to the congested vessels of the prostate afforded by the evacuation of the bladder is very prompt and complete, so that the patient can soon afterwards pass his urine as before the attack of retention. In other cases, the aspirator will be needed twice or three times, or for two or three days or even a week, before a catheter can be passed or the patient can micturate as before the attack.

In cases in which retention has become *permanent*, and catheterism is very painful, or excites urethritis; or in those in which an instrument retained in the bladder quickly becomes coated with phosphates from alkaline urine, the bladder should be tapped and drained above the pubis.

Supra-pubic cystotomy is the most suitable operation for those very severe and painful cases of large prostate for which a *permanent* drain for the bladder is required. But if the object be to drain the bladder *temporarily* for the sake of giving rest to the parts, to remove blood-clots from the bladder, to relieve the congestion of the prostate, to clear the bladder of its thick muco-purulent urine, and to restore the vesical mucous membrane to a healthy state and the urine to normal acid condition, then the perinæal incision, followed by the dilatation of the prostatic urethra with the finger, and the retention of a large indiarubber tube for ten days or a fortnight, is very efficacious, and is a better and more convenient drainage and a less serious operation than hypogastric cystotomy. It has given me very satisfactory results. Moreover, by this route a pedunculated middle lobe can be removed (perinæal prostatectomy), or the annular hypertrophy of the upper part of the prostate can be divided either by bistoury or galvano-cautery (perinæal prostatotomy). The objection to the boutonnière or small perinæal opening into the membranous urethra for permanent drainage is that the opening is on the wrong side of the prostate—*i.e.* of the obstruction—that the presence of the tube in the prostatic urethra sometimes causes such pain and spasm that it cannot be well borne, or even tolerated after a few days; but it has the advantage of providing excellent drainage and of having the retention-cannula—whether used with a stopcock, or in connection with a portable urinal worn down the leg—in a most convenient situation.

In certain exceptional cases, even for temporary relief, the hypogastric cystotomy is best. It is so in a man with a very deep perinæum, and also in cases where malignant disease of the base of the bladder co-exists with enlargement of the prostate, for under these last-named circumstances serious hæmorrhage is apt to arise from the chafing of the growth by the end of the drain-tube, especially if this tube is at all rigid.

The objection to hypogastric cystotomy as a permanent means of drawing off the urine is the inconvenience of the situation for the protection of the retention-cannula and the upward direction which the urine has to take through it. By Hunter M'Guire's operation the necessity of a permanent retention-cannula is said to be obviated. The supra-pubic opening into the bladder is made as low down as possible, and the patient passes his urine at will, and often at intervals as long as from four to six hours, through the artificial urethra thus formed. There is said to be no leak or dribbling in any position the patient might assume. (Hurry Fenwick, "Urinary Surgery.")

Radical Treatment.—For a radical cure, two things are required—namely, the removal of the prostatic obstruction, and the preservation of an efficient degree of expulsive power in the bladder; then normal voluntary micturition will be restored. Many plans have been suggested with the object of promoting the reduction in size, or of removing portions of enlarged prostates, with the view of re-establishing voluntary and normal micturition; but most of these have proved failures, and will therefore not be referred to here. As in the case of myomata and fibro - myomata of the uterus, so in these analogous enlargements of the prostate, electricity has been advocated and tried with some show of success, but is not satisfactory. The late Mr. McGill, of Leeds, introduced hypogastric prostatectomy; and his example has been followed by several of his Leeds colleagues, and by other surgeons at home and abroad, with a fair proportion of success.

Perinæal urethrotomy has also enabled the obstructing portion of the prostate to be removed in some cases.

Vignards has collected six cases in which normal voluntary micturition has been restored out of thirty-seven cases operated upon by one or the other method.

Belfield (*American Jour. of Med. Sciences*, vol. ii. p. 439, November, 1890), out of 133 prostatectomies, either perinæo-urethral or hypogastric, gives seven cases in which voluntary micturition had been maintained for two years, five cases from eighteen months to two years, three cases from one year to eighteen months, nine cases from nine months to one year, five cases for less than six months—in all, twenty-nine cases of radical cure out of 133 cases operated upon.

The cases of enlarged prostate accessible to any operation from within the bladder will always remain in the very small minority—will be always, perhaps, very rare exceptions; and of those amenable to such treatment, many are not attended by so much inconvenience or suffering as to justify the surgeon to recommend or induce the patient to submit to an operation of severity, of no mean risk, and with the chances of four to one, or rather more, that a radical cure will not after all be obtained. But though it be not justifiable to deliberately perform prostatectomy upon a patient whose condition is not so bad that his case cannot be managed with satisfaction by means of catheter and general hygienic and therapeutical treatment, it does behove the surgeon, when called upon to give relief by an opening into the bladder either above the pubes or in the perinæum, to recognise the character of the obstruction, and to remove it if it be possible. That is, he should be ready to convert a perinæal or hypogastric cystotomy into a prostatectomy if favourable conditions

are found at the time of the performance of the cystotomy. With this possibility in view, most surgeons will
prefer the hypogastric route; and if it be found impossible to
remove the obstruction, and a permanent fistula is required,
Poncet's method of stitching the cut edges of the bladder to
the cut edges of the skin can be followed.

Considering how few of the cases of enlarged prostate
can be safely or successfully subjected to prostatectomy
through the bladder, how much the operator is working in
the dark, how large is the quantity of blood often lost, and
how large the mortality hitherto has been (from 15 to 25
per cent.), and how often obstruction has been due to sub-
urethral enlargements of the prostate which could not be
removed by the supra-pubic route, I am persuaded that in the
future surgeons will come to seek a route other than any of
those now employed, and that this will be by the perinæum,
without opening either the urethra or the rectum. In a con-
versation at the Middlesex Hospital with Mr. McGill, on the
day after he read his original paper at the Clinical Society, in
November, 1887 (Trans. Clinical Society, vol. xxi. p. 52), I
advanced this opinion. I have often advocated it in con-
versation and in my lectures, and have practised it frequently
on the dead body.

Quite recently two other surgeons have independently
advocated perinæal operations—namely, Professor Dittel and
Mr. Pyle. The latter has recorded a very successful application of the median method on a patient seventy years old.
Dittel's operation is a lateral one, and the prostatic urethra is
deliberately opened. It has been tried by Kuster with some
success.

It is true that some of the enlargements of the prostate
are *eccentric*, and affect the circumference, chiefly the posterior
aspect, of the gland, and that those do not cause obstruction
to the urine: and that other enlargements affect the vesical
aspect of the prostate and result in retention. But the
concentric or vesical enlargements are by no means all alike.
Some are projections of the middle lobe into the cavity of the
bladder, and of these, some are pedunculated, and others
broadly sessile; others are projections of one or of both
lateral lobes, and of these, again, some are pedunculated and

others sessile. Another variety of prostatic enlargement presents three nodular projections towards the bladder, consisting of the middle and two lateral lobes respectively (Fig. 78, p. 299); and finally, other enlargements present a circular projection at the orifice of the bladder, and form what is commonly known as the prostatic "collar."

It is not to be supposed that each of these forms of enlargement will be equally amenable to removal by the same method of operating.

The pedunculated varieties will be always fairly readily removed with crushing forceps or the écraseur, through either the hypogastric or perinæo-urethral routes.

Mr. R. F. Tobin, of Dublin, has very successfully employed a combination of the use of an écraseur passed per urethram and hypogastric cystotomy for the removal of hypertrophied middle and left lateral lobes of the prostate of a man aged sixty years (Figs. 79, 80). The case is described in the *Brit. Med. Journal* of March 14th, 1891, p. 580, and the accompanying illustration gives a good idea of the method. It is well worthy of being employed in suitable cases. As Mr. Tobin suggests, if there was any difficulty in getting the loop of wire to bite upon the enlarged lobe, a bed for it could be made with the point of a knife or scissors within the bladder.

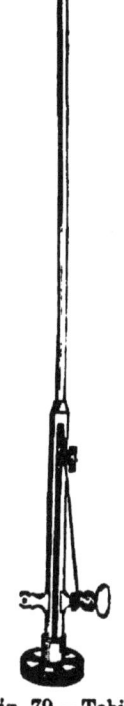

Fig. 79. — Tobin's Écraseur.

Mr. A. T. Norton has devised a prostatectome which is used through a perinæal incision of the urethra (Fig. 81). The instrument is made on the principle of a lithotrite. Both blades are cutting and fit edge to edge. The male blade has a long sloping surface to allow of its slipping back over the middle lobe of the prostate (Fig. 82). The mucous membrane is not generally cut through, and has to be divided with a knife or scissors through the perinæal incision. There is practically no hæmorrhage.

But I believe the *perinæal* method, for forms of enlargement other than the pedunculated, will ultimately prove to be the best. In spite of the interference with the prostatic plexus

U

of veins, this operation will not, I think, be attended with so great a loss of blood as either of the intra-vesical operations; whilst it possesses the advantage of not damaging the wall and mucous surface of the bladder or of the urethra.

The *perinœal* prostatectomy which I advocate for certain cases is performed as follows:—The patient is placed in the lithotomy position; the perinæum is shaved; the rectum has

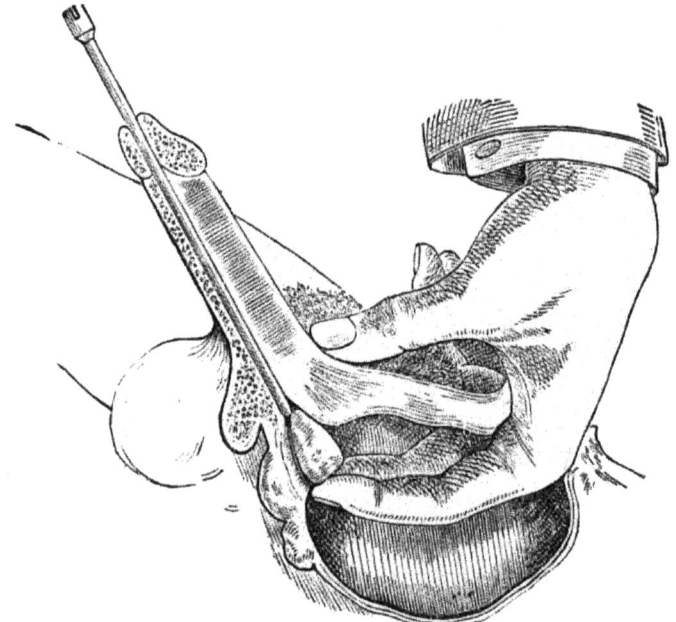

Fig. 80.—Tobin's Écraseur in Position.

been previously well cleared out.   A catheter or sound is passed along the urethra to the prostate, and if possible into the bladder, and is held in position by an assistant.   Then a crescentic incision is made about three-quarters of an inch in front of the anus from one tuber ischii to the other, and if more room is required, as it will certainly be in a fat subject or one with a deep perinæum, an incision should be made from the crescentic one forwards along the raphé of the perinæum.

The knife is now put aside, and with the tip of the index finger the tissues are easily separated until the posterior surface of the prostate is 'reached.   Whilst doing this, care must be taken (by keeping the left index finger in the rectum, and with the right index finger every now and then feeling for the catheter in the urethra) not to wound either the bowel or the urethra. A narrow-bladed, sharp-pointed knife is now passed along the index finger into the wound and made to divide the fibres of the levator ani and its fascia, and then the capsule of the prostate on its posterior aspect just beyond the apex of the gland; the finger is next pushed through the opening in the prostatic capsule, the opening enlarged if necessary, and the prostatic substance is broken up and removed either by the finger or a pair of suitable forceps guided to the prostate by the finger in the wound. In this way the glandular tissue may be completely removed, and any adenoma or fibro-myoma could be readily shelled out.

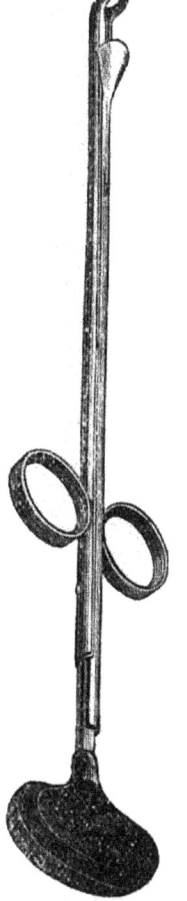

Other methods are at the present time on their trial in the treatment of very bad cases of enlarged prostate. These modes of treatment are galvano-cauterisation, castration, and the application of ligatures to the internal iliac arteries or to the whole spermatic cord, and not simply to the vas deferens. Mr. R. Harrison refers to a case in which there is good reason to believe great benefit followed the subcutaneous section of the vasa deferentia. Isnardi has recently published a successful case of division of both vasa deferentia for enlarged prostate with incontinence in a man aged seventy-one. Pavone also recommends excision of the vas deferens. Professor J. W. White, of Philadelphia, bearing in mind the

Fig. 81.—Norton's Prostatectome.

analogy between uterine fibro-myomata and prostatic overgrowth, was the first who suggested castration as likely to have the same effect on prostatic hypertrophy that oöphorectomy has upon the uterine tumours. If one lateral half of the prostate is enlarged, the corresponding testis is to be removed; if the enlargement involves the whole prostate, both testes should be excised. Besides White, W. Meyer (*Cent. für Chir.*, No. 35, September 2nd, 1893), Ramm, of

Christiania, H. Fenwick, Mansell-Moullin,* and other surgeons, have reported good results. On the other hand, Mr. A. G. Faulds, of Glasgow, has published (*Brit. Med. Journal*, May 4th, 1895) a series of seven cases of castration for enlarged prostate, all of an unfavourable nature: the patients either died, suffered from acute mania, or were entirely unrelieved. It must be in the knowledge of many surgeons that the

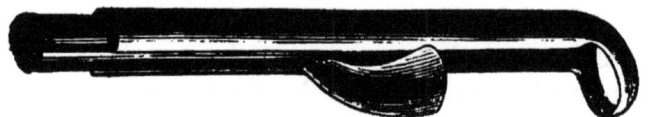

Fig. 82.—Blades of Norton's Prostatectome.

prostate remains quite unaltered after castration, and that, too, in some cases in which first one and afterwards the second testis has been excised for tuberculous or other form of disease.

Bottini's treatment by galvano-cautery through the urethra, and Watson's modification of Bottini's treatment by first opening the urethra through the perinæum and introducing the cautery through the incision, are only suitable for comparatively slight cases, and have not met with much support from surgeons as yet.

The treatment by castration is undergoing a certain amount of trial in this and other countries, the results of which will be awaited with much interest. Kummell (*Berl. Klinik*, August, 1895) has reported eight cases, with one death, of double castration performed by himself, and in seven the operation was followed by much relief. He states that in a large majority of cases of senile hypertrophy of the prostate White's operation will be followed by a more or less rapid shrinking of the prostatic tissue. He recommends the operation in very severe cases. White himself (*Annals of Surgery*, July, 1895) deals at length with the operation and gives a summary of 111. Eighteen were fatal; rapid atrophy followed in about 87 per cent., and amelioration of the most troublesome symptoms in 83 per cent. There was a return to nearly the normal conditions in 46·4 per cent.

Bier, of Kiel, suggested ligature of one or both internal iliac arteries, as the case may be, on the ground that many

* Mansell-Moullin (*Clinical Journal*, December 19th, 1894).

benign tumours disappear on cutting off their blood supply; and both he and W. Meyer report excellent results. Bier, however, had one death out of three cases. The measure is risky, and too serious to be recommended.

THE PROSTATIC BAR ; OR, THE BAR AT THE NECK OF THE BLADDER.

By this term is understood a bar formed at the neck of the bladder by the hypertrophy of some of the transverse muscular fibres which cross the trigone of the bladder. These fibres, when excessively developed, form a prominent elevation on the base of the bladder, and, when present, are always associated with prostatic enlargement, although they are not structurally continuous or connective with the prostate. It is sometimes spoken of as the "limited hypertrophy of Guthrie," and is explained by Mr. Reginald Harrison as being due to a conservative effort of Nature to empty the pouch of residual urine, which forms at the trigone when the prostate gland is enlarged. The condition is not easy to diagnose during life, nor is it of much, if any, clinical importance; it is not itself a cause of difficulty in micturition, but is the effect of the obstructiveness of the prostate; and the treatment of this "muscular bar" is the treatment of the enlarged prostate upon which it depends.

A second form of prostatic bar, or bar at the neck of the bladder, is caused by the duplication of the mucous membrane which sometimes results from hypertrophy of the lateral lobes of the prostate and the consequent transverse "plaiting" of the overstretched mucous lining of the bladder. In these cases, the end of a sound or catheter, as it enters the bladder, often catches against this bar just after it has passed the prostatic urethra, and gives the surgeon the impression of a transverse ridge or low buttress on the vesical wall.

A third variety has been described under the name of the spasmodic form of "bar at the neck of the bladder." It is quite independent of any enlargement of the prostate, and is due to an irregular or spasmodic attack of the vesical neck, when the trigone is irritated by excess of uric acid in the urine or some similarly transient functional condition. It is not a permanent or structural hypertrophy or change, and should not be described as a prostatic bar.

CHAPTER XVIII.

CONCRETIONS AND CALCULI OF INTRA-PROSTATIC ORIGIN.

It is very common to meet, in the prostates of elderly men, with a number of small blackish or brownish bodies about the size of poppy-seeds. They are most frequent just within the orifices of the prostatic ducts, and barely covered with mucous membrane; but they occur also, but of smaller size, dispersed throughout the gland. They have no relation to urinary calculi, and have received the name of **prostatic concretions** in contradistinction to prostatic calculi.

The concretions, in their earliest stages, are microscopic, oval-shaped bodies of a yellow colour, gradually acquiring a darker tint as they grow larger. They may be traced in series, from small, semi-transparent bodies to the dark, poppy-seed-like bodies visible to the naked eye. When minute, they are to be found in the fluid of the prostate, as well as filling the gland recesses and ducts, and they are composed of purely organic matter, a product of the secreting structure of the prostate. Sir Henry Thompson (who has paid great attention to these bodies) speaks, on Dr. W. S. Squire's authority, of this organic matter as belonging "to that class of nitrogenised substances sometimes termed protein derivatives, of which fibrin, gelatin, and chitin are examples." As they increase in size a considerable proportion of earthy matter, chiefly phosphate, with a little carbonate, of lime, is mixed with the superadded organic matter; and then the bodies become dense and lose their transparency. The earthy salts are precipitated upon the nucleus from the fluid secreted by the mucous membrane of the prostatic follicle, it being well known, as Thompson states, "that secreting membranes are prone to deposit opaque earthy matter under certain forms or degrees of irritation, the product in all cases consisting chiefly of the phosphate, with a little of the carbonate, of lime." In the early stage, when only just visible to the naked eye, these concretions are composed chiefly of organic matter; but the composition of the larger and darker ones is not the same, the inorganic material having increased from 46 to 85 per cent.; and in this stage the bodies may be said to have ceased to be concretions and to have become calculi. Still, they are entirely derived from prostatic secretion, and are not deposits from the urine, nor at all due to bladder derangements. Though none of the examples visible to the naked eye are observed in prostates before middle or advanced age, the microscope reveals them of a size not larger than from $\frac{1}{1000}$th to $\frac{1}{100}$th of an inch at any age after puberty. When one has attained the size of a small shot or a pea, it causes absorption of the walls of the follicle which secreted it; and thus many calculi, from many crypts, come to occupy a single space, cease to increase in size, and become faceted on their surfaces. I have removed by operation, on several occasions, between two and three hundred from the same prostate.

Prostatic calculi are in origin and composition very like prostatic concretions, except that they contain a much larger quantity of the phosphate and carbonate of lime salts. Those which have a certain amount of ammonio-magnesium phosphates, which brings them into close relationship with fusible calculi, are not entirely of prostatic origin.

Prostatic calculi occur in very different forms and sizes. The smaller are oval or rounded, about the size of sago grains or peas, or larger; they are very hard and close in texture of porcellaneous lustre, and of a white, fawn, or pale brown colour, lighter in their interior than on the surface. The larger calculi are irregular in shape, some being elongated and others branched; they consist of many fragments, fitting accurately together at their adjacent surfaces so as to form one mass. Some of the largest which have been removed have consisted of a great number of fragments, from sixteen to twenty-nine, and, when the fragments have been adjusted, have measured from five to six inches. Such calculi extend into and along the urethra, and also into the bladder. The common size is, of course, much smaller, and occupies either a separate space, or, if multiple, may occupy a common cavity in the substance of the prostate.

Symptoms.—When small and embedded in separate compartments in the prostate, they give rise to no symptoms; but when of larger size, or more numerous, and are situated close beneath the floor of the urethra, or exist in considerable numbers in a common cavity, symptoms are pretty sure to arise.

In one case under my care severe urethral hæmorrhage occurred, and continued for three or four days before the man's admission; but as, two years subsequently, I removed a small papilloma from his bladder, it is uncertain whether or not this may have existed at the first operation and been the cause of the violent hæmorrhage.   I do not, however, think it was so.

Severe irritation at the neck of the bladder, pain or some difficulty and obstruction in passing water, hæmaturia and urethral hæmorrhage, severe aching pain referred to between the anus and the bladder, a sensation of creaking as a catheter or sound passes over the prostatic urethra and also on digital examination of the prostate per rectum, and the occasional discharge of a typical calculus per urethram, are symptoms which I have witnessed in cases under my own care, and are described in some of the cases recorded by others.

In some cases they have given rise to abscess in the prostate; in others they have ulcerated as they have extended into the tissues beyond the prostate, and urinary fistulæ have resulted.   In one case of my own, complete incontinence in the standing position, and during walking and working, but not whilst sitting or lying down, followed the removal of a very large number of small calculi, through a median perinæal incision; the prostate had been riddled by them. This was due, no doubt, to the alteration in the shape of the urethro-vesical orifice consequent on the collapse of the prostate after the calculi were removed.

Treatment.—This consists in extracting the calculus or calculi, if possible, with urethral forceps, in the eye of a catheter, or by the lithotrite, after pushing the calculus back into the bladder; and if this cannot be done, or the calculi are too numerous or too large, a median perinæal incision should be made into the membranous urethra and the calculi extracted through the wound.   Care should be taken to do as little damage to the pulp of the prostate as possible, for fear of incontinence following from the shrinking and loss of the gland substance.

Where a fistula is present, and opens on the perinæum, it may be the better plan in some cases to remove the calculus by enlarging the fistula.

CALCULI OF EXTRA-PROSTATIC ORIGIN.

Prostatic calculi of urinary origin are formed in the prostate occasionally when, owing to ulceration of the floor of the prostatic urethra, the urine gains entrance into the gland and the salts of the urine are deposited amongst the tissues of the organ. Such calculi were called by Jullien " exotic " (*calculs - exotiques*). There are many conditions which lead to the formation of the requisite recess or cavity in the prostate, such as abscess, false passages, fistula, ulceration and dilatation behind a stricture, and surgical operations on the prostate. The mechanism of the formation of the calculus is the same always—deposition from stagnant urine. Generally, many years are required for the calculi so formed to attain any size.

Exotic calculi which have descended from the kidney or bladder generally gain access to the prostate by means of some surgical operation. In lateral lithotomy, for instance, a fragment of calculus broken off by the forceps and left in the wound, or gaining access thereto a few days subsequently and there remaining, will lead first to the establishment of a fistula, and later on, perhaps, to the development of a large calculus. Sometimes a fragment of stone may find its way into the prostate, as used to be occasionally the case after lithotrity at several sittings.

The symptoms and treatment of these exotic calculi—*i.e.* of calculi of extra-prostatic origin—are the same as those which have been described for concretions and calculi of intra-prostatic origin.

CHAPTER XIX.

CYSTS OF THE PROSTATE.

DISTENSION cysts of two kinds have been described as occurring in the prostate: (1) those due to obstruction and closure of an excretory duct of a prostatic *cul de sac;* and (2) those caused by obstruction and closure of the orifice of the utricle or sinus pocularis.

Retention cysts of the gland tissue of the prostate may form either in the middle of the parenchyma or project upon one of the free surfaces, especially towards the urethra and bladder. Cruveilhier, Le Dentu, and Desnos have reported such cysts of great size. In Desnos' case, the cyst was as large as a small orange, occupied all the inferior part of the organ, and communicated with the prostatic urethra by a dozen minute openings quite independent of the ejaculatory ducts.

Le Dentu found two specimens of retention cysts in the post-mortem room. One was a small, regularly spherical tumour projecting into the bladder (of a man eighty-five years of age, who had never had any urinary trouble) immediately behind the neck, and filled with a milky fluid having all the characters of the prostatic secretion; in the middle lobe of the same prostate were two small fibromata.

Dolbeau found in a man sixty years old two cysts the size of peas, situated symmetrically, one on each side of the veru montanum.

Retention cysts which result from occlusion of the orifice of the utricle have been recorded by Le Dentu and Englisch. The latter speaks of having found five in seventy post-mortem examinations of new-born children, and remarks that, giving rise to a tumour, they may explain some of the cases of congenital hydronephrosis in children at birth. Except when they attain to a moderate size, and not always then even, the retention cysts offer no clinical histories, and afford scarcely any interest other than that of a pathological character.

Sir Henry Thompson tells us that there are no true cysts known in the prostate; nothing which is at all similar to the cysts of the kidney, testicle, or mammary gland.

What have been wrongly called cysts in the prostate are not new formations, but mere dilatations of some already existing cavity, and are of three kinds: (1) dilatation of gland follicles, (2) cavities containing concretions or calculi, and (3) pus cavities. The two latter have been already referred to (intra-prostatic concretions and calculi at page 310, and prostatic abscess at page 280). The dilated follicles are generally filled with yellowish semi-fluid material, or minute yellowish, semi-transparent concretions. They never attain any size, and give rise to no symptoms; but their presence is sometimes detected during life owing to their dilated orifices acting as obstacles to the easy transit of an instrument through the prostatic urethra.

HYDATID CYSTS.

Nicaise, in 1884, collected thirty-five cases of supposed hydatid cyst of the prostate, but, on a critical examination of the evidence in each, he found only two which had, in his opinion, formed originally in the prostate gland itself—namely, Lowdell's and Butruille's. But Lowdell's case, as Sir Henry Thompson points out, was considered doubtful by Lowdell himself, who suggested that the prostate might have been destroyed by the pressure of the cyst which had grown in the tissue outside the gland. In Butruille's case the cyst was limited to the anterior part of the prostate, and, though no hooklets were found in the fluid, the character of the cyst wall and the general character of the fluid seemed to justify the diagnosis that the cyst was a hydatid.

In the great majority of recorded cases the hydatid cyst grew between the rectum and the prostate, and in its growth pushed the bladder upwards, sometimes high into the abdomen. In a case of the sort on which I made the post-mortem many years ago, the bladder was displaced as high as the left hypochondrium, and, before death, retention could not be relieved till the tumour had been evacuated through a free pre-rectal perinæal incision. This was done, and the case reported, by Mr. T. Bryant.

Why the region of the prostate especially should be selected by these parasites is not clear. By some it has been thought probably due to the proximity of the pouch of the rectum, in which the embryo echino-coccus, if contained in the fæces, sojourns for a while, and may thus easily fix itself in, or pass through, the wall of the bowel into the cellular, or the sub-peritoneal fatty, tissue. In Curling's case, a hydatid cyst as large as an ostrich's egg was situated between the rectum and bladder, and another and quite independent cyst, the size of a nut, occupied the thickened rectal wall. By other writers they have been regarded as intra-peritoneal, the embryo echinococcus being supposed to reach the neighbour-hood of the prostate by falling to the bottom of the recto-vesical pouch. The question as to the exact anatomical position of these recto-vesical hydatid cysts has recently been raised by a case read before the Royal Medical and Chirurgical Society by Mr. R. Harrison (*Brit. Med. Journ.*, April 13th, 1895). Mr. J. H. Targett (*Guy's Hospital Gazette*, April 27th, 1895), from the dissection of specimens in the Hunterian Museum, thinks there can be no doubt that in some cases at least they are *extra*, not *intra-peritoneal* as Hunter supposed ; that they are developed between the muscular coat of the bladder and the recto-vesical fascia which ensheathes it, and not in the subperitoneal fat superficial to the fascia. His reason for this opinion is that, in each of the Hunterian specimens, the hydatid cyst is springing from between the vesiculæ seminales and vasa deferentia on the one hand and the bladder on the other—in other words, " the vas deferens and vesicula seminalis of one or both sides is lying upon the wall of the cyst and not upon the bladder. To detach these structures from the vesical wall, the dis-tending force must be applied between the muscular coat and the fascia, for if the cyst were external to the fascia in the subperitoneal fat, the vasa and vesiculæ would be com-pressed against the bladder." Mr. Targett supposes that the "six-hooked embryo" reaches this position in the pelvis through the venous system, "just as hydatids occur in the epiphysial ends of long bones, and in the bodies of the vertebræ, where the vessels are most abundant."

Symptoms.—In many of the cases retention of urine has been the symptom which has drawn attention to the presence of the cyst. It has then been discovered that a catheter of ordinary length has not reached the urine, that the bladder is more or less displaced out of the pelvis, and that a large elastic tumour is felt per rectum in the situation of the prostate and bladder. Some difficulty in, or obstruction to, defæcation, or tenesmus the result of pressure upon the rectum, may be complained of. When the tumour is large and presses firmly against the brim of the pelvis, one or both ureters may be obstructed, and hydronephrosis may be the result. In the same way, pressure upon the blood-vessels and nerves as they pass through the pelvis may cause coldness, numbness, œdema, or partial paralysis of the lower extremities. In some cases there has been dysuria, or the symptoms of stricture of the urethra, increasing for months or years. In others, the tumour has been tapped per rectum, and then diagnosed by the characters of the fluid.

Diagnosis.—The clinical history will serve to exclude prostatic abscess; but if the hydatid tumour be small and not bulging, and yet lying in contact with the rectum, it may be difficult, except it fluctuates, to distinguish it from the prostate gland. If in addition to the swelling per rectum there is any elastic prominence of the perineum, if the recto-vesical pouch of peritoneum is obliterated, or if a long catheter cannot draw off urine, and there is a well-defined, dull and painful tumour felt in the abdomen, there will be good ground for concluding that the small swelling in front of the rectum is part of a large tumour, and not the prostate.

Treatment.—The best treatment is to lay the cyst freely open through the perinæum by a crescentic incision in front of the anus, and then to clear out the contents and as much of the cyst wall as will peel easily away without provoking hæmorrhage. In some cases this proceeding is urgently needed to relieve the agony of acute retention, and to save the bladder from bursting. When the cyst is large and ascends above the brim of the true pelvis, the abdominal instead of the perinæal route has sometimes to be employed. If laparotomy be adopted, great care may be needed to avoid opening the urinary bladder instead of the hydatid cyst.

CHAPTER XX.

TUBERCULAR DISEASE OF THE PROSTATE.

THIS affection occurs most frequently during the time of greatest sexual activity—that is, between twenty and forty. As a primary disease it is not common, and other organs are usually also affected. A gleet of long standing, affecting the deep urethra in a person predisposed by heredity to tuberculosis, is a common cause of tubercle of the prostate. The bacilli under these conditions find in the prostate a location of small resistance; or the urethritis, being of bacillary origin, is propagated to the prostate. When the prostate is secondarily affected, the primary disease is commonly in some part of the genito-urinary organs—testis, kidney or bladder; less frequently the primary disease is in the lungs, or peritoneum, or in a bone.

Pathological Anatomy.—This does not differ in any way from the morbid anatomy of tubercle elsewhere. The tubercular tissue occurs either as minute grey or greyish-yellow millet-seed-like bodies; or as large caseous masses which may either calcify, or soften and break down.

If the prostate has been first, or long, affected, these minute grey bodies have had time to become larger, then to blend together, and thus form caseous or cheesy masses. The mass may reach the size of a marble, or even that of a chestnut, and is then generally surrounded by a thin fibrous, uniting membrane. It tends to break down in the centre. The disease generally affects both lobes when primary; but if secondary to tubercle of the testis, the prostatic lobe of the corresponding side is first attacked. The little millet-seed-like bodies first appear in the glandular structure, in the acini of the prostate; and it is here between the epithelium and the subjacent connective tissue that the bacilli are said to first show themselves.

The prostate increases in size, but not greatly nor uniformly, and much of the increase is often due, not to the tuberculous masses, but to inflammatory œdema.

As the tuberculous masses increase towards the mucous membrane, ulcers, without any tendency to heal, form in the prostatic urethra. These ulcers become sources of septic infection and urinary extravasation. Some of the softening, cheesy masses may discharge in this direction and leave a cavity which goes on secreting pus and discharging it into the urethra or bladder (Fig. 83).

It is more common for the disease to affect the outer than the central parts of the prostate, and then when the cheesy mass breaks down, the prostatic tissue is riddled with small abscesses or the fibrous capsule is bulged out into one or several pockets. Broca refers to a case in which the whole gland was transformed into a calcareous mass. Sometimes the caseous material liquefies and becomes absorbed, and the sclerosis of the surrounding tissue leads to contraction of the gland; this is one of the well-recognised forms of atrophy of the prostate.

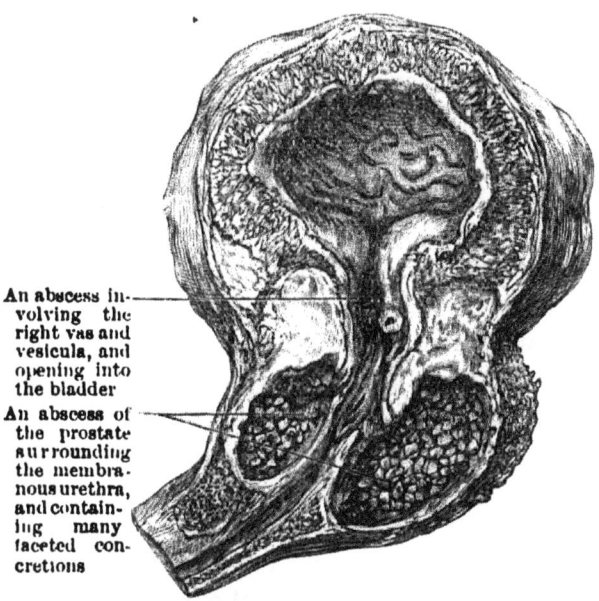

An abscess involving the right vas and vesicula, and opening into the bladder

An abscess of the prostate surrounding the membranous urethra, and containing many faceted concretions

Fig. 83.—Tubercular Disease of the Prostate and Vasa Deferentia. The testes were also occupied by tubercular abscesses. (Middlesex Hospital Museum, No. 1717.)

If time is allowed for the disease to take its course, urinous fistulæ may form and open into the rectum, or more frequently in the perinæum.

It is often most difficult to say whether the disease began in the prostate or in some other part of the genito-urinary system. The anatomical relations between the prostatic urethra, the excretory ducts, spermatic cord, vesiculæ seminales, epididymis and testis would suggest that when the bacilli gain access along the urethra, the prostate would be the first affected; but when their course is by the blood-vessels or lymphatics, the prostate may be either primarily, simultaneously, or secondarily attacked.

The prostate, as is well recognised, may be infected by the bacilli descending from the kidney.

In answer to the question, " In what proportion are persons affected with tubercle of the prostate also the subjects of pulmonary tubercle ? " there are the figures of Reclus, who out of one hundred pulmonary cases found only two with tubercular disease of the genito-urinary organs; but, on the other hand, in fifty cases of tubercular disease of the genito-urinary tract, clinical examination showed sixteen had pulmonary disease, and fourteen not. Other statistics by Jullien and Desnos supply very nearly the same proportion.

Symptoms and Diagnosis.—The symptoms are not characteristic. In the more common form—namely, when the disease affects the outer or peripheral part of the gland—it goes on for a long time unrecognised. The patient may complain of a weight in the perinæum, of some rectal tenesmus, or pain when at stool, but he probably comes under treatment on account of a urethral discharge, a lump in the epididymis, or an attack of cystitis. On digital examination per rectum, the prostate is found enlarged in part or throughout; or it may present nodules; or a soft, flaccid spot, caused by an abscess; or its surface may be granular, giving the sensation of grains of rice in its capsule; or, if the greater part of the gland is destroyed, and the liquefied material has been discharged or absorbed, it may feel small and atrophied.

If the disease affects the central part of the gland and involves the urethra, the symptoms are those of chronic inflammation of the deep urethra attended by a discharge of muco-purulent fluid in which the bacilli of tubercle may be found; there is pain with frequency in passing water, especially when the disease encroaches on the neck of the bladder; there may be urethral hæmorrhage or some blood-stained strings of muco-pus discharged with, or just after, the urine; pains may be complained of in the thighs, loins, and groins; cystitis may occur; and if there should be any inflammatory œdema or congestion around or about the tubercular deposits, complete retention of urine may supervene.

The catheter or sound, though sometimes used to clear up any doubt as to the presence of a vesical calculus, affords little or no information. If the disease is central, the instrument by its passage over the prostatic urethra will cause pain, and there is just the possibility of withdrawing in the eye of a catheter a little discharge or *débris* in which the bacilli of tubercle are found.

Prognosis and Treatment.—No regular course is followed by the disease; it may become arrested and dry up, as is the case sometimes in the lungs. When secondary, it may not have advanced far at the time of death from tubercular disease in other organs; or the disease may have existed long enough to have completely riddled the prostate, the patient being worn out after some months, or perhaps not till after a few years, by suffering or hectic.

The general treatment consists in attention to diet, exercise, fresh air, warm clothing, and regulated temperature; and in taking tonic medicines, cod-liver oil, and, if necessary, narcotic drugs in the shape of suppositories.

There should be as little use of instruments upon the urethra as possible; they cause great pain, irritate the prostate, aggravate the disease, and do nothing but harm.

No caustic or astringent applications to the deep urethra are of any use.

Surgical interference is sometimes justifiable when the lungs and kidneys are not affected, and the local disease is not too far advanced. It has taken the form in some instances, of incising and scraping away the diseased parts of the prostate, either through a median, perinæal, or crescentic wound. In other cases, fistulous tracts have been freely laid open either by incision or the thermo-cautery, or a deliberately planned perinæal incision has been made, and tuberculous masses have been scraped away and the cavity dressed with iodoform gauze.

Bowlby made with success a very radical operation of this kind.

CHAPTER XXI.

MALIGNANT DISEASE OF THE PROSTATE.

MALIGNANT disease affects the prostate very rarely either as a primary or secondary disease. Secondary cancer of the prostate is even more rare than primary, and takes place commonly as an extension from the bladder, more rarely from rectal cancer, and occasionally in association with cancer of the stomach. Sir Henry Thompson mentions having once "seen it follow encephaloid cancer of the penis, itself a very rare affection." Reboul showed a prostate in which were tumours secondary to sarcoma of the humerus. Primary cancer of the prostate occurs probably much more frequently than Tanchou's tables would lead one to suppose—viz. once in every 450 to 500 cases of cancer in the male. It is commonly of the encephaloid variety; but John Adams and Thompson have verified the existence of scirrhus, though this form of carcinoma of the prostate must be very uncommon.

Epithelioma is unknown in the prostate so far as I am aware. Melanotic deposit is said to have been found in two cases—one in a child, the other in an adult, associated with encephaloid of the prostate. Sarcoma has been found in a few instances in both the round and spindle-celled varieties. Mr. Boyd has published a case of colloid degeneration of a scirrhus of the prostate in a man aged fifty-nine, the walls of the bladder and the vesiculæ seminales being likewise involved.

Malignant disease of the prostate chiefly affects individuals at the two extremes of life—that is, before the fifth year and after the fifty-ninth. Only *six* out of twenty-three cases tabulated by Sir Henry Thompson occurred between these years. Of these, one patient was nineteen years, another twenty-one years, and a third twenty-nine years old; the remaining three were forty-one, forty-two, and forty-five years of age. Cases collected by Jolly and Engelbach and others show the same thing. Jolly says that, except the eye, no organ of the body shows so strong a tendency to cancer in children as the prostate. The progress of the disease (like malignant disease in other organs and structures) is much more rapid in children than in adults. The average time from start to finish in children is from three to nine months; in adults, according to Stein, between one and two years; according to Thompson, the duration of the disease varies from one to five years. As in some of the cases encephaloid has been engrafted upon chronic non-inflammatory enlargement of the prostate, the period between the commencement of urinary symptoms and death more than represents the duration of the malignant affection in these cases.

In children the disease is limited to the prostate and the lymphatics; in adults other viscera are usually affected. This difference is no doubt due to the slower rate of progress in adults, which affords time for diffusion and secondary growths.

Pathological Anatomy of Carcinoma of the Prostate. —Few opportunities have been afforded for the study of the morbid anatomy of the disease in its earlier stages, as the gland is generally in great part destroyed at the time of death. The disease begins as a rule with one or more deposits in one of the lateral lobes. Very occasionally it commences as a general infiltration.

It grows slowly at first, but after a while it rapidly enlarges, and may form a large mass either confined within the limits of the capsule of the prostate, or sprouting as a fungous excrescence into the tissues around.

The mucous membrane of the prostatic urethra is generally perforated at length by the growth, either in the way of fungus, or by ulceration, followed by sloughing or breaking down, or occasionally by suppuration, of the cancer. Nodules of new growth may project the mucous membrane of both urethra and bladder, the lymphatic vessels and glands are invaded, and, according to Thompson, the veins of the prostate sometimes contain cancerous material.

The naked eye and microscopic appearances are much like those of the respective variety of malignant disease in other organs. The glandular structures of the prostate are the primary seat of the disease, the prostatic stroma becoming secondarily and to a less extent involved. The form of carcinoma may be either tubular or acinous, and either may undergo colloid degeneration. In the fungus outgrowths there is no trace of prostatic tissue.

Diagnosis and Symptoms.—Besides the symptoms of obstruction common to all forms of enlarged prostate, there are others which serve to distinguish malignant disease from the acute and chronic inflammatory, and the chronic non-inflammatory enlargements—the rapid growth, the intense pain, the frequent, easily provoked, and often severe hæmorrhages; the rapid emaciation and general ill-health of the patient, unaccompanied by feverishness and lasting too long for the acute inflammatory swellings, yet progressing far too quickly for the non-inflammatory enlargements, proclaim the nature of the disease. From cancer of the bladder or of the anterior wall of the rectum, from tubercular disease of the prostate (which affects men of young adult life chiefly), and from large vesical calculi, cancer of the prostate can be diagnosed by the history and symptoms. Pain is an uncertain symptom, and in the early stages may not be more than that due to retention or obstruction. Hæmorrhage is the most certain and most constant symptom throughout the whole course of the disease. It is sometimes alarming in amount and the blood may escape either unmixed with the urine, or during micturition.

The hæmorrhage may be continuous if the disease has invaded the bladder, or is sending a fungous outgrowth into the urethra; otherwise it is intermittent, but readily excited by exertion, or by even the gentlest catheterism. The urine is not generally mixed with pus or mucus unless the bladder is implicated; but careful and repeated microscopical examination will probably lead to the detection of fragments of detached growth which have been washed out with the stream, and will throw light on the diagnosis. On examination per rectum the prostate is found hard in the early stages, and generally nodular or irregular in outline; but it is not always painful or tender, and may be quite insensitive to touch. As time goes on and fungous outgrowths form, or the tumour tissue softens and breaks down, it becomes irregular in consistence as well as outline. The obstruction caused to the urine may lead to hydro- or pyo-nephrosis and uræmia; the obstruction occasionally produced in the rectum may necessitate colotomy. The bladder may be invaded by continuity, and all the symptoms of cystitis may arise, and the tumour-mass as felt per rectum will probably then be found to extend far beyond the upper limits of the prostate. The lymphatic glands along the brim of the pelvis, and sometimes also the inguinal glands, are enlarged, and there may be evidence of secondary deposits in the lungs, kidneys, spinal column, or elsewhere.

Prognosis and Treatment.—The termination is always fatal; the treatment is only palliative. For the relief of retention the soft catheter must be used, and that with scrupulous gentleness; otherwise, and even despite all care, hæmorrhage is excited. Catheterism should be avoided as long as possible—that is, till retention makes it necessary. In some cases death has occurred within a very short time after the first use of the instrument from ascending suppurative pyelo-nephritis. Opium, or the subcutaneous injection of morphia, must be liberally administered to relieve the neverceasing misery, amounting often to agony, of these patients. In some cases of retention, relief by catheter has not been possible, and supra-pubic or perinæal puncture has been employed, but not always with success. Colotomy has given relief and prolonged life in some few cases recorded by Barwell, Fenwick, de Brault and others. Reginald Hrrrison has recorded a very successful case of excision of a cancerous growth projecting into the bladder by perinæal urethrotomy; and Czerny scraped away a growth which he reached by means of hypogastric cystotomy.

Since Kuchler, in 1866, suggested extirpation of the prostate, and Billroth first performed the operation on the living, several surgeons, by a fairly considerable number of operations, have put the treatment to the test. The record of these cases is not pleasant reading. In some nothing could be done; in others only parts of the growth could be removed; in several, hæmorrhage was excessive; and in most, death followed within periods varying from a few hours to two or three weeks.

With Thompson and Guyon I agree in thinking that little or nothing can be done beyond palliating the sufferings and ministering to the necessities of these patients.

In the early stages the diagnosis is uncertain and the risks are enormous; in the late stages, when the cancer is fungating and the lymphatics are enlarged, operation is out of the question. Partial removal when the orifice of the bladder is occluded by the growth may give temporary relief. For persisting retention, and also on account of excessive hæmorrhage from catheterisation, I have employed suprapubic drainage with great advantage.

Part III.

URINARY BLADDER.

CHAPTER I.

MALFORMATIONS AND MALPOSITION OF THE BLADDER.

THE congenital defects of the bladder are absence, malposition, exstrophy, and supernumerary bladders.

Absence of the Bladder.—Only a few instances are on record. When it occurs, the ureters open either into the urethra, the rectum, the vagina, or on the abdomen generally in the median line.

In a case reported by Raphael, of New York, the ureters terminated in a sac which contained intestines, and protruded at the umbilicus; in this child there were also an imperforate anus, undescended testes, and absence of the colon.

In a case seen by Todd, of London, the ureters opened on the abdomen, one on each side of the pubes; only about one inch of the large bowel existed. Agnew quotes a few other cases, in some of which the individuals lived to adult age, suffering little or no inconvenience. Raphael's and Todd's cases survived only a few days.

Supernumerary Bladders.—Most of the cases which have been recorded as supernumerary bladders have been either sacculated bladders or bladders bisected by a membranous partition.

In some of the sacculated bladders the coats of the sacculus or supernumerary bladder have been complete. In one case of three so-called bladders, two of the sacculi were continuous with the ureters and were probably dilated lower extremities of those ducts.

In some of the cases in which the bladder has been divided into two, there has been an opening of communication between them; in others not. One ureter opens into each division.

Fantoni and Mollinetti (Phil. Trans., vol. vii.) have described cases of true multiple bladders. That of the latter was a woman who had five bladders, five kidneys, and six ureters. Four of the ureters emptied each into separate bladders, the other two into the largest bladder.

MALPOSITION OF THE BLADDER. CYSTOCELE.

The bladder may be protruded in a hernial form when the linea alba is weak or deficient, or the expansion of the oblique muscles of the abdomen is absent.

If the whole of the front wall of the abdomen is deficient in the hypogastrium, but the bladder is properly developed, the bladder will protrude at the opening. This is not the same thing as exstrophy.

In most of the cases of protrusion or displacement of the bladder the condition is not congenital but acquired.

Etiology and Morbid Anatomy.—Great protrusions are sometimes met with in the middle line at the scar of a laparotomy wound or of an abscess. Over-distension of the abdominal walls from ascites, pregnancy, fat followed by emaciation, or the flaccidity of age, are conditions which lend themselves to hernial protrusions of the bladder as of the other viscera. The inguinal, femoral, obturator, and ischiatic foramina have all been the site of cystoceles accompanied or unaccompanied by a portion of bowel or omentum.

Vaginal cystocele is by no means uncommon in fat, flabby women who have borne several children, and in these cases it sometimes projects beyond the vulva.

The protruding part of the bladder is uncovered by peritoneum except when accompanied or preceded by an ordinary hernia of large size, or where a great portion of the bladder is involved.

Besides the weakened condition of the abdominal walls or vagina, or the easy patency of one of the natural openings in the parietes, two other conditions are requisite for cystocele, namely a dilated bladder, owing to frequent and considerable distension, and frequent straining efforts at micturition. As soon as the bladder has once escaped at a hernial protrusion it acquires a more or less sacculated or hourglass form, and urine, by being constantly retained therein, decomposes at length, and may lead to ulceration, calculous formation. or sloughing.

Symptoms and Diagnosis.—Cystocele has been mistaken for hernia, undescended or diseased testes, and abscess.

Pott speaks of the urinary bladder having been wounded in two cases of operation for strangulated hernia, and he himself opened a scrotal swelling which he mistook for a diseased testicle, but which was, in reality, a cystocele. Cystoceles in the groin have been mistaken for abscesses.

A cystocele increases with retention or accumulation of urine, and diminishes in size, though it may not quite empty, or become flaccid, by urinating or the use of the catheter. It may form a soft, flaccid, or a dull, tense, fluctuating swelling, according to the quantity of urine it contains. It is neither doughy, like an epipocele, nor resonant, like an enterocele.

In doubtful cases, Agnew recommends the grooved needle and an examination of the fluid withdrawn. A fine trochar and cannula would serve the same purpose much better and with no more risk. But it should be remembered that the urine in a pouch of the bladder like this may be septic even though the bulk of the urine is not so, and that the escape of such urine into the soft tissues might cause severe local trouble, or even general septic infection. Before resorting to any form of puncture it will be well to see the effect of injecting the bladder to moderate distension with warm boracic fluid.

If a cystocele becomes strangulated, the symptoms may simulate very closely a strangulated hernia; but, in addition, there will almost certainly be other symptoms special to the bladder, such as blood in the urine, painful and frequent micturition, and pain specially referred to the hypogastrium and neck of the bladder.

Petit says that in strangulated hernia of the bladder, vomiting is always preceded by hiccough, whereas in hernia of the intestine vomiting precedes hiccough.

Treatment.—The pouch of bladder should be kept empty of urine, either by voluntary micturition or by the catheter, and the application of a truss. If irreducible, an attempt should be made to return the protruding part, and close the opening of exit by an operation similar to the radical cure of hernia. If this is not feasible, or the patient declines an

operation, a well-fitting, well-moulded truss and pad should ·
be worn to prevent the protrusion increasing. A vagino-
cystocele should be treated by an operation for tightening
and shortening the anterior vaginal wall.

**Prolapse of the bladder mucous membrane through the
uretho-vesical orifice** is very rare in men, and does not extend
beyond the membranous urethra. In women it is less uncommon, and should be treated by applying the actual cautery
to the vesical orifice whilst the wall of the bladder is kept
in place by a catheter.

CHAPTER II.

EXSTROPHY OF THE BLADDER.

ECTOPION VESICÆ is characterised by a failure in development of the anterior wall of the bladder and of the abdominal wall in front of the bladder, whilst the posterior wall of the bladder projects at the hypogastrium, where it is continuous with the anterior abdominal parietes.

Etiology.—This malformation is more frequent in boys than in girls in the proportion of eight or nine to one. Of 141 cases collected by John Wood, Earle, and Agnew, seventeen were in females—*i.e.* 8·5 males to 1 female.

Its cause is still unknown. Many theories have been advanced to explain it, but none are satisfactory. Two, however, receive most support. One of them regards ectopion as the consequence of a rupture of the bladder owing to imperforate urethra. The other explains it by an arrest of development. The rupture theory is quite untenable. as the effect of urethral obstruction in the fœtus is distended bladder, urachus, ureters and kidneys, or patent urachus—but not ectopion. Besides, this theory does not explain the cases of ectopion associated with patent intestine (artificial anus) at the same level.

The theory of arrest of development is generally accepted. The coexistence of epispadias, the absence or non-union of the symphysis pubis, and other associated malformations of the genital organs, are arguments in its favour. If the ventral lamellæ are wanting in front of the bladder, and the bladder is well developed, hernia of the bladder occurs at this level; whereas if defective development of the anterior part of the allantois, from which the bladder is developed, coexist, ectopion vesicæ is the result. This hypothesis, however, requires scientific embryological proof, and does not give a satisfactory explanation of epispadias.

It is interesting to note that in some few cases, true dermoid cysts have been removed from the anterior wall of the bladder. Is it not possible that these have developed from a portion of

the epiblast which has closed in and made good a deficiency
of the bladder, which, had it not been for the epiblast, would
have formed an ectopion vesicæ?

Morbid Anatomy.—Ectopion vesicæ appears as a florid
red body in the hypogastric, or hypogastric and pubic regions.
In very young subjects it is not larger than a nut; in adults,
the size of an apple.

It is, in outline, irregularly oval or circular; in colour, florid
red; and presents a moist mucous membrane which generally
bulges, more or less, like the rind of half an orange turned
inside out; it sometimes forms
a depression; at others, presents
two lateral prominences separated
by a vertical groove. When of
large size, it may be pedunculated.
It expands during respiration and
coughing, and can be partially reduced by compression. Gurgling
is at times to be heard behind
it. Its circumference is sharply
defined and indurated, being
formed by the aponeuroses of the
abdominal parietes.

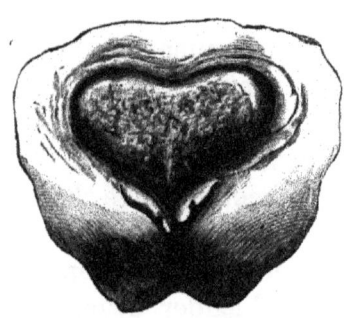

Fig. 84.—Ectopion Vesicæ. The
posterior wall of the bladder
with the opening of the two
ureters is seen.   (*Mansell
Moullin.*)

The surface bleeds readily, and is often painful; the lower
part is always moister and more vascular than the upper, and
there are upon it two small, round projections, representing
the orifices of the ureters, and on watching them one sees
urine flowing from them—not drop by drop, but by a sort of
feeble and irregular ejaculation.

At the margin, the epidermis is continued insensibly into
the epithelium of the mucous membrane, and little islands of
it are situated on the mucous surface—in fact, there is a
tendency for the epithelium to change into epidermis.

Around the ectopion the cutaneous surface is marked by
irregular cicatrices which are considered to be relics of the
allantois. Above the ectopion is a median depression, due to the
want of the linea alba, as high as the umbilicus. The umbilicus
may indeed blend with the ectopion, and, if not, is generally
very close to it. The umbilical vein is consequently elongated;
the urachus and umbilical arteries proportionately shortened.

Below, the ectopion is continuous in the male, with a rudimentary penis, on which runs a median groove, bounded on each side by the cavernous body; these are terminated by a flattened glans, and below the glans is a large pendulous prepuce. The ejaculatory ducts and prostatic sinuses open upon the penile groove.

The scrotum is flattened, and may exceptionally contain the testicles. It may be entirely absent. The testicles frequently occupy the inguinal canals, and are normal in size and structure.

In the female there is a separation of the labia majora, of the two sides of the clitoris, and of the labia minora. The external orifice of the vagina is a mere antero-posterior slit, and in some cases the sex of the infant is doubtful. The vagina and uterus are sometimes bifid. The anus is often placed further forward than normal. One of the most important features is detected by pressing upon the pubic region, when it will be ascertained that there is a wide separation of the pubic bones varying from 1½ to 6 inches (3 to 12 centimetres). It is quite exceptional for the pubes to be united at the symphysis.

By rectal examination much is learnt—viz. the absence or rudimentary state of the prostate and vesiculæ seminales, and the very forward projection of the sacrum, whereby the antero-posterior diameter of the pelvis is diminished. With the finger in the rectum and the other hand on the hypogastrium, one feels that the rectum is close up to the posterior surface of the ectopic bladder, and can make out still more distinctly the separation of the pubes.

Dissection shows the perinæal muscles to be ill-developed, and the sphincter vesicæ muscle to be absent—at least, in one instance only does it seem that a sphincter of the urethro-vesical orifice has been found. In place of the symphysis is a fibrous band of varying thickness and resistance.

Nothing but a layer of cellular tissue, and not always that, separates the vesical mucous membrane from the peritoneal coat.

The condition of the ureters is very important. Following them from the bladder wall, they dip down into the pelvis before turning up towards the kidneys. They are frequently elongated, curved, dilated even to the degree of forming large tumours prominent in the loin, such as I have described in a case of complete retention, with universal dilatation of the ureters owing to torsion of the penis. (*See* pages 162 and 163; also *Lancet*, June 8, 1895.) The walls of the ureters are hypertrophied as well as dilated, and often, especially in the adult, their mucous membrane becomes inflamed. There are many gradations of malformation between complete ectopion and simple epispadias. Tuffier, quoting from Hache, gives in progressive series no less than nine degrees of the malformations.

Symptoms.—Individuals with ectopion vesicæ may be otherwise well formed and robust; but most frequently they are thin, weakly, and constantly suffering, as the slightest friction from their linen inflames the vesical mucous membrane. Thus they often die from ascending inflammation ending in suppurative pyelo-nephritis.

As a result of the constant trickling of urine, they are always wet and in discomfort, and frequently affected with erythema, excoriations, erysipelas, or more deeply-seated inflammation of the skin and tissues around. In this way they are always in danger of getting mischief ascending to the kidneys. Sexual appetite does not, as a rule, exist in men; still, Pousson has collected several cases in which masturbation was practised, and in a case recorded by Gerdy the man was capable of coitus. In the female, conception has occurred (Drs. Huxham's and Thiebault's case), the offspring being naturally formed; but Tuffier adds that delivery is often difficult, and confinement almost always followed by prolapse of the uterus.

Many malformations of other organs have been found associated with ectopion, especially those connected with atresia ani and abnormal anus. Double inguinal hernia is very common. Sometimes the ileum terminates in the bladder. Other associated abnormalities are prolapse of the rectum or uterus, club-foot, hare-lip, anencephalus, and spina bifida. Ectopion vesicæ is, happily, very rare. Neudorfer makes it out to occur only in two out of 100,000 infants, and nine-tenths of the children so affected die within a few days of birth.

Exstrophy is not incompatible with long life. Flagani mentions a case living aged seventy; Quatrefages, another aged forty-nine; and Agnew refers to a man annually exhibited to the classes at Philadelphia, forty years of age.

Treatment. — Many appliances have been invented to collect the urine and to prevent the irritation of the sensitive mucous membrane of the bladder. They are not very successful in their object. The best are those designed by Earle, of London; Jurine, of Geneva; and Bonn, of Amsterdam. They consist essentially of a sort of cup, applied over the exstrophy, communicating by a tube with a reservoir fastened to the thigh, and may be provided with a valve at the top and a tube and tap below.

Many and ingenious operations have been devised to remedy this deformity, rare though it is. This is readily understood, because of the continual pain and danger these persons are in from the chafing of the mucous membrane and the inflammation consequent thereon; and also on account of the disgust excited by the excoriations of the skin and the soaking of the clothes with ammoniacal urine and muco-pus.

The results of these operations are only palliative, and only partially successful even to that extent. The reason of this is the absence of the vesical sphincter, which renders the patients unable to retain their urine after even the most successful operation. This strikes at the root of all such efforts as those made formerly by Dubois and Dupuytren, and recently by Trendelenburg and Passavant, to obtain a *radical* cure by bringing together the pubic bones and suturing the two sides of the extroverted bladder; and it has, perhaps, been the means of leading surgeons (Sir John Simon, *Lancet*, 1852, vol. ii. p. 568, and Mr. Sidney Jones and others) to divert the urine into the large intestine by establishing communications between the ureters and the rectum. Other surgeons (Lloyd, Johnson and Holmes) tried to accomplish the same end by establishing a direct communication between the bladder and rectum. These attempts—right in principle, having regard to the absence of a vesical sphincter and the prevention of incontinence—failed, however, to turn the urine into the rectum, and the operations of Lloyd and Johnson ended fatally in peritonitis.

Recent experiments by Narvarro, Bardenheuer, and Tuffier lead the latter to hope that this method may yet be made successful. It is the only method that has a claim to being considered *radical*.

An important question in relation to these operations has reference to the tolerance of urine by the rectal mucous membrane. This seems to have varied in different cases of recto-vesical fistula, but it forms, probably, only a theoretical objection on the part of Pousson. Agnew, who says that in a patient of his it was a source of great discomfort, states that the urine was retained for two or three hours at a time. A patient of Thiersch held urine for a certain length of time in the rectum without any inconvenience.

Probably the reason it has not been more thoroughly tested in practice is because about the same time that Mr. Simon proposed the method (1852), Roux, of Toulon (1853), introduced the autoplastic method. This is only palliative in its aim, not radical; and, as Tuffier satirically describes it, consists in hiding rather than in closing the bladder by cutaneous flaps taken from round about it and easily drawn over it. Different operations are suitable to different degrees and varieties of exstrophy, so that probably no one operation will ever sweep away others.

That which is most in vogue to-day is the *autoplastic* method—*i.e.* closure by means of cutaneous flaps. It was introduced by Roux and Richard in 1853, and adopted, with slight modifications, by Pancoast of Philadelphia, and Daniel Ayres of Brooklyn, in 1853, each of whom succeeded in closing a case. Since then, several French, and some few English and American surgeons have followed this treatment, with the following results, according to Ashhurst:—Of 55 cases, 43 recovered, 4 failed, and 8 died—a death-rate of 14·6. What is of almost equal importance, however—viz. the degree of relief afforded from the dangers, sufferings, disgust, and disabilities of the deformity—is not furnished by these figures. By "hiding, not closing," the bladder, its sensitive mucous membrane is protected from incessant friction of the clothes, and this is a great point gained; but it must not be overlooked that some of the patients, as they have reached puberty, have suffered great irritation and distress from the growth of hair upon the skin used for covering the extroversion. Though there is no control over the urine provided by these flap operations, the escape is limited to a single spot, at which, by means of an adjustable urinal, the urine can be much more effectively and securely collected, and the abdomen and limbs thereby protected from contact with it.

The dangers which attend the operations are purulent infection of the urinary mucous tract, hæmorrhage, erysipelas, and sloughing of the flaps. Space does not permit of a description of the several operative methods, and of the more or less important modifications of them, which have been practised. It must suffice here to name the classes of operations performed :—

1. Establishing a fistulous communication between the ureters and rectum.

2. Making a fistula between the bladder and the rectum. The mortality of these two methods has been 40 per cent.

3. The autoplastic or flaps method. Mortality, 14·6 per cent. This method has in several cases cured the coexisting inguinal herniæ.

4. The removal by dissection, or by the destruction of the mucous membrane of the bladder, except around the orifices of the ureters. Sonneburg, after dissecting off the bladder mucous membrane, sutures the mucous membrane to the base of the epispadias.

5. Closing the bladder by suturing its two margins. This method is sometimes combined with closure of the interval at the symphysis pubis by approximating the bones.

Mr. Greig Smith, in one case, kept the patient in bed for six weeks, covered the extroversion with green protective, coated with dextrine, and over this boracic lint, with the result that the upper part of the mucous membrane, down nearly as low as the ureters, became covered with epidermis almost as white as the surrounding skin.

According to modern views the methods of choice are as follows :—When the case is one of epispadias, with a small fissure at the inferior area of the bladder, the urethra and neck of the bladder should be closed by uniting the edges of the parts in the immediate neighbourhood. If the defect of the bladder extends somewhat higher, the edges of the

w

bladder should be freshened after dissecting up the mucous membrane without damage to the ureters. If the exstrophy is complete and the separation of the pubes considerable, the urine should be diverted into the rectum.

In a young and vigorous patient Dubois and Dupuytren's method should be employed. This consists in suturing together the 'margins of the bladder either directly or after dissecting up the mucous membrane or approximating the symphysis pubis. If the genital organs are atrophied, or the patient weakly or affected by other malformations, the mucous membrane should be sutured to the root of the urethra, or a recto-vesical fistula should be established and the mucous membrane of the bladder destroyed.

As regards the autoplastic methods, the single flap is inferior to the methods by several flaps, and the method whereby the flaps are superimposed is better than that by which they are simply joined together. (*See* papers by J. Wood, Mayo Robson, Thiersch, and others, and works on the operations in surgery.)

CHAPTER III.

FUNCTIONAL DISORDERS OF THE BLADDER.

THE great progress made of late years in the study of nervous diseases by physicians, both at home and abroad, and especially in the school of Charcot at Salpêtrière, has had its effect on surgery, and there are now known to be many vesical disorders of neurotic origin, both with and without lesions of the spinal cord. In the following account I shall closely follow an excellent article by M. Tuffier, in which he has analysed and described the functional troubles of the bladder due to some defect in the innervation of that organ. These M. Tuffier classifies as follows:—

1. Functional disturbances due to actual structural disease of the nervous system.

2. Those connected with such neuroses as epilepsy and hysteria.

3. Those connected with congenital malformations of the urinary organs.

4. Those connected with lesions of the neighbouring parts.

5. Functional disturbances of the bladder due to local lesions of this organ.

6. Those due to the composition of the urine.

7. Idiopathic sensory and motor disturbances.

8. Functional troubles of the bladder due to mental conditions (d'origine psychopathique).

If the functional disturbance is on the side of excess, we have hyperæsthesia and undue contractions of the muscular coats; if on the side of insufficiency, we get anæsthesia and muscular paralysis.

1. Functional disturbances of the bladder dependent upon structural changes in the nervous system, such as ataxy, lesions of the spinal cord and brain, localised sclerosis, general paralysis and insanity.

In *ataxy* there are many and various disturbances; they are sometimes quite the earliest symptoms of tabes, and they are noted by Fournier in ninety out of two hundred and

eleven ataxic patients.   There may be on the motor side: (1)
Paralysis without retention.   This paralysis shows itself in a
delay varying from a minute to a quarter of an hour in
starting to micturate, then in the stream stopping, to go on
again after an interval; and within an instant or two after
thinking he has finished, urine is passed into the clothes.
(2) Paralysis culminating in complete or partial retention.
(3) Incontinence which may be intermittent, and due to
overflow of urine from the bladder, or may be caused by a
peculiar irritability of the bladder, which leads to a slight
discharge of urine directly the patient makes a move to
urinate.   (4) An urgent necessity to pass water, due to
tenesmus, accompanied perhaps by cystalgia.

On the sensory side are, in the "excess" direction, urethralgia,
cystalgia, vesical colic; in the " insufficiency " direction, anæsthesia of the urethro-vesical mucous membrane, and the loss of
muscular sense of these organs.   The vesical colic, analogous
to the gastric colic, preceded by crises of variable duration and
intensity, is attended by excessive pain.

The anæsthesia of the urethro-vesical mucous membrane and
of the muscular sense is manifested by the want of feeling the
passage of urine or the distension of the bladder.   These
patients urinate in a routine manner at stated intervals, not
because they have a sense of necessity or desire to empty their
bladder.   They are obliged to watch to know whether they
are passing water or not, and when they have finished ; some
of these patients cannot urinate in the dark.

Pott's disease, and injuries to the brain and spinal cord, by
interfering with the vesico-urethral nerve centres cause paralysis
with retention, and the "incontinence of retention" or overflow.
The disturbances from these causes are very familiar.   So, too,
are the similar disturbances from serious injuries to the brain.

In *general paralysis,* according to Geffrier, there is retention from urethral spasms during the stage of excitement,
and retention from paralysis during the period of depression.

In certain cases of *insanity* the retention is voluntary, the
patients refusing to pass water just as they refuse to take food.
In *patchy sclerosis* retention due to spasms of the urethra
is caused by the irritation of the lumbar centre for the
sphincter of the bladder.

2. Functional disturbances of the bladder connected with epilepsy, the principal of which is incontinence. It differs from common nocturnal incontinence by occurring at longer or shorter intervals, and by the patient awaking with a feeling of extreme weakness, exhaustion, and weight in the head, and with the tongue sore or bleeding. Incontinence sometimes occurs during a fit of hysteria. In hysteria there is occasionally anæsthesia—*i.e.* loss of the desire to urinate, and of the sensation of passing water. These patients micturate at stated intervals in routine fashion; if this is not done, retention occurs. Tuffier refers to a case of hydronephrosis from this condition. Sir W. Roberts tells me he has met with secondary renal changes the consequences of hysteria.

In hysterical subjects with simulated spasmodic affections such as coxalgia, vaginismus, œsophagismus, etc., there may be spasms of the neck of the bladder; there is a great difficulty in commencing to micturate, and this may go on to complete retention. In some hysterical subjects there is involuntary discharge of urine under strong emotion, due to spasm of the detrusor fibres of the bladder.

Hysterical retention, due to paralysis of the bladder, is frequent, and is sometimes accompanied by hysterical hemiplegia, or more often paraplegia. If the paralysis affects both the detrusor and the sphincter vesicæ, these patients get incontinence of retention.

3. Functional troubles connected with congenital malformations and (4) those due to lesions of the neighbouring organs are what are often described as the *irritable bladder*.

The sensory symptoms are cystalgic pains; the motor symptoms, frequent spasms of the bladder and urethra, which cause frequent, but slow and painful micturition, urgent calls to pass water, and sometimes actual retention.

The causes of the symptoms are contracted external urinary meatus, tight foreskin, fissure of the anus, hæmorrhoids, oxaluria, operations on the anus; and in women, uterine and ovarian, vaginal and vulvar troubles, and operations on these parts.

Civiale, Otis, Guyon, and Reliquet, have quite established the fact that a congenitally narrow meatus is sufficient to cause all the symptoms of irritable bladder, and that it is only necessary to divide the meatus to cure these cases. I can fully endorse this statement, and can go further and say that I have seen attacks of acute cystitis brought about by the obstruction caused by a tight meatus. Beard, of New York, has seen congenital phimosis produce the same reflex phenomena on the bladder as a contracted meatus.

Nocturnal incontinence is well known to be another effect of narrow meatus and tight prepuce.

5. Functional vesical troubles due to lesions of the bladder. The reflex irritation caused by vesical calculus or tumour, and by fissure of the urethra in women, produces vesical tenesmus analogous to rectal tenesmus from anal fissure. A deep-seated but slight urethritis near the neck of the bladder often causes cystalgia. These causes of painful and irritable bladder must be recognised in order to treat them successfully.

6. Functional vesical troubles caused by the condition of the urine. The limpid urine of hysterical women, the excess of urates in gouty, and of phosphates in neurotic persons, and extremely acid urine, are· well-known causes of irritable bladder.

7. Idiopathic functional disturbances of the bladder. On the sensory side we find cystalgia ; and on the motor side, spasms of the vesical muscular tissue and the urethral sphincter—*i.e.* the compressor or constrictor of the membranous urethra.

Cystalgia is characterised by the functional symptoms of cystitis without inflammation, and without the changes in the urine. Before concluding that the condition is one of idiopathic cystalgia, we must be quite sure that there is no existing slight lesion of the urethra or bladder of which the cystalgia is symptomatic.

True idiopathic cystalgia, Tuffier writes, occurs in individuals whose parents are the subjects of migraine, nervous or rheumatic, and who are themselves liable to migraine and different nervous disorders. The determining causes of cystalgia are cold, damp, changes of season, prolonged resistance of the desire to pass water, constipation, excessive coitus, masturbation, prolonged erections. The anxieties of the patient aggravate his condition and plunge him into the deepest hypochondriasis (of which the celebrated Jean-Jacques Rousseau was an example).

8. Functional vesical troubles of méntal origin. The enormous influence of the mind over the functions of the bladder are proverbial. The remarkable experiences of Mosso and Pellacani have proved that every thought, every emotion, as well as every sensory excitation, determines an immediate contraction of the vesical muscular tissue ; and Janet has shown that if the thoughts have reference to micturition, the consequent contraction of the bladder is the more intense. They are powerful excito-reflexes of the nerves of the bladder.

The cause of these psychological troubles is an over-anxiety about micturition, which may exist quite independently of the least physical basis, or may have as its foundation some slight but real urethro-vesical trouble. As a result of this mental condition, the bladder becomes irritable, micturition is very frequent, and there is an abnormal amount of urine secreted. That the polyuria, as well as the frequency of micturition, is due to mental influence is proved by the fact that if the mind is engaged and interested, both cease as they do during sleep. The patients may pass water fifty times a day, yet sleep all through the night. A greatly increased capacity of bladder is proved to exist in these cases by injections of warm water; and yet a catheter left in the bladder as a drain tube does not remove the desire they have to pass water.

When this condition proceeds to an extreme, the polyuria occurs at night, and they either sleep lightly and rise frequently to pass urine, or they sleep soundly and pass urine into their bed. This is one of the varieties, probably the commonest, of nocturnal incontinence of urine in children.

This incontinence is not diurnal as well as nocturnal, no matter how frequent the desire to urinate, or how much urine is secreted. If there is diurnal incontinence, the condition is of a different nature, it is not due to psychological causes only.

Another form of functional disturbance from mental causes is urethral spasm manifested either during micturition or during the introduction of an instrument. If during micturition, we have the condition so happily described by Paget as "stammering of the bladder," which renders the person incapable of micturating in presence of others, or even in a ·place where the flow of their urine can be heard.

This urethral spasm may occur in private by the individual watching himself too closely to see if he has a stricture, or it may render the stream thready and corkscrew shaped, and his alarms are thereby increased till the passage of a full-sized instrument convinces him how groundless they are.

The dread of the introduction of an instrument may provoke the spasms, and thereby obstruct the easy passage of it, unless a solution of cocaine is injected, or chloroform is given previous to using the sound. These patients often have, too, other troubles connected with the generative organs, and fancy they are the victims of impotence or spermatorrhœa, and between the two sets of imaginary weaknesses they may pass into profound hypochondriasis.

The best treatment is to give them confidence, to prove to them the groundlessness of their fears, to prescribe douches and exercise in the open air, and tonics; and to cocainise the urethra and pass a full-sized instrument into the bladder.

In direct opposition to the above functional vesical troubles of nervous origin are what have been described as **nervous troubles of vesical origin.** Many writers, such as Sir W. Gull, Le Dentu, and others, have quoted cases in which some vesical lesion has been supposed to have produced nervous disorders, and in particular paraplegia; and several hypotheses have been advanced to explain this. (1) Ascending neuritis; (2) irritation of the nerve plexuses, producing, by reflex action, congestion of the spinal cord; (3) exhaustion of the nerve elements, owing to violent and prolonged irritation, are the three chief hypotheses which have found supporters. But neither the theories nor the cures on which they have been erected are generally received. Siredey says he has never seen paraplegia occur in the course of uterine affections except in hysteria, or dependent upon inflammation of the cord; and he is of opinion that it is the same in the case of vesical affections.

M. Guyon has not been able to find a case of myelitis of vesical origin, and desires to do so before he can believe in its occurrence.

INCONTINENCE OF URINE.

This is but a symptom, the causes of which are many; and the treatment must be as varied as the causes.

Even when there is no ascertainable lesion about the urinary organs to explain this troublesome condition, there are still many other causes of incontinence both in children and adults for which search must be made.

Incontinence of urine assumes two most distinct and very different forms—(1) the incontinence of the drop-by-drop kind, the incessant, continuous dribbling; and (2) incontinence in the form of intermittent large evacuations of urine·

Incontinence which occurs at night may affect adults as well as children; but, with the exception of epileptics and those who have had their vesical and urethral sphincters over-stretched by retention of urine, the nocturnal incontinents are almost entirely children.

Trousseau states that every adult nocturnal incontinent is an epileptic; but this assertion is, of course, only approximately true, and takes no account of the numerous cases of incontinence, during night and day, which are caused by organic affections of the urinary or nervous systems.

It will convey some idea of the various causes of incontinence other than organic lesions, if we group the cases into different classes.

1. The "continual" incontinence consisting in incessant dribbling of urine. This is due to paralysis of the vesical and urethral (the membranous urethra) sphincters. It may or may not be associated with retention. If it is, the incontinence is merely the overflow of the bladder and is the "incontinence of retention." If it is "incontinence without retention," the bladder is no longer serving as a reservoir, but has become merely a part of a conduit placed between ureters and urethra. This is a state of absolute incontinence. Continual incontinence, if it has not been caused by over-distension and its effects on bladder and sphincter, is probably always hysterical. Incontinence from retention due to stricture and other mechanical obstructions has been discussed in previous chapters.

2. Some children have nocturnal incontinence whose urinary functions during the day are quite normal in every respect.

These are the subjects of incontinence of a psychopathic mental) origin, and they constitute the majority of cases. It is intermittent incontinence of large quantities of urine. It arises from the child having a besetting dream of passing water, and it is aggravated by the fear that he will wet his bed. If he dreams of rain pattering against the window, of water running from a tap, or of some object he may have seen during the day, such as a horse staling, a dog crouching, or of any other animal urinating, the same result happens.

This form of incontinence always ceases at puberty, if not before; because at puberty the sexual fire commences to be awakened, and a different turn is given to the thoughts and dreams of these incontinents.

3. Another class of case is that in which incontinence of the intermittent form occurs at night only; but during the day these children have frequent and pressing calls to pass urine, and must give immediate relief to their bladders, otherwise they wet their clothes.

This form is due to irritation either of the spinal cord, of the intestines, or of the genito-urinary apparatus. Phimosis, contracted meatus, oxyluria and lithæmia, and intestinal worms play an important *rôle*. Nor, in this connection, must we forget the important observations, already referred to (page 343), of Mosso and Pellacani, who state that thoughts or dreams of micturition cause a veritable contraction of the bladder.

4. In another class of case the children have both diurnal and nocturnal incontinence. They never think for an instant of trying to prevent it. They pass water in the day-time with the same unconsciousness as they do at night. This form of incontinence is due either to defective contractile power of the urethral sphincter, or to urethral insensibility.

With such feebleness of the sphincter, the pressure of a distended bladder cannot be resisted; the patient has not the time to reach the closet in the day-time, nor to rouse himself and reach the chamber vessel in the night.

This feebleness may be congenital, and then due to malformation, or excessively small size, of the sphincter muscle; or to rudimentary or imperfect development of the external genital organs — *i.e.* hypospadias. Again, it may affect a well-developed sphincter muscle, and it is then a consequence of hysteria or of over-stretching of the sphincter by too large an instrument, or by digital examination.

In the anæsthetic form the sphincter is strong enough, but it is not warned by reflex action to prevent the flow of urine along the urethra. It occurs as a consequence of spinal lesions and also in hysteria.

Wagner has noticed that, as the result of certain forms of spinal disease, the vesical sphincter is so weakened as to allow of urine being discharged from the bladder merely by pressure on the hypogastrium. He states that in tabes, tabetic general paralysis, and spinal injuries with loss of knee-jerk, the bladder can be completely emptied by this kind of pressure. In cases in which the knee-jerk is increased, the vesical sphincter retains its power.

5. Incontinence during epileptic seizures. This takes place at the end of the epileptic attack, and occurs, as these attacks themselves do, either by day or night. It is succeeded by a feeling of extreme prostration on waking, and by the evidence of the tongue having been bitten during the seizure.

Prognosis.—The above-mentioned forms of incontinence, though most unpleasant, are not dangerous. Except in the epileptic cases, cure will be obtained sooner or later. The psychopathic incontinence will cease at, if not before, puberty. The incontinence due to irritation will be cured by removing the cause. The incontinence of atony of the sphincter, which seems at first the most hopeless, is often the most easily removed. This remark does not, of course, apply to atony of the bladder from spinal disease.

All forms, except the epileptic, have a tendency to disappear at puberty. It is quite exceptional, if not altogether unknown, to meet with them after twenty-five years of age. Spontaneous cure sometimes unexpectedly follows an attack of fever or some other illness. In some cases, after the incontinence ceases, the individuals are obliged to pass water once or twice during the night, and this necessity may continue even throughout life. Many of these patients, however, get cured of their incontinence, only to enter upon some other nervous affection, such as spasm of the bladder, irritable bladder, or to become confirmed hypochondriacs.

If proper treatment is not adopted, any form of the affection may become very troublesome.

Treatment—In the psychopathic form, moral treatment is the only useful one. The little patient must not be scolded, or punished, or reproached, or made a laughing-stock of. He should be encouraged, reassured, and even told not to mind the accident. Let him not go to sleep with a final instruction that he must not wet himself, whereby his last thought is made a connecting-link with his habitual dream. On the contrary, coax him, if possible, into the belief that he is cured, and assure him he ought not to be troubled if he should find he is not. Much is gained if a few nights pass without an accident, and this is sometimes obtained by waking the child just before the hour at which the nurse has ascertained micturition takes place. Means are sometimes recommended to lighten sleep and increase the irritability of the neck of the bladder. A hard bed, a little tea or coffee taken late before going to bed, are calculated to obtain the one aim, and the passage of catheters or sounds will sometimes accomplish the other.

For incontinence due to irritable bladder the treatment consists of the removal of the cause; thus circumcision, division of the meatus, vermifuge remedies, improvement in dietary to correct oxyluria or lithiasis, are the means which should be employed.

Incontinence from atony, or from paralysis, will be often rapidly cured by electrolysis applied to the hypogastrium, or even within the cavity of the bladder.

For the incontinence of the epileptic, the general treatment suitable for that disease is what is required.

CHAPTER IV.

WOUNDS OF THE BLADDER.

SIMPLE contusions of the bladder are probably very rare, and hardly ever come under the surgeon's observation. Wounds of the bladder, like wounds of other organs and tissues, are appropriately considered under (1) punctured, (2) incised, and (3) contused wounds, including wounds by firearms.

The bladder is most easily wounded when distended; especially is this true of all kinds of wounds inflicted upon the bladder through the abdominal parietes; for when not distended, the bladder is contracted behind, and protected by the symphysis and rami of the pubes.

There are four routes by which the bladder can be reached by accident. One, however, is very rarely taken—namely, that through the obturator foramen. The other three routes are through the abdominal wall, the perinæum, and the rectum. Each of these three have been made use of by surgeons for the performance of operations upon the bladder.

PUNCTURED WOUNDS

inflicted by sharp instruments are of the nature of incised wounds, and vary in importance according to their size, the condition of the urine contained in the bladder at the time of the injury, and the promptitude and completeness with which treatment is employed. Punctured wounds inflicted by blunt bodies are of the nature of contused wounds, and are of much more serious import.

Punctured wounds caused by minute sharp instruments, such as a needle, pin, or an aspirating trocar, are of no importance provided a blood-vessel is not punctured, that ulceration does not occur around the point punctured, and that the wounding body and the urine in the bladder are quite aseptic.

INCISED WOUNDS

are often inflicted by the surgeon—intentionally, in hypogastric cystotomy; unintentionally, during the removal of adherent abdominal tumours, in opening abscesses in the pelvic cellular tissue through the vagina, or through the rectum of a man. Such wounds, when made in the course of an abdominal operation, if recognised at once, and efficiently closed by sutures, do quite well. They might often, though certainly they cannot always, be prevented by emptying the bladder immediately before commencing an operation; but the presence of a sound in the bladder, moved about from time to time as occasion requires during the dissection, is the greatest safeguard. Accidental incised wounds are particularly rare.

CONTUSED WOUNDS

are by no means infrequent, if we include amongst them "contused punctured" wounds, such as are made by a broomstick, a stake, the horn of any animal, or by firearms.

In these latter, the projectile may of course, take any line to the bladder, and when it breaks its way through the bony wall of the pelvis, extra damage is done by the splinters of bone which are carried before it. In some gunshot wounds the projectile has passed right through the body from pubis to sacrum, wounding both bladder and rectum, and allowing urine to escape in front and fæcal matter through the posterior wound.

When boys or men have fallen on iron railings, or upstanding poles or sticks, the bladder has been reached through the anus and rectal wall, or through the perinæum. Larrey and Demarquay mention cases in which the vulnerating body, such as a Cossack's lance, the barrel of a gun, or a bull's horn, has entered the bladder through the obturator foramen. The anterior abdominal wall is the rarest route for accidents of this kind.

Wounds of the bladder may be either penetrating or non-penetrating. Some wounds are inflicted from within outwards, such as those caused by surgical instruments or foreign bodies within the bladder.

Non-penetrating wounds may concern either the outer or the inner surface. Those affecting the outer wall may be inflicted by spent bullets. Bartels and Larrey have recorded four cases in which the projectiles had been encysted for several years; but they are more frequently the result of surgical operations, as when adhesions of the bladder have to be separated in the course of operations on the abdomen and pelvis.

Non-penetrating wounds of the inner surface of the bladder are made necessarily during the removal of vesical growths; accidentally, by the clumsy use of the lithotrite, by the frequent impact of a catheter on the same spot of mucous membrane, by foreign bodies, and by the rough sharp edges of calculi.

Penetrating wounds are either intra- or extra-peritoneal, or both—*i.e.* when the wound involves the bladder wall at the line of reflection of the peritoneum.

In these cases the urine escapes and the bladder contracts immediately it is wounded, unless, as in the corresponding condition of the intestine, the wound is very small, and is plugged by the bulging mucous membrane, and then there will be little, if any, extravasation.

If the bladder empties and contracts, the relations of the wounded part of the viscus to the wound in the surrounding soft parts are at once altered; and the edges of the wound in the different layers of the bladder wall behave differently; those of the peritoneal coat become loose flaps, those of the muscular coat are irregularly contracted, whilst those of the mucous coat pucker into soft rolls or pads, and may bulge between the lips of the wound in the other layers. The bladder may be penetrated from within outwards by unskilful manipulations with the lithotrite, by catheters, or by foreign bodies introduced along the urethra.

Several ways in which the bladder is penetrated from without inwards have been mentioned above.

Symptoms.—With penetrating wounds, besides the usual symptoms of shock, with or without the signs of hæmorrhage, there are others which are special to the organ involved. Thus urine may escape at the wound, blood may be mixed with the urine, or there may be great desire and straining to pass water without the discharge of any through the urethra, or of only a little largely mixed with blood. Or there may be a history pointing evidently to the discharge of the urine into the peritoneal cavity, as, for instance, when the patient had gone several hours before the injury without micturating, and the bladder is found empty immediately or soon afterwards. If urine escapes by the wound, it may do so continuously or in an intermittent manner. If the wound in the bladder wall is valvular, urine may only escape through it when the patient micturates; if it be small and plugged by bulging mucous membrane, it will only escape when the bladder is distended and the mucous membrane is again on stretch. These are important facts to remember in the treatment of such cases.

The later or secondary symptoms will depend upon whether the wound opens into the peritoneum or not. If it does not, the prognosis and symptoms will be less grave and of an altogether different type from those which occur when the peritoneum is implicated.

At first there may be a discharge of more or less blood and urine from the wound, but subsequently urinary infiltration must be looked for. If the wound is small or tortuous, the quantity of blood and urine escaping may be small, but the liability to the serious consequences of extravasation arising from the decomposition of fluids retained in the tissues will be the greater.

It is now well known that it is not the mere presence in the peritoneum, or the tissues, of normal urine which is the source of danger, but the subsequent decomposition of the mixture of secretions from the wound, of the urine, and of the extravasated blood, which gives rise to fever, rigors, septic infection, and it may be even to death.

Blood-clots may accumulate in the bladder and by causing obstruction at the urethro-vesical orifice may hasten and increase the extravasation of urine, and aggravate the sufferings of the patient.

If the bladder is wounded through the vagina or rectum, and the peritoneum escapes, the consequences are much less severe, as the urine and blood will most likely escape directly into these passages, and thus extravasation into the cellular tissue will be avoided.

In gunshot injuries, or injuries inflicted with blunt or septic weapons there are all the risks attendant on inflammation and suppuration excited by the traumatism quite apart from those of urinary extravasation; and where the catheter has been required there are the risks of infection through it also. It is most likely that, owing to the aseptic precautions now always observed, the statistics of these wounds in the future will be less unfavourable than those of the past.

If the wound penetrates the peritoneum, the symptoms which follow in the course of several hours, or of a day or two, are those of acute infective peritonitis. It is rare but not unknown for the peritonitis to be limited, and the fluid to become encysted by adhesions of the surrounding peritoneal surfaces.

In non-penetrating wounds there are not usually any marked symptoms. Those which involve the outer surface are generally quickly covered by granulation or unite directly with an adjacent peritoneal surface. Those which involve the inner surface heal somewhat slowly by granulations, and leave inextensile fibrous cicatricial tissues; but in healthy persons they do well. In some, there may be a sudden elevation of temperature with a rigor indicative of urinary fever; in others, acute or subacute cystitis may arise, but this is not often the case.

Gunshot wounds of the bladder are very frequently complicated with other severe injuries, often of a fatal kind.

In 285 cases Bartels found 131 fractures, 98 wounds of the peritoneum or intestines, 18 wounds of the large vessels, and 26 in which there was rupture of some other organ; altogether 273 cases in which other grave lesions were associated with the wound of the bladder.

Prognosis.—Surgical wounds of the bladder, if recognised at the time of injury and appropriately treated by immediate suture, heal well, and can scarcely be said to prejudice the result of the operation in the course of which they have been inflicted. The consequences are rather more grave if there has been a considerable loss of substance; and they become very serious indeed if unhappily the bladder is wounded, and the accident is not recognised or detected at the time.

Bartels', Stein's, and Rivington's statistics show that death has almost invariably occurred when the peritoneum has been wounded. The employment of immediate sutures has made a great change for the better in the prognosis of these cases; but it is very important to recognise the fact that wounds of the bladder can heal without being united by

x

sutures, as was proved beyond question by a case I published in 1887, and which is unique in the completeness of the evidence it affords.

Extra-peritoneal wounds show also a high mortality—highest in cases of gunshot wounds. Wounds through the rectum and vagina are less serious than those which pass through the perinæum and hypogastrium; and in gunshot wounds those with a double orifice, one of entrance and one of exit, by giving freer vent for discharges, are less likely to be followed by extravasation and septic absorption than those with only an orifice of entrance. The extravasation of purulent urine, or of urine which becomes purulent, into the tissues or the peritoneal cavity, is the source of one of the greatest dangers.

Other conditions which make a grave prognosis still more unfavourable are hæmorrhage, acute peritonitis, acute cystitis; and damage to other viscera, to the blood-vessels, or to the bones of the pelvis, simultaneously inflicted. If the patient recovers from the immediate injury, he may suffer long from some of the complications, such as fistulæ, foreign bodies in the bladder upon which calculi may form, and permanent injury to the pelvic bones or hip-joint. I have removed a large phosphate of lime calculus, having a spicule of bone for its nucleus, from a young middle-aged man who four years previously had fractured his pelvis.

Diagnosis.—This will be made clear by the escape of urine at the wound and by the blood-stained urine passed per urethram, or drawn off through a catheter; by the tenesmus of the bladder, and, if the wound be intraperitoneal, by the catheter passing through an empty bladder into the peritoneal cavity and thence withdrawing urine with the jerky flow caused by respiratory movements. With aseptic precautions and gentleness, a probe may be passed along the wound, when it may be brought into contact with a sound in the bladder; or if the wound is non-peritoneal, a little weak turmeric solution may be injected at the wound and its colour detected in the urine. But neither of these procedures is to be recommended, nor are they often needed.

There is much greater difficulty in diagnosing between intra- and extra-peritoneal wounds, and, indeed, sometimes the diagnosis cannot be made without an exploratory laparotomy. In some cases the wound crosses the line of peritoneum and is thus at once intra- and extra-peritoneal. Yet it is important to make the diagnosis at once ; and for the surgeon to act forthwith, and not wait to see whether or not peritonitis will ensue. The situation and direction of the wound come to his aid here, though they do not in subparietal ruptures. Careful but thorough exploration of the bladder with a sound or silver catheter will show whether the end of the instrument passes into the peritoneum or the recto-vesical space.

In some cases a fluctuating swelling felt per rectum has revealed the escape of urine into the peritoneal cavity and its accumulation in Douglas's pouch. In others, the history of a distended bladder suddenly relieved and all evidence of it vanished is in itself proof enough of the escape of a large quantity of urine into the general cavity of the abdomen. Again, one or other or both loins may be dull in certain positions, and resonant when the patient lies with the same side upwards.

Failing other means, laparotomy with the view to actual inspection of the bladder is not only justifiable but right, and is the necessary step towards suturing the bladder if the wound should prove to be intra-peritoneal.

In gunshot wounds or fractures of the pelvis, the track of the wound and the cavity of the bladder should be searched for foreign bodies.

Treatment.—In all cases of intra-peritoneal wounds, when the patient is seen before peritonitis has set in, laparotomy should, if the circumstances permit, be performed, the toilette of the peritoneum properly attended to, and the wound in the bladder closed by sutures. Care should be taken that the sutures should be applied close enough and carried sufficiently far beyond each extremity of the wound to prevent any escape of urine. The mucous membrane should not be included. The sutures should be applied by Lembert's method. The bladder should be drained for the first two or three days by catheter. Even when peritonitis has commenced, this should be the procedure of choice. But in country practice with only one, or perhaps no reliable assistant, suturing the wound cannot be wisely attempted.

The introduction of the sutures in the postero-inferior parts of the bladder-wall is a task of great difficulty, requiring for its successful performance good light, proper appliances, and skilled help; it would be worse than useless to attempt the operation without these. What, then, is to be done? Of course hæmorrhage must be stopped, and if to accomplish this the abdominal cavity has to be opened, the bladder should be inspected and the wound closed, if possible, with such aid as is attainable; but if it is not necessary to open the abdomen to stay bleeding, then it would be best to trust to a catheter *en demeure* as a continuous drain, or to drain the bladder through a median urethrotomy or a lateral lithotomy wound.

The case I have referred to above (p. 354) conclusively shows that by thorough drainage through a catheter retained in the bladder, an intra-peritoneal wound can be closed by a fibrous cicatrix. It may be repaired by the direct union of the edges of its peritoneal coat or by the formation of adhesions with the bowel, mesentery, or omentum.

In extra-peritoneal wounds, if inflicted upon the front wall during the state of distension of the bladder, the edges of the wound should be brought together by sutures, and the bladder drained by a catheter. In wounds inflicted upon the posterior wall and base of the bladder, free drainage should be provided by means of a large catheter retained in the bladder; or if this is inefficient, by enlarging, if necessary, the wound, or by establishing a drain not only for the bladder but for the extra-vesical tissues as well, through a median or lateral perinæal incision.

Hæmorrhage in these cases must be managed on the general principles applicable to all cases. In every event, the most scrupulous care should be used to keep the wound aseptic; and this is best done after the insertion of a drain tube, by packing the wound with iodoform or carbolised gauze, and having an ample quantity of absorbent iodoform cotton-wool, frequently changed, in contact with the perinæum and buttocks.

The question of removing any foreign body introduced into the bladder, at the time or subsequently, ought to be settled by the condition of the patient and wound. If the patient is suffering much from shock, and there are no other indications for immediate active interference, it may be left till he has rallied. Voillemier and Le Dentu advise this course. The nature of the foreign body will almost surely be such as the lithotrite cannot remove, and it must be taken away either through the wound or by cystotomy.

When the wound is large enough, or when the bladder has to be incised at once for drainage, or when an operation for closing the wound by sutures is undertaken, then the foreign body should be removed at that same time. In some cases of doubt, the presence in the bladder of a foreign body may determine that an operation should be undertaken, and even the precise character of the operation.

The treatment of the subsequent complications of bladder wounds, such as urinary infiltration, urinary fistulæ, cystitis, and the associated functional troubles, is considered under their several headings.

CHAPTER V.

RUPTURE OF THE BLADDER.

RUPTURE of the bladder is very rare, very likely to be over-looked, or to be mistaken for peritonitis, or some other lesion, and is very fatal. Indeed, to be treated properly and with any hope of success, it must be seen early and diagnosed promptly.

The literature of the subject is very abundant, and ad-mirable and exhaustive monographs have been written by Dr. Harrison, of Dublin; Houel, of Paris; Stephen Smith, of New York; W. Rivington, of London: A. W. Stein, Max Bartels, and others.

W. Rivington, in his exhaustive monograph, published in 1884, has analysed 322 cases thus :—

1. Simple fatal intra-peritoneal ruptures	152
2. Complicated fatal intra-peritoneal ruptures	30
3. Fatal extra-peritoneal ruptures, simple and complicated ...	90
4. Reported cases of recovery	40
5. Fatal ruptures of uncertain position	10
	322

Besides these, cases of intra-uterine rupture in the fœtus have been recorded.

Etiology.—Ruptures of the bladder are of three kinds : traumatic, idiopathic, and pathological.

The *traumatic* are caused either by violence from without or by violent muscular efforts on the part of the patient himself. The *pathological*, result from ulceration, sloughing, thinning, and sacculation of the parietes. The *idiopathic*, occur from the spontaneous yielding of the distended bladder, independently of any form of violence, or of previous ulcera-tion or sloughing, or of tunicary herniæ.

There are certain predisposing conditions which render the bladder more likely to be ruptured when violence is applied to it. The *occupations* of men render them more liable than women. Of 288 cases, 240 were men and 48 women. Age is a factor of importance, men in their active life, from twenty to fifty, being the most frequent sufferers; but I have had two cases in boys, one with and the other without fracture of the pelvis; and Rivington gives five (out of 159 cases) under ten years of age. Distension of the bladder is very favourable to rupture; and though this state is not necessary for extra-peritoneal ruptures, nor for ruptures caused by fracture of the pelvis, it is generally the condition under which intra-peritoneal ruptures occur. Distension brings the bladder into contact with the abdominal wall, and stretches and thins the wall of the viscus. Intoxication, by increasing the action of the kidneys, deadening the sensation of distension of the bladder, and rendering the muscles of the abdominal parietes more flaccid and less excitable under reflex irritation, is a powerful predisposing cause. Falls or blows on the abdomen are more likely to cause rupture during intoxication or insensibility of any kind than when the abdominal parietes are in full activity and vigour. Old adhesions abnormally fixing the bladder to surrounding parts facilitate rupture in certain cases.

The exciting causes of traumatic rupture are blows or falls upon the abdomen; crushes, as by cartwheels passing over the belly; forcible muscular contractions, and fractures of the pelvis. All these are forms of *direct* violence to the bladder. There are other cases in which the bladder has given way by falls upon the feet, upon the tuberosities of the ischia, or on the back, which tend to show that the bladder may rupture from *indirect* violence; though the effect of violent muscular action to save the fall must not be forgotten in considering such cases.

When the pelvis is fractured, the broken end, or a loose fragment of bone may penetrate the wall of the bladder; or the bladder may be torn by separation at the symphysis, or by the drag of broken and displaced bone to which the ligaments of the bladder are attached. Violent muscular contractions cause rupture, such for example as straining at lifting or pushing, forcible blowing of wind instruments, struggling under anæsthesia, or during labour, or during forcible defæcation (Rivington, p. 14); or violent efforts to empty the bladder in retention from stricture, enlarged prostate, or other obstruction.

In straining at·stool, men with stricture or enlarged prostate are very likely to rupture a distended bladder because, owing to the urethral obstruction, the bladder does not empty readily or rapidly, and at the commencement of the act of defæcation. Such patients should be warned as to this, and told to empty their bladder before going to stool.

In all these cases of rupture from forcible muscular contraction, the bladder gives way when it is distended.

In the case of rupture during distension from obstruction, the contractions of the muscular layer of the bladder wall (probably hypertrophied) together with the muscles of the abdominal parietes are the rupturing forces. It is much more common in these cases, however, for the dilated urethra behind the stricture·to give way than the bladder to rupture. In rupture during labour, the distended bladder is compressed between two strong muscular forces— viz. the contracting abdominal parietes and the contracting and enlarged uterus. In rupture during the struggles under anæsthesia, and during powerful muscular efforts, as in lifting or pushing, the bladder-wall is passive and the rupturing force is the abdominal parietes.

Traumatic ruptures form the bulk of the intra-peritoneal and of the partly intra- and partly extra-peritoneal cases.

True *idiopathic* ruptures, or those which occur when there is no disease, and where no violence is used, are very rare. In most cases of rupture during urinary retention the bladder gives way under forcible muscular efforts as explained above; so in cases of rupture during heavy lifting, parturition, and muscular spasms. So that this class is restricted to certain cases of rupture from *simple over-distension* from stricture, prostatic enlargements, tumours, retroversion of the gravid uterus, etc.; to spontaneous rupture during alcoholism, erysipelas, fever, and other serious illnesses, and in hysteria (Dr. J. B. Wilmot's case), and in the fœtus in utero.

It has always been a disputed question whether the bladder ever ruptures from over-distension alone, and the answer has been generally given in the negative. Certainly in many reputed cases of this sort, the bladder-wall has been previously softened by fever or by fatty degeneration, or weakened by tunicary herniæ; but there are recorded cases (*see* Rivington's work, pp. 20 and 21) in which, undoubtedly, spontaneous rupture has occurred in bladders healthy except for the effects of the distension.

In other cases it is quite open to question how far the changes in the bladder-walls, found after death, preceded, or were the effect of, over-distension.

Idiopathic rupture is generally intra-peritoneal; or sub-peritoneal at first, becoming intra-peritoneal subsequently. It is astonishing to what a very extensive degree the peritoneum in the pelvis and along the front of the abdomen can be stripped off, and how large an extra-vesical cavity containing urine can be formed in untreated cases of this sort. (*See* Path. Trans., vol. xxxvii. p. 305.)

In Rivington's list of fatal cases, 59 out of 282 were idiopathic, and 223 were traumatic; and of these 59 cases, 46 were intra-peritoneal, 11 extra-peritoneal, and 2 uncertain. But Rivington, following Houel, includes under the idiopathic a large number of cases in which the ruptures were undoubtedly caused by the violence of muscular contractions. The truly idiopathic cases are very rare; and as they are all preventable by catheterism or aspiration of the bladder, they are generally a cause of reproach to the medical attendant. The possibility of their occurrence ought always to be remembered. I have recorded a case in which spontaneous rupture of the cicatrix, seven years after a former intra-peritoneal rupture, occurred owing to the thinning and elongation of the scar tissue which was adherent to the bowel. (*See* Roy. Med.-Chir. Society's Trans., vol 70.)

The *pathological* ruptures are caused by the bladder weakened at certain spots by ulceration or tunicary herniæ, giving way under distension, or by the bladder sloughing as the result of pressure or inflammation. Rivington collected 9 cases of intra-peritoneal rupture from retroversion of the gravid uterus, and 2 from extra-uterine fœtation, both intra-peritoneal; and 7 cases (3 intra-peritoneal, 3 extra-peritoneal, and 1 doubtful) due to ulceration.

Dr. Johnston of Bolton (*Brit. Med. Journal*, vol. i. p. 1003, 1893) has recently recorded a case of pathological rupture due to the giving way of a simple ulcer 3 inches in diameter.

The patient was a hale man of seventy-five, without any symptoms until thirteen days before his death, when he began to pass a little bright blood in his urine, and had to micturate every two hours; fourteen hours before death, whilst trying to pass water, he was seized with a sudden violent pain, caused by the giving way of the posterior wall of the bladder and the discharge of over a pint of blood, from a large artery, into the peritoneal cavity.

Krukenburg, who has collected ten cases, and added one observed by himself, of rupture from retroversion of the gravid womb, considers the pathology of rupture of the bladder and gangrene of the vesical wall, to be identical. In some cases, protective adhesions on the peritoneal surface are formed during the progress of the gangrenous inflammation of the coats of the bladder, and then the gangrenous parts may be cast off entire or broken up; otherwise, perforation attends the separation of the slough, even without over-distension of the bladder. Rupture may also take place suddenly from over-distension before the separation of any slough, or may result from even the most gentle and careful efforts to replace the uterus. Krukenburg adds that when retention of urine persists for ten days or longer, either gangrene or rupture of the bladder may occur, but more frequently rupture. He also gives the warning that if gangrenous portions of the vesical wall have been cast off, no attempt should be made to replace the uterus, but that abortion ought to be induced. The pressure of a retroverted gravid uterus has caused gangrene of the walls of the bladder in several instances.

Pathological Anatomy. The Character of the Rent.— There is a difference in the character of the rent in the bladder walls depending upon the cause of the rupture. Rivington writes, " In the idiopathic cases the aperture is small, often circular or triquetrous, but in the traumatic cases it is generally a rent from an inch to two inches long. This corresponds with the results of experiments on the dead body." This difference holds good for pure idiopathic or spontaneous rupture, but not for the whole group of mixed cases (spontaneous, pathological, and traumatic from muscular violence) which are included in Rivington's and Houel's idiopathic class. The rent in several of the cases so included, of rupture from muscular violence, has the same character as in rupture from external violence, as is notable in the case recorded by Mr. Reginald Harrison. In some idiopathic cases the rent is valvular, the edges sloping from within outwards. All the coats are not always torn to the same extent, and the mucous coat may be herniated through the rent in the muscular and peritoneal coats. In pathological ruptures, the character of the rent varies with the disease. In ulceration, there is a small aperture with ulcerated and ragged edges in an inflamed area, and purulent matter may be adherent about the edges of the ulcer. In gangrene there may be a hole as large as the finger tip in the centre of a gangrenous area; or a large hole with irregular edges, if the whole of the gangrenous mass has separated. In rupture of a tunicary hernia, the pouch of mucous membrane will show signs of inflammation, ulceration, or may be simply of softening of the tissues.

The Situation of the Rent.—The posterior surface of the bladder is the common site, and the more or less vertical the common direction of the simple intra-peritoneal traumatic rupture. This, however, is subject to many variations. In spontaneous ruptures, the rent is commonly behind; in traumatic ruptures, behind and above. The rent may be oblique or transverse; but the transverse is very rare as compared with the vertical: Rivington gives only eight out of 110 cases. There seems to be no difference in position and general character of the rents from direct and from indirect violence. But if the violence, instead of at once rupturing the bladder, pushes it forcibly backwards, it is most likely that the rent will be found in front, and just above the prostate gland. Out of 100 cases in which the position of the aperture was clearly noted, according to Rivington:—

44 presented the rent on the posterior aspect
22 on the posterior and superior aspect
22 at the superior fundus
3 superiorly and anteriorly
4 on the anterior aspect of the superior fundus
4 behind and below
1 at the side.

Max Bartels gives the situation of the rent in eighty-two intra-peritoneal cases as follows:—

> 24 at the fundus
> 14 in front, near the fundus
> 39 posteriorly
> 5 at the side.

As to the comparative frequency of intra- and extra-peritoneal, Rivington's figures show 182 fatal intra- to 90 fatal extra. The extra peritoneal ruptures affect the anterior surface, the neck, the posterior surface, and the sides.

It is probable, however, that extra-peritoneal rupture is much more common than appears from these figures, but is not so commonly reported. Thus in a series of ten cases occurring at the same hospital (St. George's), and reported by Sir Prescott Hewett (Path. Soc. Trans.), six were extra-peritoneal associated with injury to the pelvis, two were simple extra-peritoneal, and only two intra-peritoneal. The figures of other writers show the same thing. Thus, Bartels gives fifty-nine extra-peritoneal out of one hundred cases, Ullmann eighty-five out of one hundred cases, and Fenwick eighty-eight out of one hundred. Ruptures from fracture of the pelvis are extra-peritoneal in seventy-six per cent., according to Ullmann; and one-half of the ninety fatal extra-peritoneal ruptures collected by Rivington were associated with fracture or displacement of the pelvis.

As a rule, there is only one rent in the bladder, but in a few cases two have been found. In Gruber's case there was a complete intra-peritoneal rupture one inch and a half long, and lower down a second rent limited to the mucous and muscular coats. (*See* Thorp's paper, *Dublin Quarterly Journal*, vol. xlvi. p. 313.) The three coats are not always equally ruptured; most frequently the peritoneal is torn to the greatest extent. The peritoneum may be stripped up around the opening, or hang loosely over it, and this condition is indicative of secondary rupture of the peritoneum.

The peritoneum may give way subsequently in both extra- and subperitoneal ruptures. The point which yields may be either the peritoneal coat of the bladder, as was the case in a patient under Mr. Hulke at the Middlesex Hospital (*Lancet*, 1892, vol. ii. p. 197); or the peritoneum of the abdominal wall at a considerable distance from the bladder. Thus in a case of Sir Everard Home, the rupture was on the front aspect of the bladder, and did not involve its peritoneal coat; but the urine was extravasated into the areolar tissue and travelled up to the umbilicus outside, and then burst through, the peritoneum. The opening in the mucous membrane was the size of a goose quill only; that in the muscular coat an inch in diameter.

In extra-peritoneal rupture, instead of the peritoneum giving way, the urine may infiltrate the areolar tissue, and an abscess may form and kill the patient after many days. In Dr. Gouley's case this happened, and the patient did not die till the forty-fourth day.

There is often a very large amount of blood effused. In some of the intra-peritoneal cases as much as three pounds of clotted blood (Dewar's case), and between three and four pints of fluid blood have been found (B. Cooper's case).

Very frequently in intra-peritoneal rupture the bladder is found contracted. In one it was described as contracted " into a firm ball"; in another, " like a scirrhus uterus," and so on. This is no doubt the result of the violent expulsive efforts made.

In some cases of extra-peritoneal rupture the bladder is capable of holding many ounces of urine. In one of Sir Everard Home's cases a pint was found in the bladder at the post mortem, and a quart had been drawn off through the rectum during life.

The quantity of urine contained in the peritoneal cavity varies, and increases as life is prolonged. If death occurs within three days, a large quantity may be present without there being any signs of peritonitis. Surgical casualties in operations on the abdomen have repeatedly shown that healthy urine is harmless to the peritoneum, especially if it can find an exit, and also that it may be rapidly absorbed. Experiments, too, show the inoffensiveness of a small quantity of urine injected into the peritoneum, that the injections may be repeated with impunity, but that the persistent effusion excites peritonitis (Tuffier). On the other hand, when life has been prolonged, and septic elements have been introduced by the catheter, or have developed about the inflamed and contused edges of the wound, the evidences of peritonitis will be well marked.

Symptoms.—If the individual is intoxicated when the injury happens, he may be unaware of the accident, and only realise that he has sustained a serious injury after the lapse of several hours. If he is sober at the time, he will suffer at the moment of rupture intense pain in the abdomen, will have a sense of something having given way within him, and perhaps will vomit or faint. Thus, if intoxicated, he may be found unconscious from drink; if sober, from syncope and collapse. On the other hand, he may stagger home a mile or more; or, though conscious, may yet be unable to walk, or even to stand, or rise after falling.

In the majority of cases the power of locomotion is impaired, if not lost entirely; even if he can stand or walk, it will probably only be with assistance, and in a stooping posture. Certainly, walking, if possible, will almost always be a slow and painful performance; but there are a few remarkable exceptions on record of patients who, either immediately after the accident, or the next day, or even for a day or two, have retained the power of walking (*see* Rivington pp. 28, 29 and 30).

It is a question whether, in these cases of retained power of locomotion, the bladder was completely ruptured through all its coats at the time of the injury, or whether the peritoneal coat remained intact at first and gave way subsequently. Another explanation for some cases may be that the urine is extravasated into the recto-vesical pouch, not diffused over the general peritoneal cavity, and retained there by adhesions between the viscera. And another is probable—namely, that the urine at first extravasated, being aseptic, is inoffensive to the peritoneum, and that subsequent effusion is prevented by protruding mucous membrane of bladder or adhesions about the edges of the rent.

If the individual, before the rupture took place, had been suffering the discomfort or pain of retention, he will, as soon as the first symptoms of pain and collapse occasioned by the rupture have passed off, experience a feeling of relief. This will be of but brief duration, for soon he will be distressed by intense pain in the hypogastrium, at the umbilicus, in his groins, or "all over"; and by frequent and urgent desire to pass water. On attempting to micturate, nothing, or only a few drops of blood, or a little urine mixed with blood, will come away. On passing a catheter there is the same result; a variable quantity of urine mixed with blood, or a little blood, or nothing at all may flow through it.

If there is urethral stricture, enlarged prostate, or fractured pelvis, there may be difficulty in introducing the catheter; not otherwise. As soon as the end of the instrument has entered the bladder it may be found difficult to move or rotate it; and then, on withdrawing it a little or moving the hand to one side or the other, or up or down slightly, the catheter suddenly passes on without resistance, and water begins to flow drop by drop, or in a limpid stream, quickened by inspiratory movements, or flowing and stopping with the respiratory movements.

This means that the catheter has found its way through the rent into the peritoneal cavity. With a long catheter, it is possible that the point of it may be felt through the abdominal parietes of a thin person.

In cases of extra-peritoneal rupture, the end of the instrument has been felt in the cellular tissue between the rectum and bladder by the finger in the rectum.

The quantity of urine drawn off by the catheter, either from the cavity of the bladder itself or from the peritoneal cavity, varies very much—from nothing to five or six ounces may be found in the bladder, and twenty to thirty ounces or more in the peritoneal cavity. Blood-clots may block the catheter and prevent urine flowing, though it be present.

It is by no means rare for the patients to be able to pass urine voluntarily, either at the outset or during the course of the case; but the rule is that they cannot do so. In a few exceptional cases there has been incontinence of urine, or the urine has been passed frequently, but in small quantities. This is much more likely to occur in extra-peritoneal ruptures. In one case (Hamilton's) of incontinence, however, the rent was a transverse intra-peritoneal rupture at the upper front part of the bladder; in two others (Rivington's and Tay's) the rupture was just above the prostate. In intra-peritoneal cases there may be a more or less defined tumour, fluctuating, perhaps, and simulating the bladder, between the umbilicus and pubes, or in the recto-vesical *cul de sac*, in either case caused by the urine limited by the disposition of the coils of intestine. In extra-peritoneal rupture the urine may collect and form a doughy, asymmetrical swelling. If the rupture be anterior, this swelling will be in front of the bladder and extend above the symphysis; if the rupture be posterior, the swelling will be felt between the bladder and rectum, or more or less towards one side as the case may be.

Instead of forming a tumour the urine may be diffused in the cellular tissue, and mount up outside the peritoneum to the umbilicus or the iliac fossæ, or through the obturator foramina or the inguinal rings to the scrotum, or along the femoral canal to the thigh. Abscess, diffuse suppuration, or sloughing of the tissue may follow. In both intra- and extra-peritoneal ruptures with the symptoms above described, and which are more or less special to the organ injured, there will probably at first be the general symptoms of shock and collapse, with or without hæmorrhage. In the intra-peritoneal ruptures, sooner or later, but generally not before the third day, all the symptoms of peritonitis will supervene. In one case, on the sixth day, there were frequent seminal emissions (Cusack's); in a few cases there has been stercoraceous vomiting; and in one case a coil of intestine entered the rent in the bladder and gave rise to symptoms of intestinal obstruction which masked the symptoms of rupture of the bladder (Rivington, p. 38).

In extra-peritoneal ruptures, the symptoms of suppurative cellulitis set in after several days, with pains about the perinæum and rectum and neck of the bladder, in the hypogastrium, groins and thighs; and septic infection will show itself by rigors, elevation of temperature, vomiting and extreme depression. Death may occur at any time between fifth day or sixth week.

Diagnosis.—In intra-peritoneal rupture, the most certain evidence is the entrance of a catheter, through the rent in the empty bladder, into the peritoneal cavity. In extra-peritoneal rupture, signs of urinary extravasation may soon appear, but they do not do so in some cases for many hours.

The injection of a warm antiseptic solution into the bladder may be of great use. If the bladder is sound, the usual swelling of a distended bladder will be formed, and will disappear on the return of the fluid through the catheter. If there be an intra-peritoneal rupture, the warm fluid will be felt by the patient in the groins and abdomen, as in Mr. Christopher Heath's case; the usual swelling caused by a distended bladder will not be formed, but the fluid will be recovered through the catheter. If the rupture be extra-peritoneal, the bladder may become distended, but the injection causes pain, a sense of warmth about the pelvis, and a doughy swelling will probably be detected in the hypogastrium or by the finger in the rectum. A word of caution, however, is required about these test injections. It should be remembered that in not a few cases the mucous and muscular coats are rent, but not the peritoneal; and the repeated injections to a decided degree of distension of the bladder, which are advised by Weir, are dangerous from their tendency to cause the peritoneum to give way. The inflation of air, even of only two or three cubic inches, if it passes into the peritoneal cavity, gives rise to profound and dangerous disturbance in the patient's general condition.

A satisfactory history of the patient having, previous to the injury, had a distended bladder, and subsequently to it having made frequent and painful but fruitless efforts to pass water, with the discharge only of a little blood, or blood-stained urine, will greatly assist, especially if, on passing a catheter, the bladder is found empty or nearly so.

If the nature of the injury was a fall or blow on the hypogastrium, or a fracture or dislocation of the pelvis, the probability of rupture of the bladder is greatly increased.

Between intra- and extra-peritoneal rupture the diagnosis is often very difficult, and in some cases cannot possibly be made with certainty in the early hours after the injury, except by examination of the bladder digitally through a median perinæal incision, or by an exploratory laparotomy.

Laparotomy—in doubtful cases, and if the patient's general condition does not forbid it—is quite justifiable, considering that almost the only chance of saving life is by closing an intra-peritoneal rupture at the earliest possible moment.

When the pelvis is fractured or dislocated, the probabilities are all in favour of extra-peritoneal rupture.

The exploration of the bladder with a long, firm catheter,

Y

together with the differences above enumerated in the symptoms of the two sets of cases, will frequently enable us to form an accurate diagnosis between the intra- and extra-peritoneal ruptures.

By the same means, too, we can exclude rupture of the urethra on the one hand, and injury to the kidney on the other.

Prognosis—This is most serious. Fractures of the pelvis, or dislocations, add enormously to the dangers, and these cases, complicated as they so frequently are by other severe injuries, are generally quickly fatal. The old Hippocratic dogma condemned as fatal every case of rupture of the bladder, and almost to the present day this view has been maintained. In the opinion of many able surgeons it was deemed conclusive evidence that the bladder had not been ruptured if the patient recovered. This extreme position has, however, been rendered quite untenable since the publication of one of my cases, in the Roy. Med.-Chir. Transactions (vol. lxx.), for in this case, many years after an intra-peritoneal rupture had been successfully treated by early and continuous catheterism and a restricted supply of fluids, the cicatrix gave way, and an opportunity was thus afforded us of examining the condition of the bladder.

Two most important things in the modern management of these cases are likely to reduce the mortality considerably. These are strict antiseptic treatment of the bladder and the early closure by sutures of intra-peritoneal ruptures. Already the employment of sutures in these cases has saved some lives; out of 14 cases collected by Tuffier, 6 recovered and 8 died—a mortality of 58 per cent. as compared with 87 per cent. of cases in which this treatment was not adopted. Walsham (Roy. Med.-Chir. Soc., June 11th, 1895) has collected 28 cases of intra-peritoneal rupture of the bladder treated by sutures since 1888, and of this number 11 recovered and 17 died. In only 1 out of the 11 successful cases was peritonitis present at the time of the operation, whereas in 8, and probably in 9, out of the 17 unsuccessful cases peritonitis had set in before the operation was commenced. The causes of death in the 8 cases in which peritonitis did not precede the operation were shock or hæmorrhage, or both combined, in 5, peritonitis from leakage in 2, if not in 3. In 4 out of the 17 cases the rent had not been securely closed, and leakage occurred.

In fatal cases death occurs much earlier in intra-peritoneal rupture than in the simple extra-peritoneal — *i.e.* extra-peritoneal rupture uncomplicated with fracture of the pelvis. In 107 cases in Rivington's list of intra-peritoneal ruptures, 82 died within five days and 25 between the fifth and sixteenth days. In 52 cases of extra-peritoneal rupture 24 died at periods varying from five days to a month or six weeks.

The mortality of intra-peritoneal ruptures is said to be nearly, some say quite, cent. per cent.; of extra-peritoneal ruptures, 20 to 27 per cent., but these figures cannot include all the cases of extra-peritoneal ruptures complicated by fractured pelvis.

Treatment.—The first thing in many cases will be to attend to the condition of extreme shock by the application of warmth, gentle stimulation, etc., requisite in all such cases. Next must be the prompt local treatment with the object of preventing the further escape of urine into the peritoneum or pelvic cellular tissue by providing a ready exit for the urine as it reaches the bladder, either by catheter, or median urethrotomy, or lateral cystotomy, and catheter, and by closing the wound in the bladder by sutures when this is possible. And here everything depends upon an early and an accurate diagnosis. If the case is one of intra-peritoneal rupture, no time is to be lost (where sufficient assistance and proper convenience can be obtained for the operation) in performing laparotomy, clearing out the urine and blood from the peritoneal cavity, and securely suturing the opening in the bladder wall. It must often be a most difficult and tedious task to accomplish the last part of this programme successfully, and it has been in this respect—viz. the inefficient closure of the opening—that some of the operations have failed. (*See* page 370.) Another cause of want of success of sutures is in the too long interval of time which has elapsed before the operation was undertaken; and a third cause has been, no doubt, the contused and ragged edges of the wound. It is this last condition which has led some surgeons to contemplate better results, after cleansing the peritoneum, from leaving the wound in the bladder to close up of itself, and retaining a catheter in the bladder. The arguments for this course are, to my mind, most unsatisfactory, and, if valid, go to show that, *providing the patient's urine is aseptic*, there is no need to submit him to laparotomy at all. A catheter retained from the first in the bladder might just as likely bring about a happy result in other cases, as it did in mine.

Not to close with sutures the bladder rent and yet to perform laparotomy is only justifiable on the ground that all urine is septic—or, as Ullmann would say, contains bacteria in its physiological state and which are to be found on the vesical mucous surface—and offensive to the peritoneum, and must therefore be removed therefrom. This we know it is not, unless there is a considerable quantity of blood as well as urine effused. As regards the contused edges, they might be dealt with by inverting or removing them, as is done in similar cases of operation for ulcer of the stomach.

Abdominal section with the view of sewing up the rent in the bladder was discussed by Benjamin Bell and warmly advocated by Dr. Blundell. Indeed, the latter, except for the method of closing the wound in the bladder (a most important detail), proposed precisely the same operation which has of late years been undertaken with a degree of success amounting to from 38 to 42 per cent.

Dr. Vincent, who for a long time paid much attention to this subject, advocated cystorrhaphy by means of a double set of sutures, some passed through the muscular and serous coats and others applied in Lembert's way, through the serous only. Opinions will differ as to the precise method of suturing, but most will agree, I think, in the importance of completely closing the rent.

To Sir William MacCormac belongs the honour of having been the first who successfully operated on ruptured bladder. In most of the fatal cases the operation was not done till twenty-four hours or more after the injury, when inflammation had attacked the edges of the wound.

In all cases, in hospital and elsewhere, where proper assistants, antiseptic precautions, and suitable appliances are at hand, laparotomy and closure of the rupture ought to be performed. When the surgeon is single-handed, and cannot get assistants or appliances within twenty-four hours, let him employ anti-septic drainage of the bladder from the outset and reduce to a small limit the quantity of fluid given to the patient for the first three or four days. Paracentesis of the abdomen or recto-vesical *cul de sac* need hardly, if ever, be performed.

In extra-peritoneal ruptures a catheter should be retained in the bladder with the most rigid antiseptic precautions, taking care that the instrument is sufficiently large, that the urine is run off into a vessel under the bed containing a solution of carbolic acid, and that the glans penis is covered with an iodoform gauze dressing. Great care must also be assidu-ously bestowed upon the permeability of the catheter, and the moment it becomes choked by blood or mucus it must be changed with as much promptitude as a tracheotomy tube. If, on account of such obstruction, it is necessary to make an opening into the bladder, this may be either by supra-pubic cystotomy, median urethrotomy, or lateral cystotomy.

Different surgeons will elect different operations. Many think the hypogastric the method for choice. Personally, I prefer the median perinæal operation for exploration or simple drainage of the bladder. If it were necessary at the same time to give relief to extravasated urine, separate incisions into the cellular tissue would also be required, or lateral cystotomy might be performed if the extrava-sation was chiefly on one side. When there is reason to think that the mucous and muscular coats, but not the peritoneal coat, have given way, an attempt should be made to save the integrity of the peritoneum by retaining a catheter in the bladder for some days.

If the symptoms of extravasation in a case of extra-peri-toneal rupture are present, the perinæal operation should be done at once.

CHAPTER VI.

ACUTE CYSTITIS.

CYSTITIS, whether acute or chronic, is always a complication of some other disease, or accident, or morbid state. It is never an idiopathic, independent affection. It has always some ascertainable cause. It is a symptom like jaundice, œdema, or dropsy.

We do not speak of " idiopathic jaundice, idiopathic œdema or dropsy," neither ought we to do so of " idiopathic cystitis."

We know nowadays that inflammation is due to microbic infection, and that bacteria are the cause of cystitis as of inflammation of other organs and tissues ; but admitting the bacteria to be the actual agents which provoke the inflammatory process, what we want to know are the conditions under which these agents set to work upon the mucous membrane of the bladder—in other words, " what are the secondary causes of cystitis."

Etiology.—There are predisposing and exciting causes of acute cystitis. The predisposing are either general or local.

General predisposing Causes.—Certain constitutional conditions favour the development of the disease. These are commonly stated to be rheumatism, gout and tubercle. As to the latter, there can be no doubt ; but as to gout and rheumatism, there is room for scepticism ; and the student will do well to remember the words of Sir Henry Thompson with reference to gout: " A very refuge in time of trouble for practitioners of feeble diagnostic power is gout, particularly ' suppressed gout.' Therefore, beware of it. And while I think it must be admitted that inflammation, either of the urethra or of the bladder, may be sometimes a mere local development of the ubiquitous influence so named, I am sure that this cause is of exceedingly rare occurrence."

Cold, improper food, and defective hygiene are also regarded as predisposing causes of a general kind. Highly-savoured dishes, alcoholic drinks, and everything which increases the acidity of the urine, or the amount of urates it contains, increase the tendency to the affection. The continued fever and general infective diseases play an important part sometimes; but whether they act as causes of infection, or simply create a latent local tendency, is uncertain.

The *local Predisposing Causes.*—Every cause provocative of congestion of the bladder predisposes to cystitis; in this way pregnancy and parturition, as well as all the above-named general causes, act. It is by producing congestion that retention of urine from stricture and enlarged prostate, the too rapid evacuation of the bladder after prolonged retention, the presence in the bladder of a calculus, a foreign body, or a new growth, also act. In the same manner diseases of the spinal cord, fractures of the spinal column, and wounds of the bladder lead to cystitis. To masturbation, excessive coitus, menstruation, and hæmorrhoids is imputed a similar tendency. Retention of urine, from stricture of the urethra and chronic enlargement of the prostate, acts with special intensity, frequency and rapidity.

The composition of the urine sometimes predisposes to cystitis; it is in this manner, no doubt, that gout is a cause. The toxic state of the urine in fever patients, as well as the retention of urine which often affects them, induces congestion of the bladder. Cantharides and some other drugs which are eliminated by the kidneys, by passing over the mucous membrane of the bladder have a distinct power to cause frequency and pain in micturition. Sir Henry Thompson says he has seen "cystitis," severe in character, and lasting from ten to twenty hours, produced by an ordinary blister. That cantharides has an irritating effect upon the bladder mucous membrane is beyond question; but it is not, I believe, established that this effect is attended by the development of micro-organisms and pus—in other words, that it is a real cystitis.

Determining Causes.—These are catheterism, gonorrhœa and urethritis in the male, and vaginitis and other infective processes about the vulva and external urethral orifice in the female. They all produce cystitis by provoking a direct microbic infection of the vesical mucous membrane, by means of the secretion and discharges conveyed to the bladder from the urethra.

Cystitis is extremely frequent as a result of a deep-seated urethritis. Under the influence of any of the predisposing causes above named, or after some slight injury, great fatigue, sexual intercourse, horse exercise, dancing, or anything, in fact, that can favour the movement of micro-organisms upwards along the urinary tract, men with deep urethral discharge are liable to get acute cystitis.

In reference to the subject of exciting causes, and in apparent contradiction to the microbic origin of cystitis, is the fact that the mucous membrane of the bladder is very tolerant of certain infective products, such, for example, as the pus of pelvic abscesses, and pus or muco-pus from the ureters and renal pelves, which in many cases passes over the bladder mucous surface for a very long time without exciting inflammation in it.

Pathological Anatomy.—Not much is known about the morbid changes of acute cystitis, because the opportunities of studying them are happily not frequent. The affection is not often fatal. The trigone, the part of the bladder sometimes spoken of as the pathological area, is the chief seat of inflammation. The mucous membrane is commonly alone affected, very rarely the muscular or cellular layers of the parietes.

When inflammation attacks the cellular tissue between the muscular and peritoneal coats of the bladder, it is spoken of as *pericystitis.*

The first changes in cystitis are a pronounced injection of the blood-vessels of the mucous membrane, especially about the ureteral orifices and the neck of the bladder. As the inflammation advances the mucous membrane swells, becomes a bright crimson colour, and the distinct outline of the distended arborescent vessels disappears. Microscopically, the epithelial cells are swollen, their nuclei broken up, and the rete mucosum is infiltrated with leucocytes and embryonic cells. The muscular coat is sometimes similarly infiltrated. Occasionally, but rarely, small abscesses are formed in the mucous membrane, and, after breaking into the bladder cavity, leave small ulcers on its surface. Morgagni and others have seen cases of gangrene of the mucous membrane; and, as a consequence of cantharides, and of cystitis from severe and continued fevers, "false membranes" or casts of the bladder have been thrown off. Mr. Reginald Harrison refers to an interesting case of acute cystitis in a man aged forty, with old stricture of the urethra, under Mr. Heycock, where the entire mucous membrane of the bladder was exfoliated and withdrawn in the form of a loose bag through a perinæal incision. Such a case is quite different from those where a false membrane forms in the bladder and keeps up a cystitis.

The bacteriological study of cystitis goes to show that several forms of pyogenic bacteria are capable of exciting the inflammation; but the microbe which has been most generally met with is the *bacterium coli commune*. Other forms are the *uro-bacillus liquefaciens* and the ordinary agents of suppuration, and very much more rarely the *bacillus griseus*, *micrococcus albicans amplus*, and the *diplococcus favus*. In men and women it is the coli bacillus which is most frequently found, and which is, indeed, in men the agent of almost all cases of cystitis; but in females the staphylococci, as the elements exciting puerperal and post-partum cystitis, are met with almost as frequently as the coli bacillus. In cystitis from gonorrhœa, as well as from other causes, the same bacteria are found, and it is quite the exception to meet with gonococci.

Symptoms.—Acute cystitis appears in two very different degrees: one, almost insufferable to the patient and alarming to witness; the other, much less severe and dangerous. The type of acute cystitis is that which sometimes occurs in the latter weeks of an attack of gonorrhœa. The onset of the disease is then sudden and distinct. In other instances it commences more insidiously, and is merely a slightly exaggerated episode in the course of a chronic cystitis, or of a chronic discharge from the deep urethra.

When it occurs during gonorrhœa, it is frequently provoked by an injection, or by the passage of a catheter, and sets in at once with urgent desire to micturate every fifteen or thirty minutes during the day, and nearly as often at night. Micturition excites a most violent pain behind the pubes, radiating along the urethra, and the urine contains a distinct quantity of pus. M. Guyon points out that cystitis is characterised by three constant symptoms: frequency in micturition, painful micturition, and pyuria.

The *frequency* is very variable; it may be so great as to be almost continuous, and thus to justify the expression "false incontinence." It may vary from fifteen to 120 times in twenty-four hours.

Besides the frequency there is irresistible impulse to pass water when the desire comes, so that the patient pisses his breeches if he cannot immediately get to the pot.

The *pain* may be agonising. It is worse at the beginning and at the end of micturition; but it ceases almost immediately after finishing the act.

It is, therefore, in a way proportionate to the frequency; if the frequency is almost incessant, so is the pain. The situation of the pain is behind and above the symphysis, but radiates along the penis to the groins, testicles and loins. Some patients, to relieve the pain, squat down to pass water or assume some other unusual posture, others have rectal as well as vesical tenesmus, and are obliged to discharge the contents of their bowels each time they empty their bladders; thus engaged, they pass hours on the night commode.

The *pus* may not be present at first; when it appears, it is diffused throughout the whole of the urine, but the first and last portions passed at any one act of micturition contain more than the intermediate portion.

Microscopically, the purulent deposit consists of leucocytes mixed with irregular and agglutinated epithelial cells.

In the very acute forms of cystitis, blood as well as pus is contained in the urine, which then has, as Mr. Reginald Harrison describes it, the appearance of thin prune juice. When the urine is allowed to stand, a greenish thick sediment of pus, or of blood and pus forms, the supernatant fluid being relatively clear. Small clots of blood are often mixed with the sediment. The urine is neutral or alkaline.

Besides the above functional symptoms there are certain *physical signs* due to the condition of the bladder. These are: (1) pain and tenderness over the trigone felt on digital examination through the rectum or the vagina; this pain is much accentuated if at the same time pressure is made over the hypogastrium. (2) Intra-vesical tenderness. Usually in passing a catheter the discomfort experienced by the pressure of the beak of the instrument along the urethra increases as it goes over the prostatic urethra, but ceases at once after its entrance into the bladder ; but when cystitis exists, pain is aggravated by the presence of the instrument within the neck of the bladder. (3) Distension of the bladder with an antiseptic solution. If this is attempted, intense pain accompanied with uncontrollable desire to empty the bladder follows the injection of a very small quantity.

As regards the question of temperature, M. Guyon has pointed out that there is no fever in acute cystitis, that the most painful forms of the disease show no elevation of temperature whatever, and that as soon as there is a fever temperature developed in a patient with cystitis, it is certain that there is some prostatic, perivesical, or, much more commonly, some uretero-renal inflammation.

Diagnosis.—The affection as a rule is easily diagnosed by the three classical symptoms of Guyon: frequency of micturition, painful micturition, and pyuria. The presence of all three of them is necessary. Either taken alone go no way towards establishing a right diagnosis.

It is not by the amount or character of the sediment, but by the pain and tenderness on pressure per rectum or per vaginam, and the fact that the first and last portions of the urine contain most pus, that we diagnose the cystitis to be of the neck and trigone of the bladder. When the whole of the bladder surface is equally involved, the pus is uniformly diffused through all the urine.

The cause of the cystitis ought always to be ascertained, and this can easily be done in the case of stricture, calculus, new growth, or enlarged prostate. The chief difficulty consists in distinguishing tubercular cystitis in its early stage from cystitis due to a chronic urethral discharge. The family history of the patient, the bacteriological tests by means of the microscope, tubercle bacilli culture, and the presence of tubercular deposit in the testes, epididymis, prostate, and vesiculæ seminales, will give the clue to the cause.

Pericystitis will be diagnosed by the high temperature, by the tumefaction felt through the rectum or vagina or above the symphysis pubis, which is not relieved by using the catheter, and by the signs of deep-seated suppuration. It is very rare.

Dr. Englisch, a year or two ago, collected thirty cases of

idiopathic prevesical cellulitis. The cellular tissue of the cavity of Retzius immediately behind and above the symphysis pubis was the site of the inflammation. A tumour suggestive of distended bladder, sharply circumscribed and of a wedge shape, with the base upwards, was formed in the hypogastrium. Most of the patients were adult males. If suppuration occurs the abscess may burst into the bladder or peritoneal cavity, or into the urethra or bowel; in the female the abscess may break into the vagina.

Pyelitis and suppurative pyelonephritis are to be distinguished by the temperature chart, the dry, red tongue, the thirst, dry skin, loss of appetite, and the pinched, sallow face. Moreover, the urine is, as a rule, acid, whereas in cystitis it is always neutral or alkaline, and generally very alkaline.

Prognosis.—Cystitis from urethritis is readily cured, often in a week, by appropriate treatment; if neglected, it will pass into chronic cystitis. When caused by calculus, stricture, new growths, or foreign bodies, the removal of the cause is often followed by a very rapid, almost magical cure. Cystitis is often very difficult to relieve when due to enlarged prostate, and still more so when of tuberculous origin.

Patients with enlarged prostate are very prone to get relapses.

Grave complications occur in the form of (1) ulceration, which may be followed by infiltration of urine, or peritonitis; (2) gangrene, which is more especially frequent in puerperal cystitis.

The prognosis depends chiefly on the cause of the affection, upon the length of time it has existed, and as to the degree to which it is "painful," "purulent," and "hæmorrhagic."

Treatment.—The cause of the disease must be removed as soon as possible. In many cases cystitis is the indication for an immediate operation, as for instance when it is excited by the presence in the bladder of a foreign body, calculus, growth, or by urethral stricture.

Preventive measures ought always to be taken against exciting cystitis by catheterism, or by forced injections, in cases of gonorrhœa, or deep urethral discharges.

For the rest, the treatment consists in palliating pain by hot baths, hot fomentations to the hypogastrium and perinæum; morphia suppositories of half, to one grain in very acute cases, or by subcutaneous injections of morphia; all articles of diet likely to make the urine irritating, such as highly-spiced food, coffee, alcohol in all its forms, etc., must be avoided. Irrigation of the bladder, so good in chronic cystitis, must, as a rule, be shunned in the acute; although benefit follows in some cases from the injection of a few drops of a solution of nitrate of silver, gr. j to ʒ iv, increasing to gr. j to ʒj, as recommended by Sir Henry Thompson.

Cystotomy may be required to relieve tenesmus and to give rest by drainage to the bladder. Mr. R. Harrison relates that in the case mentioned above, in which the entire mucous membrane was exfoliated, perinæal cystotomy was rendered necessary by the fetid character of the urine, and the recurrence of retention from impaction of the detached membrane in the urethro-vesical orifice. A drainage-tube was placed in the bladder. Immediate relief and rapid recovery followed.

Dr. Cabot, of Boston, successfully treated by supra-pubic cystotomy a case of what he calls pachydermia vesicæ— namely, cystitis attended with the formation of false membrane (*Amer. Journ. Med. Sciences*, 1891).

CHAPTER VII.

CHRONIC CYSTITIS.

Etiology.—Any of the forms of acute cystitis just described may terminate in chronic cystitis.

The *predisposing causes* enumerated under acute cystitis (page 374-5) are of great pathogenic importance in, and must be duly considered when forming a prognosis of chronic cystitis.

In old men, especially prostatic subjects, inflammation of the bladder assumes an indolent, chronic form, very different from the acute inflammation so often seen in young and middle-aged men with stricture. Acute cystitis does occur from enlarged prostate, but it is the exception. As a rule, cystitis in the female is of the chronic form, though some of the most acute cases I have witnessed have occurred in women after parturition.

The cystitis attributed to rheumatism and gout, as well as tubercular cystitis, is of a slow and persisting kind.

The *exciting causes* (determining) are the same as those enumerated under acute cystitis (page 375-6). Catheterism becomes a factor of the first importance because of the frequency of its requirement in these cases and the possibility it affords of reinfection. The bladder should be emptied slowly, gradually, and with every antiseptic precaution.

In the cases in which the disease seems to be spontaneous it is necessary to bear in mind that either gonorrhœa or any of the forms of deep-seated urethritis may have left behind some latent source of infection in the pouches, recesses, or glands of the urethra. Occasionally, but very rarely, cases are seen in which there is no urethral trouble, in which the catheter has not been used, and in which neither retention nor any organic disease of the bladder is present. Thompson refers to such cases, and Tuffier states that he has met with one, but only one, and in that the coli bacillus was found in the urine.

Morbid Anatomy.—The mucous membrane of the bladder is of a slate colour, ecchymosed in places, and marbled, purple, black, or green, and covered with an adherent layer of muco-pus. Sometimes there are large or small ulcers on the surface. The changes in the mucous membrane affect the bladder throughout, but are most marked about the trigone, and are least so about the base of the bladder. The mucous membrane is softened, thickened, and swollen, and sometimes small abscesses are present both in the membrane and beneath it. Such abscesses are rarely larger than a pea, and tend to open into the cavity of the bladder. The epithelium disappears, or is reduced to its deepest cylindrical layer. The basement membrane is infiltrated with embryonal cells, and the capillaries are hypertrophied. The mucous membrane is detached from the subjacent layer, the muscular coats are thickened, but modified in this respect by stricture or enlarged prostate ; the perivesical tissue has generally undergone fatty degeneration.

The different conditions presented by the mucous membrane have given rise to differential names. Thus there are described ulcerative cystitis, gangrenous cystitis, "croupous cystitis"—*i.e.* cystitis attended with the production of false membranes—and the villous form of cystitis (cystite fungo-vasculaire). It is only necessary to name these varieties to indicate the different aspects the mucous membrane may present.

Mr. Reginald Harrison refers to an interesting case under Mr. Teale of the villous form, in which the whole mucous membrane was in a velvety or granular condition, lined by a membrane (diphtheritic) like soft writing paper. As seen through a supra-pubic opening, the mucous membrane at the neck of the bladder was fringed by feathery warts and elongated papillæ, the greater part of which Mr. Teale removed by forceps and scissors.

Dr. S. Alexander, in his excellent article on Cystitis in the "System of Genito-Urinary Diseases," edited by Dr. Prince, refers to a form of cystitis which he has since more fully described. He points out that there are a number of lymphoid foci in the normal mucous membrane of the bladder, as well as in that of the renal pelvis, ureters, and prostatic urethra ; that in some cases of cystitis an exaggeration of these lymphoid foci occurs ; and that thus a peculiar type is given to these cases which makes them worthy of being regarded as a special variety, to which he gives the name of "Nodular Cystitis." This is a pathological distinction, but not a clinical one, so far as symptoms and treatment go.

In the croupous cystitis, the false membrane is of a yellowish colour, and composed of fibrinous material, containing in its substance leucocytes and epithelial cells, and having its surface sometimes encrusted with phosphates. This membrane, which is frequently formed in very acute cystitis, and in the cystitis of lying-in women, may invade the ureters and the renal pelves.

In other cases the false membrane is made up entirely of epithelium, from fifty to one hundred times as thick as the normal vesical epithelium.

In gangrenous cystitis the false membrane may be mixed with some of the constituent parts of the bladder mucous membrane more or less destroyed.

Bacteriological investigations have proved the presence of the same organisms in chronic as in acute cystitis (page 377) —namely, the coli bacillus most frequently, staphylococci occasionally, and micrococcus uræ rarely.

Symptoms.—Chronic cystitis may come on slowly and insidiously, as is often the case in old prostatic cases in which the catheter is daily or frequently used; or it may succeed to acute cystitis. Conversely, intercurrent attacks of acute cystitis occur in the course of a prolonged chronic inflammation. The symptoms are the same as those of acute cystitis, but in a very much milder degree. The three cardinal symptoms—frequency of micturition, painful micturition, and pyuria—are present together. The degree of pyuria is extremely variable. It is always most abundant at the commencement and finish of micturition, indicating its chief source as being the mucous membrane in the neighbourhood of the neck of the bladder. It differs, too, much in appearance in different cases, being sometimes yellowish, or greenish; in others having a tenacious, glairy, stringy character, adherent to the bottom of the vessel, like a gelatinous coating of greater or less thickness, which, on pouring off the urine, cleaves for some seconds to the vessel, and then falls from it like a solid or semi-solid mass. It is the abundance of this last-named secretion occurring in patients with but slightly increased frequency of micturition, and little or no pain, which caused the name "catarrh of the bladder" to be given to such cases of chronic cystitis. In stricture cases retention of urine is often caused by the blocking of the narrowed portion of the urethra with this tenacious, gluey secretion. Even if it does not cause retention, it gives rise to great pain and difficulty from the efforts required to make it pass through the urethra.

The urine of chronic cystitis is alkaline, and has a strong offensive odour when it is not actually ammoniacal. When the mucous membrane is sloughing, the urine has an odour characteristically offensive.

The *physical* symptoms of chronic cystitis are very slight; and the general good health is maintained by many patients for a long time, even when the quantity of muco-pus is very large. After a time, however, the patients become feeble, lose flesh, look pale and sallow, get a dry skin and furred tongue, and their digestion becomes difficult or painful. In a large number of cases, chronic pyelo-nephritis is gradually induced ; in others, an acute attack of suppuration throughout the higher urinary mucous tract carries off the patients.

Diagnosis.—Before making a diagnosis, we should inquire as to the three coexisting cardinal symptoms. viz. the frequency and pain of micturition, and the presence of pus or muco-pus in the urine. The conditions with which chronic cystitis is most likely to be confused are neuropathic states of the bladder, tuberculosis of the bladder, and pyelo-nephritis.

In neuropathic conditions, pus is generally absent, though pain and frequency of micturition may be present. The bladder is not over-sensitive to the catheter, nor to vesical injections. With even the smallest trace of pus we ought to exclude simple neuralgia.

In pyelo-nephritis there is a uniform turbidity of the urine, and the turbidity remains even after the urine has had time to deposit; the general health is impaired, there are feverish attacks, and the urine is acid if the bladder is unaffected. If the bladder is carefully washed out, the urine which flows away through the catheter immediately after is turbid with pus.

If there is polyuria, with but little or no pain, or undue frequency of micturition, but a large quantity of pus from

z

the neck of the bladder, the case may be mistaken for suppurative pyelo-nephritis, unless it be remembered that the urine in the renal affection is acid, and, that though it deposits a large quantity of pus, much remains diffused throughout its volume.

In the absence of other known causes, the cystitis will most probably be of tuberculous origin; but the inflammation in some cases is started by a urethral discharge, and subsequently only becomes tuberculous. Bacteriological investigation may quite clear up the diagnosis by the discovery of the tubercle bacilli.

Prognosis.—Chronic cystitis threatens life through its liability to lead on to pyelo-nephritis.

When the determining cause can be removed, as in stricture, foreign body, calculus, etc., the prospect is much more favourable than in chronic prostatic disease, or other conditions which act permanently. Tuberculous cystitis is very unfavourable, though it is sometimes very prolonged if acute exacerbations do not occur. Pain and increased frequency of micturition are much more serious than the pyuria, because the broken rest which they cause soon wears out the patient; whereas with free suppuration, attended by little or no pain or frequency of micturition, rest is unbroken, and the health is maintained for a long time.

Treatment.—The surgeon's first thought should be how to prevent cystitis; it should be an after-thought how to cure it. He will have comparatively little cystitis in his practice if he attends to three preventive methods: (1) To be scrupulously careful as to the perfect aseptic condition of all instruments, injections, and lubricants for his instruments; (2) to remove as soon as possible all determining causes, such as stricture, calculus, foreign bodies, etc.; (3) to destroy all micro-organisms contained in the bladder or urethra.

With the view of accomplishing the third object, many drugs have been recommended of a germicidal character which, by being eliminated by the kidneys, are thought to act upon the micro-organisms of cystitis and urethritis. But it should be borne in mind that, to be effective these drugs require to be taken in such large and frequently repeated doses that they cannot be borne by patients whose digestive functions are, as in these persons, greatly impaired.

Nor are all the numerous family of demulcent decoctions, which at one time and another have each found its special advocate, of the least good in cystitis, beyond furnishing a more or less unpleasant beverage, whilst in barley water or linseed tea we have much more readily obtainable and equally beneficial substitutes. Most of these drugs found favour before bacteriology threw the proper light upon the pathogenic treatment of suppurative diseases, and now that we know that micro-organisms of some kind are the essential exciting causes of the commencement, continuance, and recurrence of cystitis, it may be questioned whether these bland mucilaginous decoctions do not do harm rather than good by adding to the urine a suitable nutrient medium for the development and growth of the microbes.

It is in the daily irrigation of the bladder by suitable antiseptic solutions that the proper treatment of chronic cystitis resides. This irrigation must be conducted on a careful and systematic plan, not only as regards the details of antiseptic precautions, but in other respects as well. It is harmful to throw in too much fluid at a time, or to inject it with too much force. A tender inflamed bladder must be irritated, not improved, by such treatment. It should always, where possible, be a soft flexible catheter of No. 8 or 9 size which is used, the solution to be injected should be of the temperature of the body, and should not be too strongly impregnated with the antiseptic substance. Only from two to three or four ounces at a time should be injected, and then, after being retained for a few seconds in the bladder by keeping the finger tip on the end of the catheter, it should be allowed to escape. This process should be repeated till the solution returns as clear, or nearly so, as when it was injected.

The best means of injecting the solution is by a four or six-ounce indiarubber bottle, fitted with a graduated nozzle and stopcock, such as are made for this express purpose. Or. instead of the indiarubber bottle, a glass irrigator, with a long tube and nozzle at the end, can be hung above the patient's head. This is, perhaps, a more convenient plan when the washing out is done by the patient himself.

Various solutions are employed, thus: acetate of lead, one or two grains to four ounces of water; dilute nitric acid, two or three minims to the ounce; dilute phosphoric acid, three or four minims to the ounce; acetic acid, four minims to the ounce. These are especially useful where there is a great tendency to phosphatic encrustation of the bladder. Sir Henry Thompson recommends biborate of soda and glycerine; his formula is two ounces of glycerine, one ounce of biborate of soda, and two ounces of water; and of this mixture, half an ounce is added to four ounces of water, to form the injection solution.

Mr. Nunn, as long ago as 1872, used and recommended a solution of quinine sulphate in the proportion of two grains to three ounces of water, the strength of which might be increased to one or two grains to the ounce. He used it as a germicide in cases where there was an abundance of mucopus. I have pleasure in referring to this fact because it shows Mr. Nunn to have been in this respect—as his colleague at the Middlesex Hospital, Mr. Campbell de Morgan, was in general surgery with chloride of zinc and sulphurous acid solutions—a pioneer in the use of antiseptic measures.

Another drug recommended to be used in solution as a wash by Sir Henry Thompson is nitrate of silver of the strength of half a grain or one grain in four ounces, gradually increasing to half or three-quarters of a grain to the ounce. Salicylic acid $\frac{1}{16}$ per cent. is recommended by Bryson, of St. Louis, as useful when it is necessary to cleanse the bladder of tenacious muco-pus before injecting other washes for the bladder. To attempt to wash out the bladder, and apply medicinal solutions to the inflamed surface until this very gluey and adhesive mucus and muco-pus is removed, is useless; so that free injection with warm water or with the salicylic acid solution ought to precede the other medicinal injections. Creolin in $\frac{1}{2}$ per cent. solution, resorcin in solutions varying from 2 to 15 per cent. when the urine is neutral or alkaline, and weak solutions of boroglyceride, are amongst the very numerous substances which may be tried. "Instillations," in the form of twenty or thirty drops of a 1 in 50 solution of the silver nitrate, of a sublimate solution 1 in 10,000, gradually increased to 1 in 5,000, or even to 1 in

1,000, are considered by many French surgeons to be the best mode of antisepticising the bladder. The "instillation" solution is injected through a catheter, the bladder being empty at the time. Even the washing out of the bladder with simple warm water is of great use by removing the last few drops of decomposing urine. Stale urine in the presence of mucus and muco-pus especially, has its urea converted into carbonate of ammonia, which irritates the mucous membrane and aggravates the inflammation. What the effect of such urine is upon the bladder can best be imagined by trying the effect of the vapour of ammonia on the eyes and nasal mucous membrane. If only a few drops of such urine is retained, it tends to the rapid decomposition of the fresh urine coming in from the kidneys, and in this way a vicious circle is established—viz. the inflammatory secretion from the bladder mucous membrane hastens the decomposition of the urine ; the decomposition of the urine aggravates the cause of the secretion. In this state the bladder, as Sir Henry Thompson puts it, is like a badly washed utensil, and the improvement from irrigating this unclean vessel is often as rapid as it is beneficial.

But there are bladders which cannot be completely emptied by the catheter and yet bear the injection of an ounce or two only of fluid at a time. Such bladders are those which have pouches or tunicary herniæ, and are often found in old prostatic subjects. Intra-vesical injections are contra-indicated in cystitis due to enlarged prostate, where injections cause much pain even if only an ounce or two is injected. In these cases much benefit is, I think, likely to follow from medicating the bladder by Mr. R. Harrison's instrument for introducing vesical suppositories, and by means of which Dr. Dunns, of New York, introduced iodoform suppositories for disinfecting purposes.

Where there is much pain, washing out cannot be well borne, but the "instillations" recommended by the French surgeons, are sometimes very useful.

Much benefit is often derived from an injection of a drachm of iodoform emulsion of the strength of two scruples of iodoform to an ounce of water. An excellent formula for iodoform emulsion is that of Bell and Co., viz.: Iodoform. præcip., grs. xliv; spir. vini rect., ♍x; pulv. tragacanth, grs. vj; aquæ, ℨj. To be carefully mixed. With this may be combined one grain of conmarin to the ounce.

The diet must be carefully regulated, alcohol forbidden, and the various agents, local and internal, employed which are recommended at pages 380-1 for acute cystitis.

Where pain and other symptoms continue severe and unarrested, after the trial of the various means above described, the bladder should be put into a state of rest for a fortnight or three weeks by draining it through the perinæum or above the pubis. I have witnessed the happiest results from opening the membranous urethra in the middle line, dilating the vesical orifice with my finger, removing in some cases a phosphatic incrustation more or less extensive, and then draining through a piece of large-sized tubing for many days.

In women dilatation of the urethra, vesico-vaginal cystotomy, or hypogastric cystotomy may have to be performed for similar conditions. The latter operation is to be preferred, except in cases where it is reasonable to expect that the drainage will not long be required. In many cases of cystitis and chronic prostatitis sanmetto in drachm doses three times a day does excellent service. So also does the solution of parsley and kola seed mixed with coca and saw palmetto made by Bell and Co. of Oxford Street, and named by them "liquor petroselini cum serenoâ compositus." Tyson recommends sandalwood oil, to be administered before meals, and an injection of sodium salicylate (a drachm to a pint) or of alum solution, 2 to 3 or 4 grains to the ounce. Minute doses of cantharidin cure many cases of cystitis quickly and completely, and will sometimes succeed where sandalwood oil fails. Even in cases in which the drug has failed to cure, it has improved the urine and relieved strangury.

Frendenberg reported favourably of cantharidin after trial of it in fifty-six cases, and arrived at the conclusion that it is approached only by sandal-wood oil in its action in cystitis, but that the latter drug is to be preferred if urethritis is present.

CHAPTER VIII.

TUBERCULAR DISEASE OF THE BLADDER.

THIS disease acquired a new importance for the surgeon with the discovery of the bacillus of tubercle and the extension of surgical operations upon the bladder.

It is a disease which affects the period of activity of the sexual organs, but is met with occasionally in children under four years of age, and also in extreme old age. It is three times more common in men than in women; and this is probably because the sexual apparatus of the male is in direct communication with his urinary organs, whereas in women the two sets of organs are quite distinct from one another.

Etiology.—There are predisposing and determining causes. The *predisposing* are both general and local; the general are the same as of tuberculosis in other organs; the local are somewhat special, and are to be found in the frequency of gonorrhœa and other urethral discharges, and of infective cystitis. There is no doubt that chronic simple inflammation is prone to pass into tubercular disease in individuals with a hereditary tendency to tubercle.

The *determining* causes:—Infection of the bladder may emanate from the kidney or from the urethra. Cohnheim, Verneuil, Fournier, and others believe that the disease is communicable through coitus by the tuberculous vaginal mucus; but, if so, it is only exceptionally the case, as tubercular disease of the anterior and middle part of the urethra is not often seen. It is believed to be more commonly secondary to renal tuberculosis, descending along the ureters to the bladder.

With the frequency with which the testes, prostate, and vesiculæ seminales are affected it is much more likely that the deep urethra—the meeting of the cross-roads to the urinary and genital system—is the starting-point, and that the disease spreads by continuity to both sets of organs. In many cases, no doubt, the disease is primary in more parts of the

genito-urinary organs than one, and two or more spots are
affected simultaneously.

Morbid Anatomy.—The bladder is generally small,
shrunken, and thickened, and surrounded by a bed of
sclerosed fibro-fatty tissue. The mucous membrane is red,
irregular, and fungous-looking, especially about the trigone
and about the orifices of the ureters; minute grey miliary
tubercles are occasionally seen, more or less confluent, but not
forming the larger cheesy masses so often met with in the
kidneys, prostate, testes and vesiculæ. Ulceration is present
in the more advanced stages; the ulcers have the typical
characters of the scrofulous ulcers in other parts, and may be
small and numerous, or several may have coalesced into one
large ulcer; their depth varies from mere surface destruction
to actual perforation. Though perforation is rare, it sometimes results in fistulous openings into the rectum, vagina, or
perinæum; or, after forming an abscess in the cavity of Retzius,
an opening may be established through the hypogastrium.
Vigneron, who has written an excellent summary of tubercular disease of the genital organs as a whole (*Gazette des
Hôpitaux*, June 24, 1893), attributes the rarity of perforation
of and suppuration outside the bladder wall to the perivesical fibro-fatty sclerosis which is a marked feature in
the morbid changes of the disease. Ulceration may extend
through the urethro-vesical orifice and invade the urethra;
and Ricord reports a case in which it reached to the external
meatus.

It is very rare for the bladder to be the only part of the
genito-urinary apparatus affected at the time of death.
M. Cornil has observed such cases, however, and Guyon
estimates that in 50 per cent. the kidneys remain intact.

In cases of pulmonary phthisis the bladder is sometimes
found in quite an early stage of tuberculosis without any
signs of its existence during life having been shown.

Symptoms.—The first symptom is frequency of micturition after meals and at night. Then the urine is tinted
more or less, and at longer or shorter intervals, with blood.
Later still, pain occurs and the urine is much thicker and
contains pus; it is then that cystitis appears, and, as Tuffier
writes, the disease, which till then was "vesical tuberculosis,"

becomes " tubercular cystitis." Even so it may last for years without very greatly affecting the general health.

The functional symptoms are (1) frequency of micturition, (2) hæmaturia, (3) pain, (4) certain morbid constituents of the urine. Each of these symptoms must receive a brief notice. *Frequency of micturition* comes on insidiously, and may exist for a long time without the patient having taken much notice of it. It is due to a slight congestion of the mucous membrane, and increases with its cause, till at length the need to pass water becomes very imperious, and occurs every hour, or even every half-hour : in the gravest cases it may be almost continuous, being tantamount to a condition of " false incontinence." It is generally worse at night than in the daytime.

Hæmaturia is an early symptom, but, like frequency of micturition, it may be so slight as to escape the patient's observation for a time. It is compared to the hæmoptysis of pulmonary tuberculosis, and is due at first, like the frequency of micturition, to active congestion of the mucous membrane, though later it may be an actual hæmorrhage from an ulcerated surface. As an early symptom it is spontaneous and slight, the urine being faintly pink or rose-tinted throughout, but there may be a few drops of pure blood at the end of micturition. As it comes, so it goes, without obvious cause, and is thus unlike the hæmaturia of calculus, but in this respect similar to the hæmaturia of tumour. There is this difference, however ; the bleeding of tumours is free and abundant, whereas the hæmaturia of tuberculosis is slight. In the middle stages of the disease the hæmaturia may cease, but in the later, if it should recur, it may be very considerable.

Pain is an indication of cystitis. It is often brought on by sounding, after which the three cardinal symptoms of cystitis occur—viz. frequency, pain and pus. In some cases the pain of tubercular cystitis is by no means severe, and certainly not incompatible with the ordinary pursuits of the patients. In others, it is frequent and intense, continuous and agonising ; preceding, accompanying, and following micturition ; and as the frequency of micturition is increased by the cystitis, there may be no cessation day or night to the terrible sufferings.

Sometimes the pains are accompanied by spasm of the membranous urethra, and thus temporary retention adds still further to the distress. In the most advanced stage, especially if the neck of the bladder has been partially destroyed by ulceration, there may be incontinence of urine.

The urine.—With the onset of the frequency of micturition the urine is often increased to three or four pints in twenty-four hours; it is then clear, pale, except when tinged with blood, and limpid. With the occurrence of cystitis it contains pus. The amount of pus, like the degree of pain and the frequency of micturition, varies in different cases. It may be slight and flocculent, and contained chiefly in the urine first discharged. When it is abundant and uniformly diffused through all the urine, it is an indication that pyelitis or pyelonephritis is also present.

Microscopically, the sediment shows blood and pus corpuscles, epithelial cells from the bladder, and often from the ureters and kidneys; there are also sometimes renal casts.

The bacilli of tubercle are not often seen in the purulent urines, but before the urine contains pus they are discovered both by the microscope and by cultivation experiments. After cystitis commences, the microbes of common suppuration are present. Tuffier states that in one case of tubercular cystitis in which no instrument had ever been introduced into the urethra he found the coli bacillus, but not the bacillus of Koch; inoculation cleared up the doubt. He mentions it as a warning against possible error occasioned by the presence of a bacillus analogous to the bacillus of Koch, and frequently occupying the groove behind the glans penis. Little information is afforded by the physical signs of the bladder beyond the general tenderness caused by pressure on that organ. The prostate, cord, and testes should always be carefully examined, as any deposits felt in them supply confirmatory evidence.

Diagnosis.—Vesical tuberculosis ought to be suspected in any case in which frequency of micturition, with slight hæmaturia, occurs in a person between the ages of fifteen and forty-five, especially if the individual has a tuberculous aspect or family history. If to these symptoms an attack of cystitis is added; or if, on examination of the prostate, vesiculæ, spermatic cord, or epididymes, a hard nodule is felt in either;

or if the lungs afford corroborative evidence of tubercle, the diagnosis becomes fairly certain.

The examination of the urine in this early stage, and before suppuration is established, will give, by the microscope and by bacteriological inoculation, positive proof.

Some of the nervous vesical conditions dependent on hysteria, epilepsy and ataxy may occasionally simulate the symptoms of vesical tuberculosis; but in the early stage of vesical tuberculosis there is no pain—none at least till cystitis supervenes—whilst in the nerve diseases there are present their own special symptoms to characterise them. (*See* Chap. III. Part III.)

Vesical calculus is sometimes simulated, by the sense of uneasiness in the bladder, of weight behind the pubes, with aching pain radiating to the groins, anus, and end of penis, by frequency of micturition and hæmorrhage, and by these symptoms being increased by movement and standing. But the character of the hæmaturia is very different in the two diseases: relief is afforded both to pain and hæmorrhage by rest and the horizontal posture in calculus of the bladder. No such relief is obtained in this way in tuberculosis; on the contrary, in the horizontal position and at night the symptoms are often aggravated.

Vesical tumours affect middle-aged and elderly people, bleed abundantly, but cause no undue frequency in micturition, and no pain till cystitis supervenes. Tuberculosis attacks young subjects, and excites frequency of micturition usually before hæmaturia; and when hæmaturia appears, it is rarely very marked, and disappears with the advance of the other symptoms. Moreover, there is the evidence of tuberculosis often afforded by other organs, and the results of bacteriological investigation.

From cystitis due to other causes, tubercular cystitis is diagnosed by the onset and course of the disease, and the result of examination of the urine. There may be some difficulty in making a diagnosis in those cases in which the tuberculosis has followed upon an old gonorrhœa or deep-seated urethral discharge.

From tuberculosis of the kidneys and ureters, the diagnosis is often very difficult. The disease in the bladder progresses very much more slowly than in the kidneys. In cystitis the urine is at first, and for a long while, much less charged with pus, and that which is first passed contains more than the rest of the urine; and there are not the digestive disturbances, the dry tongue, and the rapid emaciation, which are produced by the renal disease.

In women the diagnosis is more difficult than in men. Hæmaturia is more likely to be the first symptom noticed than frequency of micturition, the sexual organs do not give corroborative evidence, and cystitis is more often met with where there is no adequate cause to explain it. Inoculation experiments and the inefficacy of general treatment will point the diagnosis.

Terrillon (*Progrès Médical*, 1880, p. 101) drew attention to polypoid excrescences about the urinary meatus in women, mounting more or less up the urethra, and painful to the touch, as having some diagnostic value; and I am able, from my personal experience, to give some support to this. A sister of mercy under my charge for hæmaturia had a luxuriance of polypoid, warty growths around the meatus, and forming an arch over it like the handle of a basket. After snipping these away I examined the bladder through the urethra, where I felt and removed some half-dozen upstanding granulation masses about half the size of a grain of barley. Her left lung was tuberculous, her larynx soon gave evidence of the same disease, the hæmaturia was followed by pyuria, and emaciation rapidly advanced. There can be no reasonable doubt that the hæmaturia was caused by vesical tuberculosis, and the condition of the meatus in this patient was confirmatory of Terrillon's observation.

The thermometer seldom fails to assist us in doubtful cases of urinary tuberculosis, as there is nearly always a rise of temperature.

Prognosis.—It must be remembered that the course of tuberculosis of the bladder is a slow one, and though it is complicated with acute attacks there are also frequent periods of amelioration so considerable that a cure seems likely to occur. Thus the disease may last, not months only, but even several years.

If all symptoms should disappear for a time, it would be

necessary, before pronouncing that a cure has taken place, to have a thorough bacteriological examination made of the urine; otherwise we may be surprised to find, after a chill or some indiscretion in mode of living, all the old symptoms lighted up again. Tuberculosis of the bladder is, nearly always, essentially a chronic disease, probably one of the slowest of tubercular visceral affections.

Even when the kidneys are affected it may be quite a long time before the general health suffers. The progress is generally more rapid in cases in which the tuberculosis of the bladder is secondary to pulmonary tuberculosis. When the testicles and vesiculæ seminales are involved in a case in which the bladder symptoms are recent, the prognosis is more unfavourable. So too, is it, when severe and obstinate cystitis sets in, for then the strength of the patient rapidly gives way to the pain, discharge of pus, and loss of sleep and rest.

It is very rare for hæmorrhage to be severe enough to threaten life, even when due to ulceration of the bladder. The end is generally brought about by pyelo-nephritis of the common suppurative form, even if the tubercular process itself has not reached the kidneys. Occasionally, tubercular peritonitis, acute phthisis pulmonalis, or acute general tuberculosis is the immediate cause of death. Cold abscesses about the bladder or prostate, and the continued discharges from the resulting fistulæ, help to wear out the patient.

Treatment. — Surgical treatment based on the radical extermination of the microbic cause of the disease has, up to the present, been disappointing.

There are many diseased conditions which the physician would do well—which, indeed, in the future he will be compelled—to hand over for early surgical treatment. But there is one which, so far as we can tell at present, the surgeon would do wisely to leave entirely to the domain of therapeutics, and employ as little surgical intervention as possible, and that is " vesical tuberculosis " and " tubercular cystitis." Let him bear in mind the clinical distinctions between these two conditions, and remember that it is by the use of the catheter or sound, especially if strict asepticity be not observed, that the less serious is changed into the graver condition of the two. Irrigation of the bladder is worse than useless; it is often actively harmful in tubercular disease before suppuration has commenced. It is contra-indicated in all cases of ulceration or where there is a tendency to bleed; and in tuberculosis of the bladder, ulceration and hæmorrhage are both frequent. It is only in cases where cystitis has been superadded to vesical tuberculosis, and the tubercular element is not very active, that any form of irrigation treatment is admissible.

The general and medicinal treatment in the early stages of the disease are the same as in pulmonary phthisis as regards climate, diet, clothing, medicines, dry frictions, sulphur or salt baths, sea voyages, visits to the thermal springs, arsenical preparations, creasote, cod-liver oil, etc. The articles which ought specially to be avoided are those which, through the urine, irritate the bladder, such as all forms of stimulants, curries, spices, nux vomica, juniper, etc. Thus it is to medicinal, rather than to surgical means, that the patient should look for benefit.

It is when cystitis has supervened that surgical treatment, if at any time, is more likely to render some assistance. Then, so long as the disease remains limited to the mucous membrane of the bladder, it is possible we may obtain some benefit from local treatment. Nitrate of silver solutions have failed. Iodoform has been tried and found wanting at the Necker Hospital, though Mr. Harrison says he has found benefit from it when suspended in mucilages in the proportion of five grains to an ounce. Mercurial irrigation of the bladder, with solutions of 1 in 1,000 and 1 in 2,000, has proved abortive; but M. Guyon tells us that mercurial "instillations" render great service. These instillations consist of the injection into the bladder of from 10 to 40 drops of corrosive sublimate solution varying in strength from 1 in 5,000 to 1 in 1,000.

It is claimed for this treatment that it not only acts as a medicinal remedy to relieve pain, but as a germicide to kill the microbes, and that its value is realised in early stages as a means of relieving frequency of micturition.

If these means fail, and the bladder becomes very irritable and the pains severe, morphia must be liberally administered, even if required to the extent of several grains in the twenty-four hours. Of course, the dose will be commenced small, and will be cautiously and gradually increased; but very large doses can ultimately be tolerated.

Cystotomy should be the last resource, and only employed to relieve frequent and severe pain and irritability of bladder. The operation which hitherto seems to have afforded most relief has been supra-pubic drainage of the bladder, followed in some cases by the application of nitrate of silver, in others of balsam of Peru, or iodoform, or chloride of zinc, or corrosive sublimate solution 1 in 5,000 strong. Where true localised fungous masses have been seen, the curette, followed by cauterisation of the surface, or strong chloride of zinc solution, is said to have accomplished sometimes complete eradication. But in these cases also it is probable that the real cause of improvement has been the very prolonged drainage of the bladder, which has been extended in some of them to several months' duration.

CHAPTER IX.

STONE IN THE BLADDER.

Etiology.—What determines the formation of calculus in any part of the urinary apparatus? How comes it that a stone is localised in the bladder?

1. Owing to defective or imperfect nutritive processes, and to the gouty diathesis, there is a great tendency to the formation of uric acid and the urates in excess in the blood, and these substances are then excreted in such quantity by the kidneys as to be deposited either in brickdust-red or cayenne-pepper-like particles of uric-acid gravel: or as a powder of light yellow, fawn, or pink colour, being the salts formed by uric acid in combination with soda or ammonia.

It is the same with cystine and some forms of oxalate of lime gravel.

In persons with a strong phosphatic diathesis we often find such an abundant elimination of the phosphates that the urine passed by them is quite milky, or may have the appearance of a thick admixture of chalk with water. This is no doubt an extreme degree of " phosphatic gravel ": but it is quite common to find enough phosphates in the urine to cause a very dense opacity on boiling the urine, which clears up with effervescence on the addition of a drop or two of acid. In these cases the urine as it is passed is neutral or alkaline, and if there are present the symptoms of stone in the kidney, we know of what composition the bulk of the renal calculus will probably be. I have removed phosphatic calculi from the pelvis of the kidney in many cases, and in a large proportion of them there have been calculi in both kidneys. But the great majority of the cases of phosphatic calculi are formed entirely in the bladder, and are due to septic infection of the vesical mucous membrane—in other words, to cystitis.

Besides these several diatheses, calculi are ascribed to other causes, such as cold climates, too highly nitrogenised food, articles of drink or diet too rich in oxalic acid, insufficient exercise, hereditary predisposition apart from inherited gouty tendencies; and, amongst the dwellers along the Nile especially, the imbibition with the drinking water of the distoma hæmatobium (the bilharzia hæmatobia). Senator has shown that persons with enlarged spleens pass a large quantity of uric acid in their urine, and the question has been raised whether splenic disease is not therefore a cause of uric acid calculi in the kidney and bladder.

2. Sex and age are two general causes of the localisation of stone in the bladder. Vesical calculus is rare in women, because, owing to the shortness and dilatability of their urethra, calculi which can traverse the ureter can easily escape from the bladder. Gravel and gout are much less frequent in women than in men. As to age, Sir Henry Thompson points out that the most favourite period for calculus in the bladder is from fifty-five to seventy-five, the next in order is that below puberty, and the rarest period is middle life. It may seem that stone is most common in children, if the total number of cases which occur at different periods of life are compared with one another; but by comparing the number of cases of stone with the number of persons living of the same age the facts are seen to be as Sir Henry Thompson states them. He further points out that, whereas stone is common in children of the poor classes, so that the half of 1,827 cases known to him as occurring in hospital practice were in children under thirteen years of age, yet that the children of the well-to-do and rich are very rarely the subjects of calculus. Conversely, that stone in men of the poor and labouring classes is rare, whereas it is comparatively common among the well-to-do and well-fed classes.

The point with which we are now concerned is this: that stone being common at the two ends of life it is more frequently localised in the bladder, because the small size and undeveloped state of the urinary organs in the one case, and the obstruction caused by chronic prostatic enlargement in the other, offer difficulties to the escape of a stone from the bladder which do not exist to the same degree in middle age. Other causes tending to the same result are, no doubt, the greater physical activity and the more perfect condition of the digestive organs in manhood than in childhood or old age.

Local causes of the localisation of stone in the bladder are all those which tend to the stagnation of urine in the bladder and to the development of cystitis. When these two conditions, decomposition of urine and cystitis, occur, as they so often do, together, the ammonio-magnesium phosphates are precipitated. This precipitation may occur spontaneously, and thus lead to the formation of a primarily vesical calculus; or it may take place even more readily around a concretion which has descended from the kidney, and this is the process by which uric-acid calculi become enveloped in a white casing of the phosphates.

It is by this same precipitation of the phosphates that foreign bodies in the bladder become encrusted with salts, and that thus are formed calculi, with such things as blood-clots, pieces of bone, hairpins, twigs of trees, berries, and a host of others, for their nuclei. In the same way, too, the surface of vesical tumours and the ends of catheters retained in the bladder become encrusted with a white layer more or less thick of the mixed phosphates.

Aseptic bodies will remain long in the bladder without causing the precipitation of the salts of the urine, but not so septic foreign bodies. By making a section of a calculus the history of the stone formation is seen; there is the nucleus of uric acid or the urates as it was formed in the kidney, and which may have gone on growing after its descent to the bladder; then occurs an attack of cystitis, and a layer of greater or less thickness of the phosphates is deposited around the primitive calculus. Sooner or later the cystitis ceases, and then a layer of uric acid or the urates is superadded. These processes may be repeated again and again, and each one leaves its record on the calculus.

There thus exist two distinct classes of calculi: (1) those formed out of the constituents of the urine owing to some constitutional state, some diathesis; and (2) those of local origin derived from the precipitation of the phosphates, and, whether found in the bladder, the renal pelvis, or the urethra, caused by a septic state of the urine.

Physical and Chemical Characters of Stone. Number. —In children there is generally one calculus; in adults there are often several in the same bladder; in rare instances,

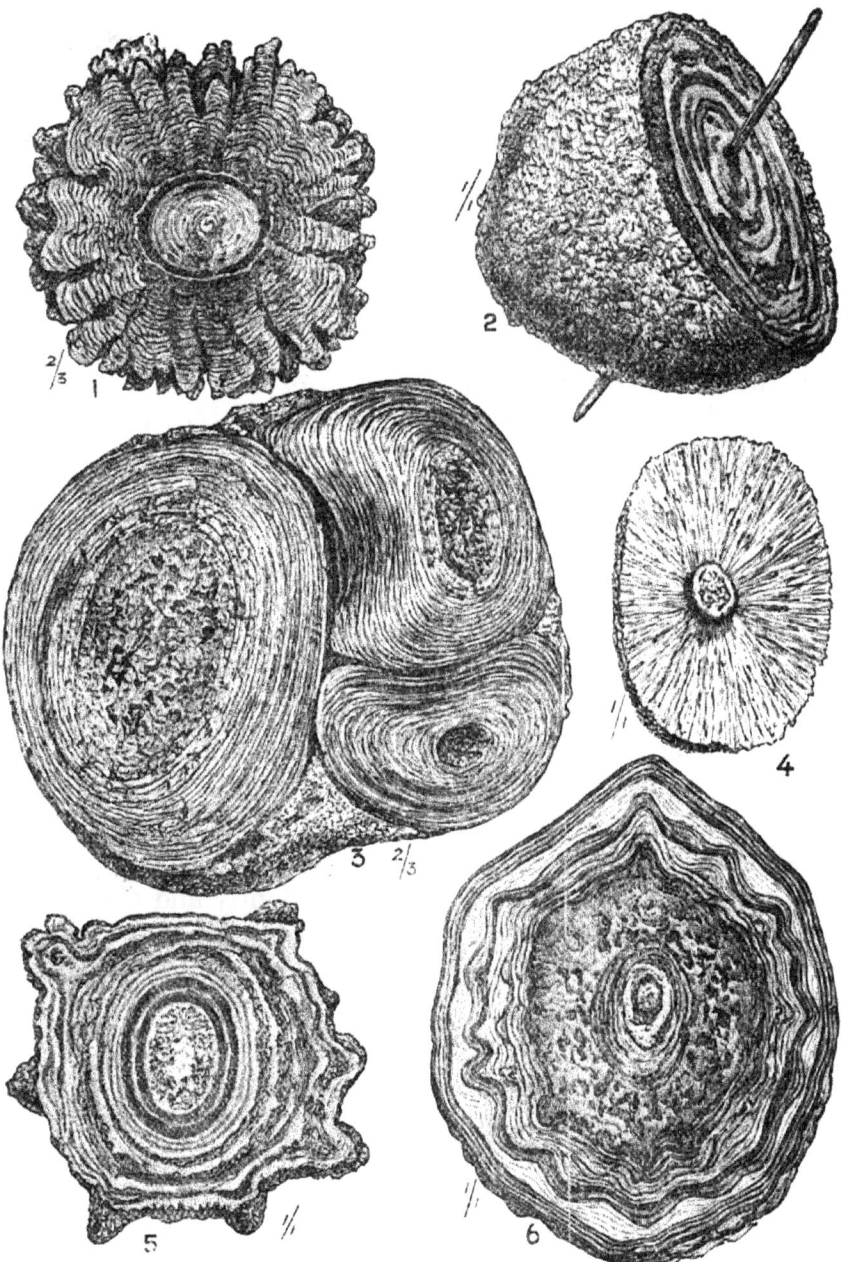

Fig. 85.—Vesical Calculi. (Hunterian Museum.)

1. Section of an oxalate of lime calculus having a large nucleus of urate of ammonia of well-marked character. The surface of the stone is thinly coated with a white layer consisting of oxalate and phosphate of lime: 2, Calculus of mixed phosphates deposited upon a piece of steel; 3, Section of a large uric calculus, consisting of three distinct calculi united by a deposit of earthy phosphates; 4, Triple phosphate calculus (in section) deposited upon a small nucleus of the fusible compound. 5, Section of a uric acid calculus, coated on the exterior with a thin layer of dark oxalate of lime. The stone has thus had given to it the external appearance of a mulberry concretion; 6, Section of an oxalate of lime calculus having a small nucleus of impure urate of ammonia. The white layers consist principally of phosphate of lime.

from 50 to 300 and more have been noted; but it is very common to remove two, or three, or four. Their *size* varies from a canary seed to an orange, or they may be even much larger. Their *weight* may be anything from a few grains to many ounces. Every pathological museum possesses one or more prodigies of its kind. As a rule, calculi are heavier than the urine, but in exceptional cases they float.

The *shape* is generally spherical or ovoid and the surface smooth, if the calculus is of uric acid or the urates; porous, friable and chalky if of the phosphatic character; rough and mammillated, heavy and very hard if of oxalate of lime. The latter are the so-called mulberry calculi, and being very prone to excite bleeding owe their dark colour to blood staining. Some calculi are deeply grooved, or hour-glass shaped, if two calculi have become united together by phosphatic concretion. Occasionally they send out a branch which fits into the neck of the bladder or into a vesical pouch.

Physical Conformation.—The construction of the calculus may be one of three varieties, as Civiale pointed out: (1) those formed in successive layers or lamellæ around the nucleus, like the layers of an onion; (2) those formed by the agglomeration of small crystalline or amorphous masses, each little mass forming and growing independently and then joining the others; (3) those formed by these two processes going on simultaneously. In the stratified (1) variety, the nucleus is either central or nearer one of the poles. Some of them are *simple* calculi—that is, composed entirely, or to a predominating degree, of one substance. Others are *compound*—that is, consisting of a combination of different substances arranged in concentric layers of different colours and density, and having sometimes irregular empty spaces between the different strata. This stratification is characteristic of vesical calculi; it is not seen in stones which have never left the kidney.

Chemical Composition.—There are three chief classes of vesical calculi. (1) The most frequent are formed of uric acid and its combinations; (2) the next most frequent are composed of phosphoric acid in combination with volatile alkali and the alkaline earths; and (3) oxalate of lime.

According to Sir Henry Thompson, uric acid and the urates form about three-fifths, a few of them having a slight admixture of phosphates; whilst nearly two-fifths are phosphates either alone or in combination with some uric acid, in which latter case they are called mixed calculi (compound);

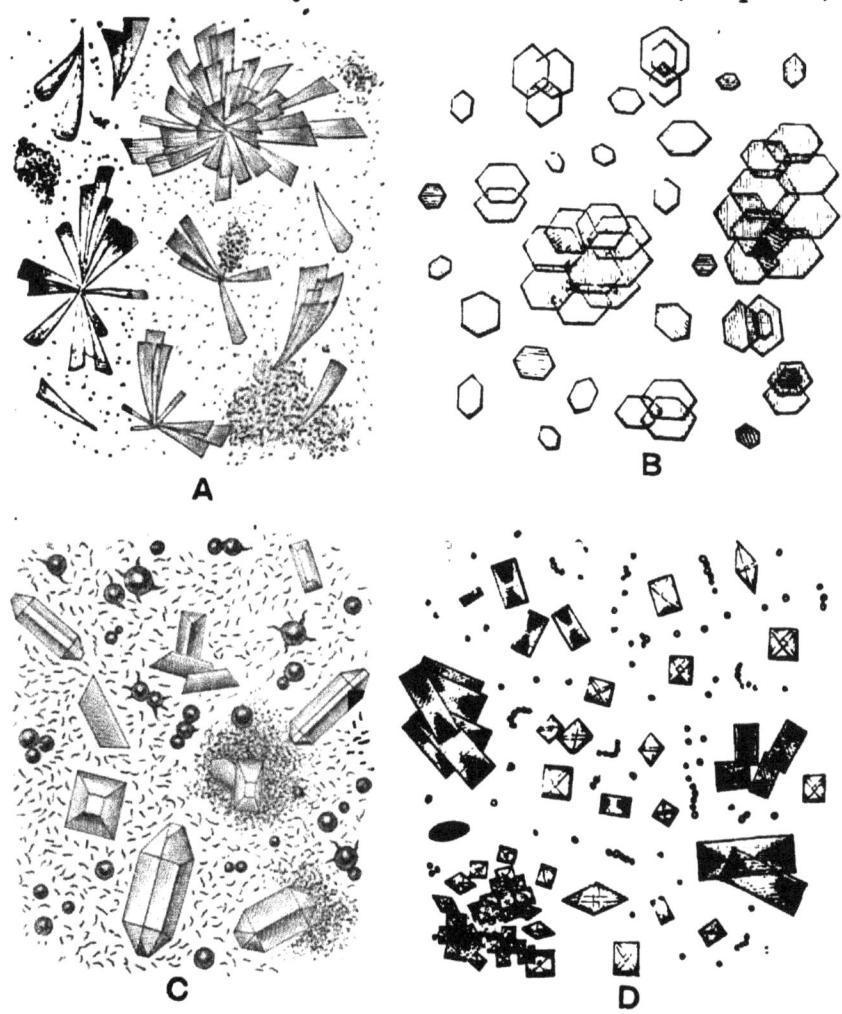

Fig. 86.—Crystals. (Modified from Ultzmann and Hoffmann.)

A, Neutral phosphate of lime, several are arranged together with their points towards a centre. The fine-grained plaques consist partly of carbonate and partly of amorphous tribasic phosphate of lime; B, Cystin, six-sided tables, which in one place are gathered together in a large six-sided rosette. C, Sediment of urine undergoing alkaline fermentation. It consists of transparent sarcophagus-shaped crystals of triple phosphate, of brown plain or pointed double balls of urate of ammonia, and of an amorphous mass of tribasic phosphate of lime mixed with bacteria; D, Sediment of urine undergoing acid fermentation. It consists of brown crystals of uric acid, of crystals of oxalate of lime and chains of yeast cells.

lastly, about 3 per cent. are composed of oxalate of lime. He has operated upon only one case of cystine and one of phosphate of lime. Xanthine, silica, benzoate, and chloro-hydrate of ammonium, uro-stearin, blood, mucus, and various colouring matters have been found in vesical calculi, but are altogether too exceptional to require more than mention here. The *colour* varies with the chemical composition. Calculi of uric acid and the urates are of a fawn colour, or yellow or yellowish pink; oxalate of lime are reddish brown. Phosphatic calculi are white or whitish grey; and those of cystine are greyish yellow.

The *relation of the calculi to the wall of the bladder* is generally free. Occasionally a calculus of the prostate projects into the bladder and there grows to a large size (*see* page 311), still remaining connected to its prostatic portion. But there are three ways in which a vesical calculus can be fixed or " set " in the bladder :—(1) When it occupies a pouch (in which, may be, it originated and grew) which communicates with the cavity of the bladder by an orifice more or less wide. (2) When it is encysted—*i.e.* is situated in a pouch which is altogether shut off from the cavity of the bladder, or communicates with it only by an exceedingly small orifice. This condition is very rare. (3) When it is adherent—*i.e.* tightly held by the projection of the mucous membrane, or of granulations on the mucous membrane, into sinuous depressions of the stone. (4) When the calculus has perforated the bladder-wall and remains fixed in it, as in Mackinder's and Farrar's case. (*British Medical Journal*, April 2nd, 1892.)

Morbid Anatomy of the Bladder.—The bladder tolerates a calculus for a long while, and remains unharmed. Frequently its muscular coat is hypertrophied owing to its incessant contractions caused by the presence of the stone. Cystitis is an occasional complication, and when it occurs is quite as often due to catheterism as to the stone. The pathological changes in the bladder due to this cause have been described in a former section. (*See* page 383.)

Symptoms.—Although in a certain number of post-mortem examinations calculi are found in the bladders of persons who have never had any symptoms whatever, yet, as a rule, there is no lack of evidence of their presence in the vast majority of those affected.

The only absolutely sure proof of the presence of a stone

in the bladder is its detection by means of a sound or metal catheter. But there is a certain combination of symptoms which leads the surgeon to diagnose their presence before he has explored the bladder. These symptoms are pain, frequency of micturition, and hæmorrhage. To these symptoms may be added—(1) the sudden interruption of the stream of urine, a symptom to which, however, undue importance is often given; (2) the patient's clinical history, especially as to the passage of gravel or sand; and (3) the previous occurrence of an attack of nephritic colic, whether followed by the escape of a calculus or not.

Perhaps frequency of micturition is as a rule the first symptom; but it is not rare for an attack of hæmaturia, especially after exercise, to give the first warning. The majority of these patients do not attach so very much importance to the frequency of micturition, and thus it is usually either hæmorrhage or pain which excites their fears and brings them under the notice of the surgeon.

Pain. — The pain varies in its situation and in its character. There is a sense of weight in the perinæum, or an aching behind the symphysis, radiating along the urethra to the end of the penis, and increased by standing, walking, horse exercise, riding in a train or carriage, especially if there be any jolting, by the shaking in coming down stairs, or in jumping down a step or off a chair. Pain is caused, too, by the contractions of the bladder, and hence it is aggravated at the end of micturition. It is lessened by, or· disappears altogether in, the recumbent position.

It may radiate to the loins and suggest the presence of renal calculus, and, indeed, in quite a number of cases the lumbar pain is actually due to renal calculus, the coexistence of renal and vesical calculi, especially of the phosphatic order, being by no means rare.

Sometimes, both in children and adults, there is an itching, sometimes a great pain, at the end of the penis, which leads the patient to squeeze the glans hard, to pull upon the penis, or to pass some foreign body, such as a leaf or fruit-stalk, etc., into the urethra. I have known this done by an elderly man, and the leaf, subsequently getting into the bladder, formed the nucleus of a second stone.

The intensity of the pain varies in different cases from a mere sense of weight or of aching to acute suffering of a burning or tearing character: it varies also very much at different times in the same person. One patient will never have had any pain at all, or may have had an attack on some single occasion only, whereas another may be in constant pain and become bedridden in consequence. The pain and consequent straining excites in some patients rectal tenesmus, and this is followed by hæmorrhoids, or prolapse, or involuntary defæcation.

Hæmorrhage is sometimes the first symptom. After a long walk, ride, or drive, the man passes water, and, to his surprise, finds it heavily mixed with blood. During the same night the urine will gradually get clear, and the next day, or even it may be at the next micturition, it will be again quite free of blood. Subsequently a similar cause will produce a recurrence of the hæmaturia. It is characteristic of calculus that hæmorrhage follows movement or shaking, but is diminished or checked by resting in bed. How often this is witnessed in the case both of renal and vesical calculi!

Another way in which hæmaturia appears is by the discharge of a few drops of blood or bloody urine at the end of micturition; and if this occurs only when the patient passes water standing up, and not when he micturates whilst lying down, it is very significant of stone. The quantity of blood is not often great, the urine may be bright red, but it is very rare for clots to be passed, especially during resting.

There are never the large quantities of blood and blood-clots passed in calculous cases as there are in cases of vesical tumour.

The *frequency of micturition*, like pain and hæmorrhage, is increased by movement. During rest, and at night, it is much diminished or is normal. .

The *sudden stopping of the stream* occurs from two causes —(1) it may be due merely to spasm of the urethral sphincter (the membranous urethra), and then it has no diagnostic value whatever; or (2) it may be due to a stone coming against the urethro-vesical orifice. If the sudden stoppage occurs during micturition in the upright position, but never does so if the water is passed when the patient is lying down, it is a very characteristic symptom. In children it may be but a very small stone which will stop the stream, and as it may at any time become impacted in the urethra, the surgeon should crush and extract it without delay.

The *characters of the urine* may for a long while remain unchanged. Though there be hæmaturia, there may be nothing which is abnormal besides the blood constituents. The microscope may reveal an undue quantity of crystals of some of the urine salts, but there may not be a trace of pus. It has elsewhere been stated (Cystitis, page 375) that a stone in the bladder is a determining cause of cystitis, but it needs some incident such as the introduction of a catheter or bruising of the bladder wall to be superadded before the inflammation is developed. The calculus alone, being an aseptic foreign body, will not excite inflammation. When this happens, the cardinal symptoms of cystitis, frequency of micturition, painful micturition, and pyuria, are added to the cardinal symptoms of vesical calculus—viz. frequency of micturition, pain, and hæmorrhage. Then it is that the sufferings become most intense, the rectal tenesmus most violent, and the urine most markedly ammoniacal. Rest and treatment may abate or cure the cystitis for a time, but relapses are pretty sure to occur, and the patient is exposed to all the risks of suppurative pyelo-nephritis.

Physical Examination.—In boys a stone in the bladder can often be felt by digital examination per rectum.

In adults this is not the case unless the stone is of considerable size, because the prostate and the depth of the perinæum prevent the finger reaching high enough.

Examination per vaginam enables us to feel stones in the female bladder, and also to judge as to their number and size, especially when firm pressure is exercised at the same time above the pubes.

Sounding.—But it is by means of the sound that we gain the most precise information.

Sounding should be done with all the scrupulous care as to asepticity of the urethra and the appliances, which has been repeatedly urged in these pages. (*See* page 236.)

The patient should be placed on his back and a catheter should be passed, and after his urine has been drawn off, his bladder, if not quite clear, should be washed out with some warm antiseptic solution. A few ounces of this solution should be left in the bladder; then the buttocks of the patient should be raised on a pillow and the sound should be introduced. A slight shock is felt by the hand of the surgeon as soon as the end of the instrument comes in contact with the stone; and if the stone be a hard one, a sound is produced loud enough often to be heard by those standing at the bedside, if not by the patient himself. If the stone be phosphatic it may be too soft to give any sound, but the little jarring of the instrument when it comes into contact with it is readily detected by the experienced surgeon. By drawing the beak of the sound over the stone we can approximately ascertain its size and the character of its surface, whether smooth or rough, whilst the presence or absence of the ring of the stone tells of its hardness or otherwise. It will not be forgotten, however, that owing to the physical construction of calculi, a stone which has a very hard nucleus may have a very soft phosphatic encrustation.

By turning the beak of the sound right and left, or pressing it forwards and backwards, we may be able to detect the presence of two or more stones by as many little clicks or ringing sounds of the instrument.

It is easy to overlook the presence of a soft stone coated with a thick layer of glairy muco-pus. I have on several occasions known this to have been done; but it will be avoided if the precaution I have given be followed of always washing out the bladder previous to sounding, when the urine is septic and the bladder secretes muco-pus. If there is still uncertainty with the sound, the bladder should be searched by a small lithotrite, whilst the rectal wall is pressed against the bladder with the forefinger or the rectal bag; and if still there remains any doubt as to the presence of a small stone, or fragment of one, the best plan is to give the patient an anæsthetic, and inject the bladder by Clover's syringe or by Bigelow's evacuating bottle. By this means any small mass of calcareous matter is washed into movement by the injecting process, and as the bottle is allowed to expand, the fluid rushing back into it brings the stone against the end of the evacuating tube. This can be felt by the surgeon holding the tube, but it can also be heard if the ear is placed near the abdominal wall at the hypogastrium.

The *growth of calculi* is, as a rule, slow and progressive. The phosphatic increase more rapidly than the other kinds, and grow from day to day. The rapidity with which these salts are precipitated can be judged of by the rate at which catheters left in the bladder become encrusted. Four or five days are quite sufficient for the portion within the bladder to become thickly coated. Uric-acid and oxalate of lime calculi probably require many years to attain the size of from two and a half to three inches in diameter.

Complications.—(1) The calculus may become impacted in the urethra; (2) certain vesical lesions may be caused by it; or, (3) other complications may be caused by renal lithiasis, of which, indeed, the calculus itself is very generally only a manifestation.

The vesical disturbances are either functional or organic. The functional are retention and incontinence. The organic are ulceration and perforation. They are all rare.

The complications due to lithiasis are sclerosis of kidneys, ureters and bladder, very frequent in these cases; and pyelitis and inflammation of the ureters caused by injury due to the passage of the calculus from the kidney to the bladder. Moreover, nephro-lithiasis tends to the constant manufacture of fresh calculi in the kidney, which may at any time travel down the ureter to the bladder. Hence patients with a strong lithic-acid diathesis should be dieted, and drink freely of diluents and solvents with the view of dislodging these calculi from the kidney and ureters.

Diagnosis.—Vesical calculus has to be diagnosed from cystitis, tumours of the bladder, and certain affections of the kidney.

1. Cystitis is the affection most frequently mistaken for vesical calculus. There are the same symptoms—namely, frequency with pain in micturition, and in very acute cases of cystitis as well as in the tuberculous form of the disease, there is often hæmaturia as well. These symptoms (except hæmaturia) are increased by fatigue and walking; and if it be also remembered that after cystitis has been once set up there is pus in the urine of calculous cases as well as blood, this confusion

in the diagnosis of the two complaints is both intelligible and excusable. The increase of the pain and hæmaturia by exercise, and their relief by resting, are very characteristic of stone.

It is, however, the clinical history and the exploration of the bladder with the sound which will clear up all doubt and difficulty. The history of lithiasis, gravel, or renal colic in the one case, and of gonorrhœa, deep urethral discharges, or frequent catheterism in the other, with perhaps the discovery of the tubercle bacillus by bacteriological examination, will go a long way towards shaping the diagnosis before the sounding of the bladder settles it.

Errors occasionally arise with regard to cystalgia, and bladder trouble secondary to spinal lesions, in which both pain on micturition and hæmaturia occur. The sound will make all clear.

2. Tumours of the bladder are to be diagnosed by their insidious onset and course, and by free hæmorrhage coming on without obvious cause, and frequently without pain.

3. Calculus of the kidney can give rise to all the three cardinal symptoms of vesical calculus, and these symptoms are aggravated and ameliorated by precisely the same means in both classes of case. There is often no fulness, no tenderness in the region of the kidney in cases of renal calculus; and no more pain there than is sometimes caused by cystitis or vesical calculus. The sounding of the bladder will alone settle the doubt. But let it be always borne in mind that many patients with vesical calculi live and die with stones in each of their kidneys. So that the discovery of a calculus in the bladder by no means proves that there is none in the kidney. Before leaving the subject of the diagnosis of stone, it should be mentioned that in former days many patients were cut for stone in whose bladders no stone was found. If these surgical catastrophes did not occur from carelessness, *i.e.* from omitting to sound the bladder immediately before the cutting operation was commenced, it must have been due to one of two causes:
—(*a*) to a small stone being washed suddenly out of the bladder with the first gush of urine at the time of the operation and so lost, or missed for the moment; or (*b*) what has been proved to happen in children with small narrow pelves must have occurred—namely, striking the bony wall of the

pelvis during the manipulations of the sound. In elderly men
the very prominent and hypertrophied muscular trabeculæ of

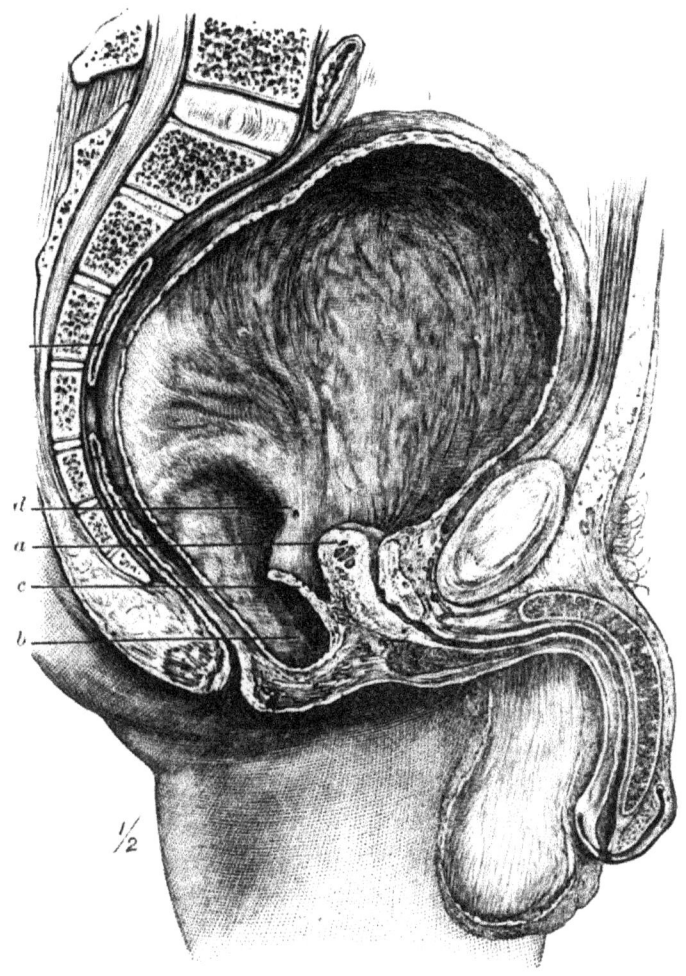

Fig. 87.—Enormously dilated Bladder from an old Man.

a, Hypertrophy of middle lobe of prostate, which contains a cystic space ; *b,* pouch
of bladder behind prostate ; *c,* ridge formed by wall of bladder ; *d,* orifice of
left ureter. The enlarged middle lobe of the prostate acted like a valve, and
so obstructed the urethral opening. The pouch *b* formed a receptacle for
retained urine. (St. Mary's Hospital Museum.) (*Pepper.*)

the ·bladder wall, especially if coated with phosphatic concretion, might give the sensation of stone ; but such an error
ought to be, and will be corrected by an experienced hand.

Causes of Failure in Sounding.—I have previously referred
(page 410) to the possibility of not recognising a stone with the

sound if the bladder wall and the calculus are covered with an abundant layer of glairy muco-pus. I have known very large phosphatic calculi to be thus overlooked by experienced surgeons. Though large, such stones are soft and do not give a distinct ring against the sound, and when they have a thick coating of gluey muco-pus it is not difficult to understand how they escape detection. To avoid this the bladder ought always to be well irrigated in such cases immediately before introducing the sound. Other causes of failure in sounding to detect a calculus are the following :—(1) The stone may lie in a pouch behind an enlarged lobe or collar of the prostate which projects into the bladder (Fig. 87); (2) the stone may be in a sacculus of the bladder, or be encysted behind the pubis or elsewhere out of ready reach of the sound; (3) a small stone may be covered over by a fold of swollen mucous membrane—a condition likely to occur if the bladder is in a state of congestion or inflammation ; (4) a stone lying loose in the bladder of a man with a slightly enlarged prostate and a thigh anchylosed in a flexed and adducted position escaped detection by several experienced surgeons until sounding was made through a perinæal opening. Where a deep post-prostatic pouch makes the diagnosis difficult, Mr. Hurry Fenwick, finding the cysto-scope of no assistance, proposes the sounding of the bladder by means of a loosely fitting blunt pilot passed through an aspirator cannula which has been thrust supra-pubically into the bladder. Mr. Buckstone Browne has designed a sound with a beak like a flat-bladed lithotrite for searching the bladder in these cases, and in a suggestive contribution to the *Lancet* (April 19th, 1891) has illustrated some difficulties attending the search for a calculus in post-prostatic pouches.

Where sounding, and the aspirating bottle and tubes, and the cystoscope have all failed, an inspection of the bladder through the hypogastric cystotomy opening is the last resource of the surgeon. There are cases of calculi in diverticula of the bladder and in retro-prostatic pouches which cannot be dealt with in any other way. *See* cases by Vincent, Jackson, and Bruce Clarke in the thirty-ninth volume of the Pathological Society's Transactions (pp. 192-3).

The best way to avoid failure is to sound with the bladder

fairly full, to have the hips raised so that the stone may fall away towards the fundus of the bladder, to change the position of the patient during sounding, to shake him by the pelvis, to move the sound in the bladder whilst the finger or rectal bag is pressing forwards and upwards against the trigone, to supplement sounding with the suction-bottle of Clover or Bigelow, and, if need be, by the cystoscope. If it is possible to avoid it, sounding ought not to be done whilst the bladder is in a state of acute inflammation.

Prognosis.—Stone in the bladder is by no means fatal in all cases. A gentleman of sixty-six first discovered he had vesical calculus by an attack of hæmaturia after a day at Goodwood races and a drive home of fourteen miles: he lived to the age of seventy-nine, and then died of carbuncle of the neck. The only treatment he adopted was a quiet, restful life, and drinking a fair daily quantity of some alkaline water. Yet he dined well, and drank moderately of port wine, travelled by omnibus and railways, and could stand through a long morning or afternoon, fishing. He never had an attack of cystitis or any other bladder symptom, and his first attack of hæmaturia was also the last. He was sounded by the late Mr. Edward Cock of Guy's Hospital, who detected the stone, and after that, no instrument was ever again used upon him. Cases of this kind are known to all surgeons of experience. The fact is that an elderly man of sedentary life, and who has no enlarged prostate and no cystitis, can live many years with a large stone in his bladder, and die of something unconnected with it. But if after years of comfortable life with a stone in the bladder, painful symptoms should necessitate an operation, the patient is only too likely to succumb from suppression of urine or from suppurative pyelo-nephritis, because the kidneys and ureters will have become greatly dilated and the renal tissue atrophied.

An illustrative case of this sort was that of an old man who for many years had carried a stone in his bladder, without suffering, but was obliged at length to have it removed by supra-pubic cystotomy. The stone weighed over four ounces and two drachms. Almost immediately his kidneys ceased secreting, and in the restlessness and semi-comatose state of suppression he constantly disturbed his dressings, the bladder again became septic, as it was before the operation, and he died on the fifth day. Similar results follow the perinæal operation and also litholapaxy.

It is the supervention of septic infection of the bladder, whether any operation has been done or not, that creates the dangers and conduces to the fatal result by exciting ascending suppurative pyelo-nephritis. It is the existence of this condition before the operation that adds so largely to the risks of surgical interference, and to which such small mortality as follows litholapaxy as now practised by skilled hands, is attributable.

The spontaneous expulsion of calculi in the case of men cannot be reckoned upon; but women pass large stones through the urethra, and others still larger sometimes escape into the vagina by ulceration of the vesico-vaginal septum.

As a rare occurrence, spontaneous fragmentation of stones is known; it is due to molecular changes which lead to their complete disintegration; and spontaneous expulsion of the fragments follows. Dr. Ord has collected several cases, and others are recorded by Mr. Sydney Jones and Mr. Clutton in vol. xxxvii. of the Pathological Society's Transactions.

Thus then, if no operative treatment is employed, some few calculi remain stationary, or at any rate quiescent throughout; some few become spontaneously expelled either after or without being first spontaneously disintegrated; but the great majority give rise to progressive troubles, and end finally in death from pyelo-nephritis. But even when suppuration in the kidneys has commenced, there is still some hope, for the affection is not necessarily fatal if not too far advanced, provided an operation is undertaken, and the bladder is thoroughly antisepticised and maintained in an aseptic condition.

Treatment.—The complete account of the treatment of vesical calculus would include the prophylaxis of the lithic, oxalic, and phosphatic diatheses; but we are concerned now only with the treatment when a calculus is actually formed and is occupying the bladder. This has passed through three distinct historical stages. The first stage reaches from Pliny and Aræteus to January 13, 1824, when Civiale first crushed a stone in the living bladder. The second stage extends from that date down to the antiseptic treatment of wounds by Lister, and the introduction of litholapaxy by Bigelow in 1878. From this time, the treatment of vesical calculus has been entirely changed, the reasons for the selection of one operation rather than another completely revolutionised, and the mortality tables happily have had to be rewritten. This is the present stage.

Otis first demonstrated how much more dilatable all parts of the urethra are than surgeons had previously regarded them as being.

Bigelow, of Boston, showed that it was possible and safe to prolong, under anæsthesia, the manipulations within the bladder, to use larger and therefore more powerful instruments than had hitherto been employed, and to wash out the fragments by the suction action of very thick, and therefore very strong, indiarubber bottles. Thus even very large stones came to be completely removed at one operation, instead of the patients being submitted, as previously, to a repetition of short crushings at intervals of three or four days, and the broken fragments left in the bladder to bruise and lacerate it, or be discharged with the urine by the expulsive efforts of the bladder, often ploughing up the mucous membrane of the urethra in their transit. It is but just to remember that, prior to the publication of Bigelow's paper (*Lancet*, 1878, vol. ii.), Clover had suggested, and Sir Henry Thompson had used, a small indiarubber evacuating bottle for the removal of fragments after crushing, and that Maunder had added to this a little well or reservoir, into which the fragments subsided as they were washed out.

The improvement in the cutting operations by the antiseptic treatment of the wounds is great, though less marked than in the crushing operation by the substitution of litholapaxy for lithotrity. Formerly, by the extraction of very large stones through the perinæal route, or by lateral, bilateral, and rectal lithotomy, injury was done to the ejaculatory ducts; to the rectum, leading to vesico-rectal fistulæ; to the artery of the bulb and the prostatic plexus leading to serious or fatal hæmorrhage; or to the neck of the bladder, resulting in permanent incontinence of urine; moreover, the suppurating and sloughing processes which often occurred in

B B

the wounds, led to pyæmia, cystitis, and fatal ascending sup-purative pyelo-nephritis by no means unfrequently.   Listerism has diminished these risks very materially: (1) by the pro-tection of the wound and the urinary organs from septic infection; and (2) by thus encouraging the substitution of the hypogastric operation instead of the perinæal for the extrac-tion of large stones.

Litholapaxy as introduced by Bigelow and modified by Sir Henry Thompson and M. Guyon is now the recognised operation for all cases (with few exceptions to be named presently) of vesical calculus in males.   Lithotomy, how-ever, cannot be banished from the category of useful and necessary surgical operations.   It is the only operation possible for very large stones—beyond six centimetres if phosphatic, and five centimetres if composed of uric acid or oxalate of lime; for calculi so hard that they resist the strongest lithotrites; for those very sensitive bladders which resent the slightest attempts to inject sufficient antiseptic solution to form a safe medium for the employment of the lithotrite; and where secondary calculi are formed, owing either to the diseased condition of the bladder, or to the fragments of a crushed stone dropping into the recesses and pouches of a hypertrophied bladder, from which they cannot be washed free, and in which they grow.   It is the operation, too, for all calculi "set" in a pouch of the bladder, or "encysted," as well as for some which are "adherent."   Some surgeons incline to the opinion that advanced renal disease is a reason for lithotomy rather than litholapaxy.   The mortality incident to both operations is enormously increased by this cause, that of lithotomy being about 90 per cent.   It seems to be the better practice to adopt litholapaxy.   Stricture of the urethra, which used to be considered a bar to lithotrity, is no longer so to the same extent or in the same way to litholapaxy; the stricture should be dilated or divided so that the urethra will readily admit the lithotrite and the evacuating tubes. If the stricture be divided, time should, when possible, be allowed for the healing of the wound in the urethra before operating upon the stone.   The objection, formerly, to lithotrity in cases of stricture was not so much the difficulty of introducing the lithotrite as the contracted size of the bladder, and the impaction of the fragments in the strictured part of the urethra during the process of their discharge with the urine.

In some extreme cases of hypertrophy of the prostate especially when the calculus or fragments of a calculus are inaccessible in a pouch behind the gland, the stone must be removed by a cutting operation. As regards the choice between the various forms of lithotomy, the operation of election with most surgeons is the hypogastric. It is almost universally preferred by foreign surgeons, and the same must, I think, be said to-day of the profession in England and America. Whether this preference will continue so general as at present, remains to be seen. The advantages claimed for it are that, (1) it allows of the complete inspection and evacuation of the bladder ; (2) the operation, and the wound subsequently, can be kept completely aseptic; (3) it avoids the danger to the ejaculatory ducts, to the neck of the bladder, to the rectum, and to important blood-vessels which are in danger, yet cannot be seen, during the course of lateral lithotomy; (4) the opening made into the bladder can be free enough to allow of the extraction of very large stones without bruising or lacerating the tissues, which is not always the case in the perinæal operations ; (5) enlargement of the prostate is no obstacle in the operation, whilst it renders the perinæal operation unsatisfactory or even impossible, and the cavity of the bladder is in some cases thereby put beyond the reach of an ordinary index finger.

There are, however, some few cases in which the best route to the bladder is through a median incision in the membranous urethra. This is specially the case where some of the stones occupy a very dilated prostatic urethra (*see* page 209), and where a prostatic calculus has extended through the urethro-vesical orifice into the bladder and there grown (as in Fig. 60, page 209). It is the best operation in certain cases of stones of medium size where there is cystitis. The vesical orifice can be enlarged by dividing the prostate if necessary, either by a vertical median cut, or by a lateral incision in the prostate on one or both sides of the median line. It avoids opening up an extensive plane of loose connective tissue such as exists in the hypogastric region, and which is very likely to become fouled by the escape into it of a few drops of septic urine after the operation is completed.

Mr. Harrison has of late years reintroduced the operation by the mixed method of Dolbeau (1862). This consists in making a median incision into the membranous urethra and crushing the stone and removing the fragments through the opening thus made. Mr. Harrison prefers crushing forceps to a lithotrite in this operation, and in Figs. 88 and 89 are shown a straight and a curved pair, which he has found very suitable for the purpose. He advances half a dozen or more reasons in favour of this mixed operation; but, though all may not agree with his reasons, it must be admitted that the operation is well suited for cases complicated with unusually troublesome stricture, for weak and permanently damaged urethra, for cases in which there is a great tendency, owing to cystitis, to the formation of secondary calculi, and in which, therefore, continuous drainage of the bladder is desirable and advantageous.

Mr. Harrison has performed the operation in twelve cases without death, and, as Tuffier's figures up to 1886 showed a mortality of 27 per cent. for the hypogastric operation for stone, and as Mr. Swinford Edwards has more recently shown (*Med. Press*, October 12th, 1892) that supra-pubic operation for stone has a mortality of 50 per cent., there is ground for giving the method the support and trial it seems to deserve.

Litholapaxy and its highly successful application to boys of all ages, on the one hand, and aseptic and antiseptic precautions on the other, have done so much to diminish mortality that the statistics of operations performed more than 15 or 16 years ago are no longer of use in a comparison of different methods of treatment. Surgeon Major P. J. Freyer states (*Brit. Med. Journ.*, 1889, vol. ii. p. 811) that out of 232 recent operations for stone up to April, 1889, he had but 3 deaths. Of these 232 operations, 177 were litholapaxies with one death; 52 were perinæal lithotomies with one death, and 3 were suprapubic lithotomies with one death. Dittel, in 1890, published the results of his last 100 cases, showing 4 deaths in 70 litholapaxies, and 5 deaths in 25 lithotomies—all the patients who died, excepting two, were hopelessly stricken, and would have died, he says, no matter what operation had been performed. Guyon's statistics in 1887 (M. Tuffier) show 41·6 per cent. on

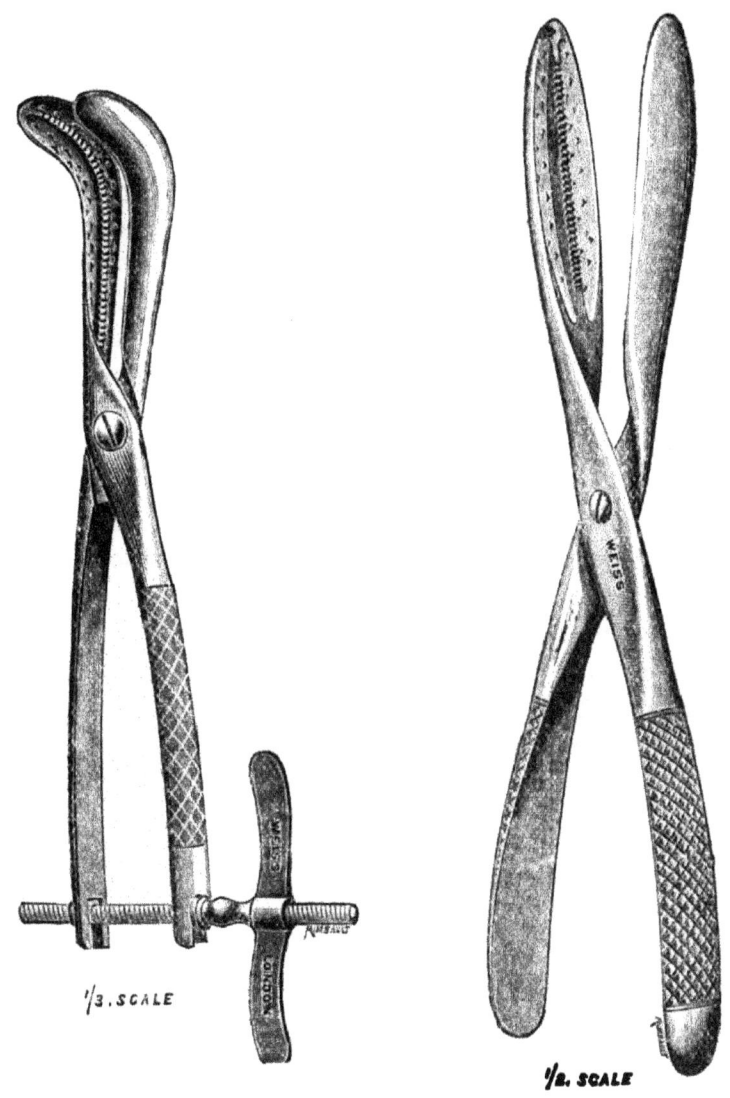

HARRISON'S CRUSHING FORCEPS (WEISS).

Fig. 88.—Harrison's curved Forceps for crushing Vesical Calculi through a Median Perinæal Opening.

Fig. 89.—Harrison's straight Forceps for crushing Vesical Calculi through a Median Perinæal Opening.

12 perinæal lithotomies, 48 per cent. on 19 hypogastric lithotomies, and only 5·2 per cent. for litholapaxy.

In females, lithotrity is said to be more difficult than in

males, owing to the want of the prostate, but this only applies
to the operation in hands inexperienced in lithotrity in males.
It is, however, rarely required in women, because of the
capacity and dilatability of the urethra. In female children,
the best operation is lithotrity by means of a lithotrite of
the calibre of a full-sized catheter (No. 12 or 14), followed
by the evacuation of the fragments with Clover's or Bigelow's
evacuating bottle (aspirator), and in adult females the same
operation, using Erichsen's or Harrison's crushing forceps
instead of a lithotrite, may be employed for stones which
are too large to be wisely extracted in their entire state
through the urethra. Or the fragments of the stone might
be removed with forceps through the dilated urethra. The
operation is allied to the mixed operation in males. In
women with stone of a large size, the vaginal cystotomy,
followed by immediate sutures, is an easier, safer, and more
satisfactory operation than the hypogastric.

In boys, lateral lithotomy has always been a most successful operation, and lithotrity in rough or inexperienced hands
is more than usually dangerous in them. Indeed, cases are
on record in which the bladder has been ruptured by the
lithotrite. But in skilful hands, and with proper lithotrites,
the results of litholapaxy are far better even than those of
lateral lithotomy, namely, as 1· is to 6·6 per cent.

The Anglo-Indian surgeons have given us ample proof
of the success, in boys, of litholapaxy in their hands.
On this subject I will quote from a private letter from
Surgeon-Major D. J. Keegan, written on July 14th, 1894.
He says :—" I performed my first litholapaxy in a boy in
December, 1881, and between that date and the 1st of April
of this year (1894) I had performed 239 litholapaxies in boys,
with five deaths. Four, if not all, of these deaths were caused
by extensive organic disease of the kidneys, and were certainly not the result of any accident or failure in the method
of operating. The average weight of the stones removed in
these 239 operations was 98·44 grains ; the time spent in
hospital after the operation averaged 4·16 days ; the age of
the boys averaged 6·40 years ; and the mortality was 2·09 per
cent." The signal success of this series of cases speaks for
itself. Surgeon-Major Freyer has performed litholapaxy in

143 cases in India on children without a death. Surgeon-Major Gimlette has had 40 successful cases in boys and children. Thus these three surgeons have done litholapaxy

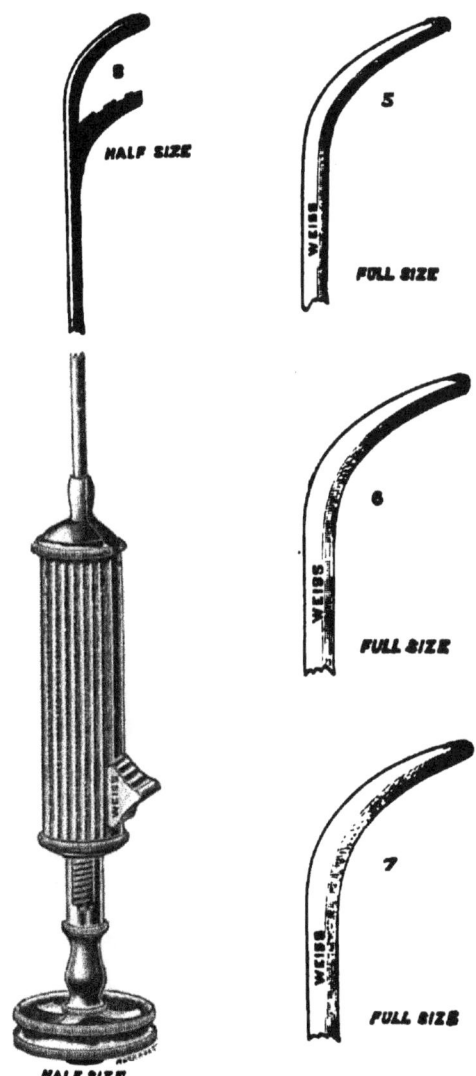

Fig. 90.—Fenestrated Lithotrites of Sizes from 5 to 8 (English gauge) for use on Boys (Weiss). The numbers indicate the size of the instruments at their curve.

for boys 422 times with only five deaths—a mortality of little more than 1 per cent. Surgeon-Major Keegan insists that the surgeon who aspires to perform litholapaxy in boys must provide himself with a large assortment of fully fenestrated lithotrites of small size, and made of superlatively good steel.

These fenestrated lithotrites should range from No. 4 or 5 at the bend of the blades to No. 8 (English scale); and the evacuating catheters, or cannulæ, should be fitted with serviceable stylets and never introduced or withdrawn without the stylets in them.

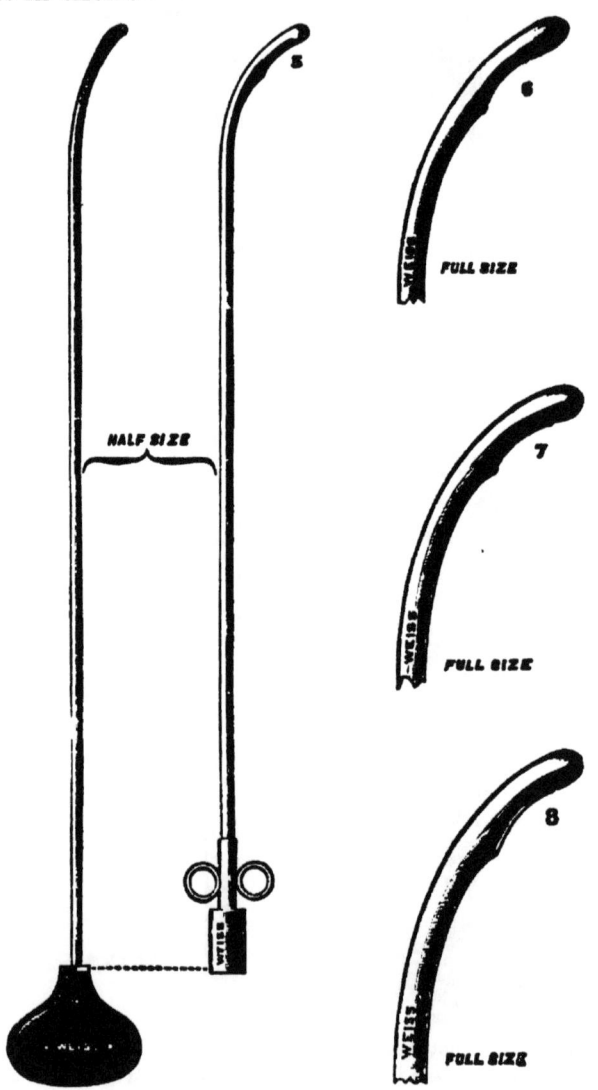

Fig. 91.—Evacuating Cannulæ with Keegan's Stylets, for use on Boys, from Sizes 5 to 8 (Weiss).

The advantages claimed are—(1) the low mortality, (2) absence of after ill-effects, (3) very quick recovery, the child often being up the next day, (4) the avoidance of cutting.

CHAPTER X.

FOREIGN BODIES IN THE BLADDER.

FOREIGN bodies gain access to the cavity of the bladder (1) through the urethra, (2) by being forced through its walls by injury, (3) by means of ulceration, or by the formation of a fistula, which is most often of cancerous origin.

1. Those which enter the bladder along the urethra include pieces of catheters, lithotrites, and filiform guides, which have been broken off during some operation, or, in the case of catheters tied in, during their sojourn in the bladder.

Besides these, and forming by far the greater number, are the substances introduced by the patients, either to allay itching or tickling in the passage, or to dilate some real or imaginary stricture, or aimlessly or for a sensual purpose. The variety of things which have been so introduced is almost endless, and comprises articles so different as the leaves or twigs of plants, eight or nine inches of indiarubber tubing, fruit berries, beads, bodkins, hairpins, a mouthpiece of a pipe, a pencil case, and a great number of other things besides.

2. Foreign bodies forced through the bladder walls, or into the ureter and renal pelvis, and which subsequently descend to the bladder, include bullets, pieces of bone or of raiment, or buttons. A case is quoted in my work on the Surgery of the Kidneys, in which a piece of the tunic of an officer, which entered the kidney, after many months passed into the bladder and through the urethra, and was subsequently discharged.

3. Foreign bodies which ulcerate into the bladder, or find their way along fistulous tracts, come either from the vagina, or rectum, or the intestines higher up, from extra-uterine gestation cysts, from dermoid cysts, or from abscesses in the pelvic cellular tissue.

In this way uterine pessaries have passed through the vesico-vaginal septum ; pieces of bone, coins, fæcal matter, and intestinal worms have entered from the bowel ; fragments of a fœtus in extra-uterine gestation ; hair and teeth from dermoid cysts; hydatids; and pus and bone from pelvic abscesses. Amongst surgical catastrophes, and miraculous recoveries there is the case of a pair of pressure forceps left in the peritoneal cavity at an ovariotomy, in which ulceration of the vesical wall occurred, and the forceps entered the bladder, and were thence successfully removed after a long interval.

Pathological Anatomy.—Allusion is made (at page 204) in reference to foreign bodies in the urethra, to the theory as to the manner in which they work their way backwards. But whatever may be the real mechanism of their transit along the urethra, it is important to remember that fruitless attempts at extraction assist them onwards in their course to the bladder.

From the observations of Guyon and Henriet it appears that when once fairly within the cavity of the bladder, they occupy most frequently a transverse position between the summit and the neck of the bladder, and rather nearer to the neck. In the empty bladder this position is more constant than in the full bladder; in the empty bladder it is the only position which bodies not longer than ten centimetres can take.

Smaller bodies can occupy any position in the distended bladder; but in the empty, or nearly empty, organ they assume the transverse diameter.

A body of twelve centimetres takes a vertical position, or, if one of its ends is buttressed near the neck, it may be an oblique direction.

Light bodies float; hollow ones, like a piece of tubing or catheter, generally lie in the base of the bladder.

Some become disintegrated and are passed in particles, sometimes even without the patients knowing it.

Foreign bodies, when in the bladder, may remain entirely quiescent, or may excite cystitis; after a time they may cause ulceration and perforation, and, giving rise to a perivesical abscess, may escape by the direction through which the abscess is either opened or spontaneously discharged. Or the foreign body, having penetrated the vesical wall, may remain partly within the bladder, and partly within the peritoneal cavity. A case of this sort is recorded by Benham and

Greig Smith (*Bristol Med.-Chir. Journal*, March, 1886). The foreign body was the end of an iron rib of an umbrella, projected for two inches into the peritoneal cavity without doing harm, and phosphatic salts were deposited for half an inch on the outside of the bladder, which suggested to the authors that the bladder wall, in emptying and filling, must have glided up and down the metal.

It is remarkable that septic foreign bodies, such as a particle of fæces, for example, by no means invariably excite cystitis.

The foreign bodies become encrusted with phosphates, however, and are thus often the nuclei of calculi. It is remarkable how quickly this deposition begins; in some instances even within twenty-four hours. The deposition commences upon the largest part of the foreign body, and proceeds thence towards the extremities, which, however, never become encrusted. Thus, even when the calculus formed upon the foreign body (a needle or pin for example) is of large size, the sharp ends of such a body remain uncovered.

Symptoms.—The urine may remain normal, no symptom whatever may appear, and the individual may go about as if nothing had happened. The same absence of symptoms, we know, attends some vesical calculi. Much depends on the shape and character of the foreign body.

But, as in the case of calculi, the rule is for the patient to have pain and frequent micturition, and possibly the discharge, at the end of micturition, of a little blood. Hard, rough, or sharp bodies are apt to excite cystitis, with its attendant cardinal symptoms. If the foreign bodies penetrate the cellular tissue and form an abscess in the pelvis, we have the local and constitutional signs of inflammation and suppuration. If they penetrate the rectum, there will probably be rectal tenesmus; if the peritoneum or small intestines, the signs of peritonitis will most likely occur. The case quoted above, however, shows that this does not invariably happen.

Foreign bodies largely encrusted and forming the nucleus of a large calculus, behave like calculi formed in the ordinary way, except that there is always the risk of ulceration or perforation by the projecting extremities of the foreign bodies.

Diagnosis.—When the foreign body has been introduced by the patient, the readiest road to a correct knowledge of the case is the frank admission of the patient; but he often denies any knowledge of what he has himself caused.

In surgical accidents, or when catheters break off in the bladder, there is no room for doubt. In traumatic cases there is the history of the injury, the presence of a wound or scar. In perforation of the rectal or vaginal septum, there is the history of local pain, and the existence probably of the ulcerated aperture or its scar. When the foreign body has passed through from the intestinal tract, there may be or may have been the escape of gas, fæces, or ingesta along the urethra.

In the case of hysterical women, however, it is necessary to bear in mind that all sorts of things are designedly mixed with the urine.

Hydatids passed with the urine will give the clue to their possible presence in the bladder.

It is of great importance, especially with a view to its extraction, to learn, if possible, the shape and size of the foreign body, and the length of time it has been lodged in the organ. In all cases of doubt, the surgeon should examine the bladder (1) with his finger in the rectum or in the vagina, (2) by sounding, and (3) by the cystoscope.

Treatment.—If the foreign body has quite recently been introduced, and it is soft and pliable, like a piece of tube or gum-elastic catheter, it can readily be extracted by the lithotrite, no matter how it is seized by the blades of the instrument. Hard, rounded bodies can also be easily extracted by the lithotrite, either without or after breaking them into fragments. Elongated substances, whether blunt or sharp, give great trouble because of the difficulty of catching them in their long axis. The cystoscope will often be of great value in this respect by informing us of the direction in which the body lies. Certain special instruments, such as Roberts' and Collins's "redressing" forceps, made something like a lithotrite, are very useful (Fig. 92). They cause a long body to rotate on itself till it rests between the blades in its long axis. Some bodies, such, for example, as a hairpin, may be luckily caught by their curved ends by means of a blunt hook at the end of a flexible stem. An instrument of this sort, such as the one devised by Guyon, will answer also for extracting flexible bodies by catching them transversely, and then, by traction, causing them to double upon themselves as soon as they meet with the resistance of the neck of the bladder. For flexible bodies of a harder or more resisting nature, instruments have been made to effect the bending process. These, in principle, consist of a male blade with a hook sliding within a female blade; the foreign body is caught by the hook of the male blade, which is withdrawn into the female blade, dragging

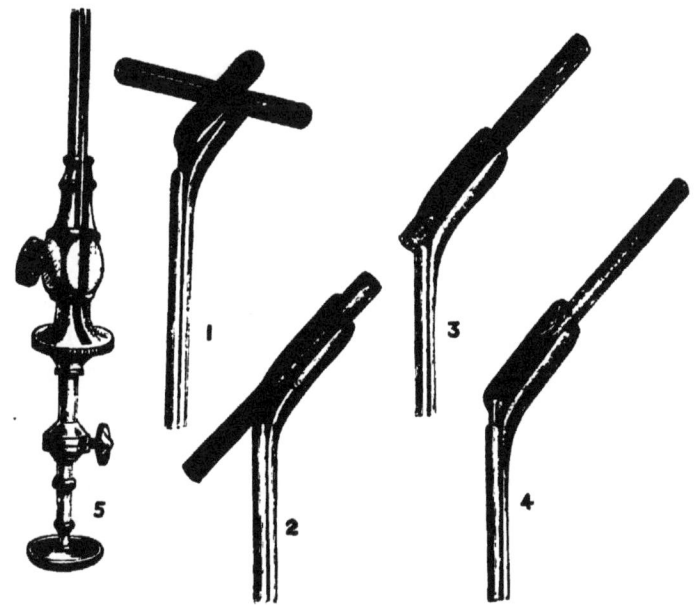

Fig. 92.--Roberts's and Collins's " Re-dressing " Forceps.

with it the foreign body. It acts on the same principle as Fleet Spier's artery constrictor.

If the foreign body cannot be readily extracted by any of these methods, there ought to be no delay in removing it by a perinæal or hypogastric operation, rather than run the risk of violent or too prolonged attempts at extraction through the urethra. The hypogastric will be best in most cases. Different surgeons will select different routes; but whether it be by hypogastric cystotomy, or median perinæal urethrotomy, the wound in the organ ought to be sutured immediately after the extraction of the foreign body, unless, owing to the presence of cystitis, there is necessity to drain the bladder.

If the foreign body has long sojourned in the bladder, and

has therefore become encrusted with calculous matter, some advise that the deposit should be detached by the lithotrite and the foreign body extracted in the same manner as if it had only recently been introduced, and then that the calculous matter should be removed as in litholapaxy.

It is, however, by no means always easy, and sometimes it is quite impossible, to detach the calculous matter thoroughly from the foreign body; and, on the whole, it is the better practice in most cases of calculous formation to remove the foreign body by perinæal or hypogastric operation, without attempting the double procedure with the lithotrite and an extraction instrument, as just described.

Such foreign bodies, as leaves, or twigs of trees, are very dangerous, as they are liable to be broken and their particles to cling to, or stick into the mucous membrane, from which they cannot be dislodged either by instruments or irrigation. Cystitis is very apt to arise and to be followed by ascending suppuration and death from pyelo-nephritis. This complication of course may occur in the case of other foreign bodies.

In women it will be rarely necessary to resort to any cutting operation, the dilatability of the female urethra allowing of the extraction of most foreign bodies which can reach the bladder by any of the methods mentioned at the beginning of this section.

After the extraction, the treatment is the same as after extracting an ordinary calculus, and will vary according as there is, or is not cystitis. Should a fistula or perivesical abscess have been formed, it ought to be treated in the manner described under these headings.

CHAPTER XI.

TUMOURS OF THE BLADDER.

Up to within the last fifteen or sixteen years, tumours of the bladder had only a histological and pathological interest; but the work and writings of Billroth, Thompson, Volckman, Kocher, and Guyon have given them an additional clinical importance by bringing them within the range of operative treatment. The literature of the subject is rapidly increasing, and the London Pathological Society's Transactions alone show with what industry these cases are being collected and reported.

Tumours of the bladder present numerous histological varieties, and considerable clinical differences. Clinically, some are benign and others malignant. Histologically, the benign comprise papillomata, myxomata, fibromata, and myomata. The malignant are carcinomata and sarcomata.

As to the relative frequency of malignant and non-malignant new growths in the bladder, Mr. W. Roger Williams, whilst Surgical Registrar at the Middlesex Hospital, made a very extensive investigation. He analysed 13,824 primary neoplasms of all kinds which had been consecutively under treatment at the Middlesex and three other large hospitals in London, and found that 90, or 0·65 per cent., originated in the bladder. They were:—

	Total.	Males.	Females.
Cancer	59	43	16
Sarcoma	6	5	1
Fibroma	2	1	1
Papilloma (villous) ...	23	21	2
	90	70	20

Ch. Féré ("Cancer de la Vessie") tabulates 82 cases in which the nature of the tumour was ascertained; of these, 52 were carcinomata, 3 were sarcomata, and 27 were papillomata (villous).

Contrary to the former belief that villous growth (papilloma) is the commonest variety of bladder tumours, it is seen from

Williams's and Féré's list that the malignant tumours are between two and three times more frequent than the benign, and that cancer alone is more than twice as frequent as villous growth. As to the relative frequency of carcinoma and sarcoma, allowance must, of course, be made in this table for the absence of microscopical examination of many of the cases.

Mr. Roger Williams also gives us an idea of the frequency with which the bladder, as compared with other organs, is the seat of new growths ; thus :—

0·65 per cent. occurred in the bladder.	5·8 per cent. in the ovaries.	
2·66 ,, in the stomach.	6·3 ,, ,, tongue and	
2·66 ,, ,, lip.	mouth.	
2·9 ,, ,, maxilla.	7·7 · ,, ,, connective tissue	
3·3 ,, ,, rectum.	9·4 ,, ·, skin.	
4·0 ,, ,, bones.	17·5 ,, ,, breast.	
5·1 ,, ,, genitals.	19·2 ,, ,, uterus.	

Galt's figures, as given by Tuffier, show bladder tumours to occur in 0·39 per cent. of tumours generally, and, according to Ulzmann, they only form 3·2 per cent. of all bladder affections.

There are some characters common to all bladder tumours. (1) Their usual *situation* is in the region of the trigone and about the orifices of the ureters; rarely, they grow from the lateral walls, and still more rarely from the antero-superior. (2) The *form* of the benign tumours is generally rounded, often polypoid or tufted ; the malignant tumours are more generally spread out. (3) Their *size* is not frequently large, but varies from that of a cherry or a nut to that of a hen's egg. Exceptional tumours have been met with as large as a cocoanut, or fœtal head, and these have generally been myomata.

Not unfrequently the cancerous tumours are multiple and, to all appearances, independent of one another. This is contrary to what is known of this disease in most other organs. Surgeons are, however, familiar with the occurrence of epitheliomatous growths on opposite surfaces of the vagina, on the apposed surfaces of the labia pudendi, on the under surface of the tip of the tongue and the corresponding part of the floor of the mouth. The explanation of all these facts is, no doubt, the same; they are instances of impregnation by contact. In the case of the bladder, the surfaces fall into contact in the contracted state of the viscus, and implantation can occur if the free surface of the primary growth is eroded or injured.

Mr. Hurry Fenwick has reported three cases of "contact carcinoma," and given reference to similar cases in the bladder and other parts of the body, in the 39th volume of the London Pathological Society's transactions.

Such is often the case in sarcoma also, and was well seen in a case under my care in 1882, of sarcoma in a diverticulum of the bladder, in which the secondary growths affected the wall of the diverticulum as well as the bladder (Path. Soc. Trans., vol. xxxiv. p. 152).

The *connection* of tumours with the vesical wall is of importance in regard to operations for their removal. They may be embedded in it, or be sessile or pedunculated, or may infiltrate it.

In the progress of tumours which infiltrate, all the coats of the bladder may be invaded, and the area affected may be much greater than is detectable by eye or finger, as is the case with malignant growths elsewhere. Any of the tunics may be the *seat of origin* of tumours.

BENIGN TUMOURS.

Papilloma.—The bladder mucous membrane has no papillæ, hence Virchow and many other pathologists, objecting to the term papilloma for these vesical growths, have named them " papillary fibromata." There is, however, no need of the presence of normal papillæ for the development of papillo-matous tumours—the conditions of their growth in a hollow cavity filled with fluid explains their special form. Moreover, the most perfect example of physiological papillary growths is to be found in the chorionic villi, and the chorion is formed by the extra-abdominal portion of the allantois, the intra-ab-dominal portion of which is the bladder. Besides, the presence of papillæ at the level of the trigone of the bladder is admitted by many observers.

There are two kinds of papillomata of the bladder, namely, the fimbriated, or " villous polypi," and the fibro-papillomata, or the " papillary tumours."

In the villous polypi the stalk sends off numerous branches and sub-branches, each consisting of a capillary vessel covered

c c

by a basement membrane, and a more or less thick layer of epithelium; in the papillary tumours the stroma is compact and has a dense fibrous or muscular structure, amongst which may be found embryonal cells and leucocytes.

The villous polypi are very frequently multiple, and form tufts or feathery bunches more or less spread over the mucous surface, of varying lengths (Fig. 93); these float in the urine. When very long their extremities are often carried into the urethro-vesical orifice during micturition and are there nipped by the sphincter. This is often a cause of considerable suffering.

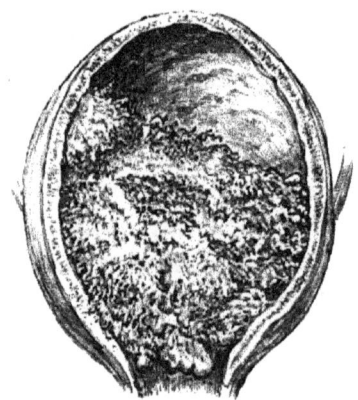

Fig. 93—Villous Polypi of the Bladder. (Middlesex Hospital Museum.) ("Manual of Surgery.")

There is no infiltration of the vesical wall about their points of attachment. The papillary tumour or "fibro-papilloma," may be single or multiple; it is generally rounded in shape, and of the size of a pea, a cherry, or a walnut. It is more often sessile than pedunculated; its surface is villous, but its consistence is firm.

Myxoma.—This is in some instances a "fibro-papilloma," or a fibroma the cell portions of which have undergone a mucoid degeneration. They are soft in texture, grow rapidly, and are met with most frequently in young children. They are probably often congenital; frequently multiple and pedunculated; their common situation is near the neck of the bladder; and they may extend into the prostatic urethra. It is possible that some of the cases formerly reported as myxomata were sarcomata.

Mucous Polypi having a texture resembling that of ordinary nasal polypi, except that the epithelial covering is squamous instead of ciliated, have been found in the bladders of children under two years of age, as well as in adults. Mr. Shattock published one such, and there are two specimens in the Hunterian Museum. The accompanying figure (Fig. 94) is borrowed from Mr. Pepper's "Elements of Surgical Pathology."

In the early stages they may not give rise to any symptoms; later, they may simulate the symptoms of vesical calculi, and, growing to a considerable size, project into the urethra (or beyond in the female) or distend the bladder with new growth as high as the umbilicus or higher.

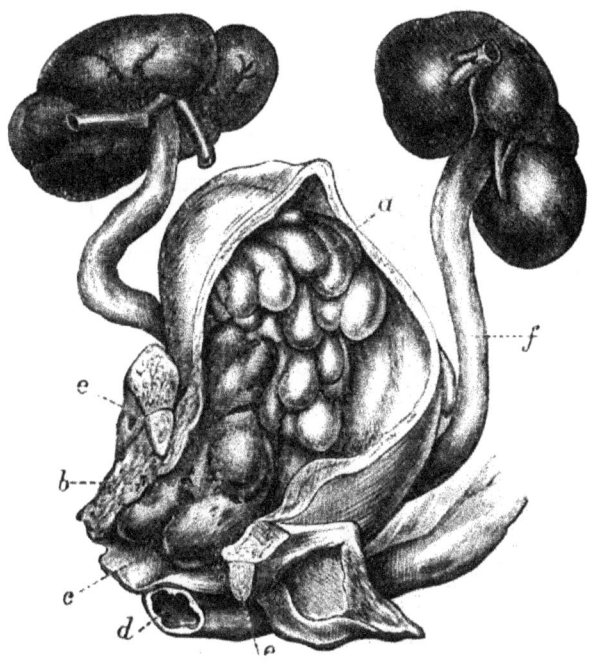

Fig. 94.—Mucous Polypi of the Bladder of a Female Child, aged 18 months.

a, Polypi ; *b*, the same prolapsed and congested from partial strangulation by the dilated urethra ; *c*, vagina ; *d*, rectum ; *e*, cut surface of divided symphysis pubis ; *f*, dilated ureter. The majority of the polypi are attached around the orifice of the right ureter. The urinary organs have been removed in their entirety, together with the rectum and a portion of the pelvis. (*Pepper.*)

Fibromata.—Fibrous tumours originate in the deep mucosa, or in the muscular layer, and are covered by normal epithelium. Like the myxomata they are pedunculated, but they occur in adults, and have not yet been found in children. They are very rare.

Myoma.—Tumours containing in their composition muscular fibres are rare, and are considered by Virchow to be outgrowths from the prostate ; but two cases reported by Belfield show indisputably their occasional origin from the vesical wall. They occur as nodules encapsuled in the submucosa ; and may be composed either of unstriped muscular fibres (myoma) or of a mixture of unstriped muscle and fibrous tissue (fibro-myoma).

Some exceptional tumours which have been found in the bladder are adenomata, angeiomata, serous cysts and dermoid cysts. Martini, Hache, and Bryant report instances of the last-mentioned tumours. Dermoids are probably due either to an abnormal development of the bladder wall, by which a portion of the epiblast fills in a deficiency, or are perivesical in origin.

Bilharzia hæmatobia sometimes causes fungating exudation masses of considerable size in the bladder. It is a not uncommon cause of hæmaturia in Egypt, along the Nile. A good example is described by Mr. Eve in the thirty-ninth volume of the Pathological Society's Transactions; and in the same volume is reported a case in which the Bilharzia seems to have caused a large sprouting epithelioma of the bladder.

MALIGNANT TUMOURS.

Sarcoma.—Malignant tumours of the connective tissue type are comparatively rare, but their rarity has probably

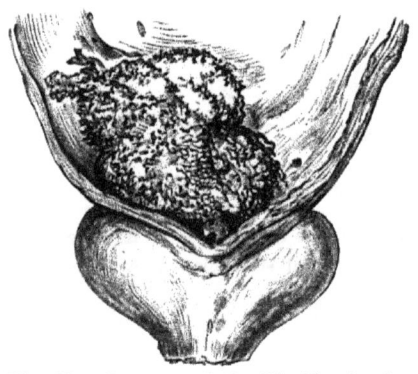

Fig. 95.—Sarcoma of the Bladder having a Villous Surface. (Middlesex Hospital Museum.) ("Manual of Surgery.")

been greatly exaggerated. Mr. D'Arcy Power in 1888 found nine preparations of sarcoma of the bladder in the London museums (Path. Soc. Trans., vol. xxxix. p. 175), and their number since then has probably much increased.

Mr. Southam, of Manchester, records six cases under himself and his colleagues. Mr. Hurry Fenwick (Path. Soc. Trans., 1888, vol. xxxix. p. 171) collected 50 cases, and found (1) that the tumours are most common in children under five and in men over fifty-five years of age; (2) that in children they are multiple, polypoid, and pedunculated or subsessile; in adults, single and sessile, only 10 per cent. being pedunculated; (3) that the average size is that of a hen's egg; the largest, the size of a double fist, was attached to the anterior wall; (4) that in 20 per cent. the tumours had a villous covering (Fig. 95); (5) that 34·5 per cent. were round-celled sarcomata, and 17 per cent. spindle-celled.

Mr. Shattock reports a case of **chondrifying sarcoma**

removed, together with multiple papillomata, from the bladder of a man aged fifty-five by Sir Henry Thompson (Path. Soc. Trans., 1887); Mr. Eve has reported a case of **lymphosarcoma** in a man sixty-eight, and Mr. Chaffey a similar growth in a boy aged three (Path. Soc. Trans., 1885).

An interesting and exceptional case occurred in my practice in 1882 of a sarcomatous tumour growing in a diverticulum of the bladder as large as the bladder cavity itself, and communicating with the bladder proper about one inch above the left ureter by a rounded opening the size of half-a-crown. The tumour could be felt through the abdominal wall, and was the size of a large apple. Where the growth came in contact with the wall of the pouch, outgrowths of a similar character were seen upon the lining membrane. The base of the growth and the parts beneath it were suppurating. Microscopically it consisted of a small-meshed fibrillar stroma, and round and spindle cells, with numerous blood-vessels throughout.

Carcinoma.—Two varieties are met with: (1) epithelioma, *i.e.* squamous-celled carcinoma, or cylindroma; and (2) glandular-celled carcinoma, either encephaloid or scirrhous. Colloid degeneration of the glandular-celled carcinoma may occur, but is rare.

Secondary carcinoma is more frequent than primary, and may be consecutive to cancer of the rectum, vagina, uterus, or prostate. Formerly cancer of the bladder was always regarded as secondary. Barling has collected 74 cases of the primary disease, 47 of which were epithelioma and 27 alveolar cancer.

They form prominent swellings, irregularly rounded, widely attached, and infiltrating more

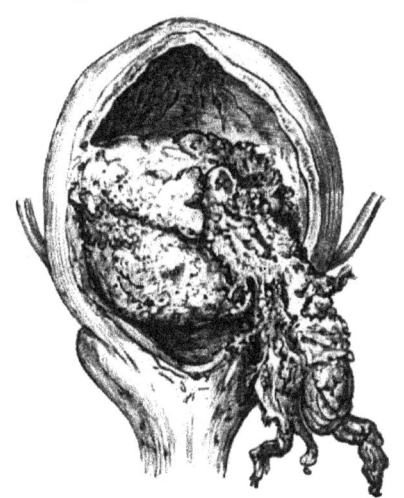

Fig. 96.—Epithelioma of the Bladder. (Middlesex Hospital Museum.) ("Manual of Surgery.")

or less deeply the vesical coats (Fig. 96). Their surface is granular, and in some cases villous and in the later stages ulcerated; occasionally they present gaping ulcers with raised and indurated walls.

These tumours are hard, but friable; and therein differ from the softer and but little friable fibro-papillomata. They are often multiple, and are most common in the trigone or base of the bladder. They develop slowly; seldom ulcerate early; and cause death before they attain any great size, sometimes even before they are followed by secondary growths in distant organs. Barling, in 27 cases of epithelioma examined after death, found the iliac or inguinal glands involved in 11 cases : the kidney, lung, or liver in 6. In 15 autopsies of alveolar cancer, M. Tuffier found 3 in which there was secondary disease in neighbouring organs, 11 in which the glands were widely involved, and one case of perforation of the bladder.

Pathological complications of bladder tumours are: (1) localised thickening of the bladder walls due to hypertrophy of muscular and interstitial tissue; (2) hydro-nephrosis; (3) calcareous deposit on the surface of the tumour; (4) occasionally a phosphatic calculus free in the bladder, the result of cystitis provoked by the growth; a portion of the growth broken away from the rest may possibly form its nucleus; (5) suppurative pyelo-nephritis with or without distension of the kidney. Barling found renal complications in 49 out of 74 cases, and in 33 of these there was either hydro- or pyo-nephrosis.

Symptoms.—Bladder tumours are met with at all ages, the sarcomata and myxomata in children; cancer between forty and sixty. They are much more common in men than in women—Roger Williams states in the proportion of 70 to 20; Féré as 62 to 20. The existence of psorosperms in the epithelial cells as described and figured by Albarran (" Les Tumeurs de la Vessie," G. Albarran, Paris, 1892) is supposed by some to be the cause of the malignant growths.

In a small number of cases tumours of the bladder have not been suspected during life and have been found as a surprise at the autopsy. But as a rule their presence is made only too apparent by hæmorrhage, pain, frequency of micturition, and not infrequently by the presence of a swelling, felt either through the rectum or vagina, or, as in a case under my care in 1882, to which reference has just been made, through the anterior abdominal wall. *Hæmaturia* is by far the most constant symptom; it is in some cases the only one, and is sometimes alone the cause of death. It is nearly always the first symptom complained of, and the one which brings the patient to his doctor. Its onset, its course, and its abundance are characteristic of tumour. It comes on spontaneously without injury, fatigue, or even movement, and is associated with difficulty in micturition only when clots accumulate in the bladder, or one for a while obstructs the urethra. It may be excited by catheterism or by distension of the bladder; and rest even in the recumbent position has no effect in stopping it. After the hæmaturia has existed for hours, days, or weeks, the urine may suddenly become quite clear. Whilst the hæmaturia lasts, the urine is not equally charged with blood at each micturition, the quantity may vary from day to day or even from hour to hour, and the urine passed at one time may be clear, whereas that voided immediately before and immediately after, may be highly coloured. More blood is passed at the end of micturition than at any other part of the flow; this always indicates that the hæmorrhage has a vesical origin.

The quantity of blood is often exceedingly great, the urine being frequently deep-red or quite black; clots—red, black, and discoloured—may be passed, and may cause great suffering in passing, or they may be retained in the bladder and require cystotomy for their removal. When the bleeding has been abundant it may disappear either suddenly or gradually.

When the attack has passed, the patient may remain weeks, many months, or a year or two, without recurrence of hæmorrhage. There is no relation whatever between the size of the tumours and the amount of blood lost; the hæmorrhage may be alarming, even fatal, from a small innocent growth— as was the case in a man aged sixty-five, brought to me in a cab, having been found blanched and faint in a urinal. He declined an operation until it was too late, and died on the third day after the fit of syncope. At the post-mortem there was found a fibro-papillary tumour the size of a small chestnut attached by a stalk not thicker than that of a pear—the very type of tumour for easy and successful removal.

When there have occurred repeated or prolonged hæmorrhages, the patient is anæmic and waxen-looking, and his lower extremities become œdematous. In some cases the urine is a yellowish-pink colour, and coagulates soon after it is voided, forming a mass which adheres to the vessel. This is caused by transudation of liquor sanguinis at the surface of the tumour; it has been recorded by Ultzmann, Stein, and Custer, but is very rare. As a rule, the examination of the urine reveals nothing except the presence of blood, though occasionally there may by chance be found some fragment of tumour tissue.

In concluding this account of the hæmaturia due to tumours, I will quote the words of M. Tuffier, who describes it as "spontaneous, capricious, abundant, lasting, recurrent, and maybe the only symptom."

Pain is not a constant symptom; it appears late, and is generally due to cystitis. When it exists it is often very intense, and is worse at the end of micturition. It is felt in the hypogastrium and at the neck of the bladder, and radiates to the penis and testicles, and down the thighs. But except from cystitis, from nipping of the growth by the sphincter vesicæ, or from retention due to clots of blood, pain occurs only when the growth is pressing upon the nerves by infiltrating the bladder wall.

Frequency of micturition, associated with strangury, is in some cases a cause of great distress; this is more especially likely to be present when a malignant growth is infiltrating the neck and trigone of the bladder.

Physical signs are those ascertained by abdominal, rectal, or vaginal examination, by the endoscope, by injecting fluid into the bladder to the degree of distension, and by the catheter. If these means afford positive signs, well and good; but if not, we must not exclude tumours from our diagnosis, when the functional symptoms, and especially hæmaturia, as above described, are present. With the patient lying on his back with his knees and shoulders raised, we can, in a thin individual, sometimes feel the tumour through the abdominal walls by palpating immediately above the pubes.

Still more frequently can it be felt by rectal or vaginal examination, especially if at the same time the bladder is firmly pressed upon by the left hand applied in the hypogastrium.

The result of this kind of examination may be positive

or negative. It will be negative if the growth is either villous polypus or fibro-papilloma, or a small pedunculated myxoma-fibroma; but if we feel an irregular, nodular, or infiltrated vesical wall, or a thickened mass above the prostate, we know the disease is malignant. Mucous polypi, when large and abundant, have also been felt through the abdominal parietes by pressing with the fingers over the hypogastrium.

It is well always to examine the urine first passed after this kind of examination, because when a tumour is present manipulation is often followed by slight hæmorrhage. This was notably the case in my patient with sarcoma of a diverticulum of his bladder, as well as in several other cases which have been under my care, and it has been very frequently noted by Guyon and others.

The catheter and sound ought to be used with the greatest care, not only as to their aseptic condition, but with lightness, so as to avoid bruising the tissue of the tumour, and provoking hæmorrhage. Instrumentation is at best an unsatisfactory adjunct, but when it imparts information it does so either by giving the sense of a slight jar as the sound strikes against the tumour; or by the feeling of hardness and irregularity of the bladder surface; or by exciting hæmorrhage, which it may do even though the instrument used be a soft rubber catheter; or by the chance extraction in the eye of the catheter of a fragment of the growth. With a silver catheter or sound, combined with a digital examination per rectum, or per vaginam, we can trace out the least thickening of the vesical wall at its base and trigone.

When these mechanical methods combine in giving nothing but a negative result, we conclude that the tumour is of a soft, more or less pedunculated, and benign nature; if, on the other hand, a tumour of some weight or volume is detected, or a general thickening or infiltration of the base of the bladder exists, we conclude the growth is malignant, and know that the prognosis is very serious.

In cases in which the catheter and digital examination fail to give information, the distension of the bladder with a solution of boric acid or weak carbolic solution, by exciting hæmorrhage as the last drops flow away, is a valuable diagnostic guide between hæmaturia of renal and of vesical origin. Sometimes, especially if the growth is near the neck of the

bladder, a drop or two of blood flows through the injection
catheter either as it enters the vesical cavity or as soon as
the injecting process ceases.

The cystoscope in some cases gives most valuable information, but it is quite useless when there is blood in the
bladder, and it ought not to be used indiscriminately upon
all patients. It is not required for women.

Diagnosis.—This can generally be made pretty accurately
(1) by the character of the hæmorrhage ; (2) and by the
physical signs described above ; (3) by the cystoscope, which
in certain cases enables the new growth to be actually inspected ; (4) in the female by digital examination per urethram,
and in the male by an examination of the bladder through a
perinæal or hypogastric incision. Absolute certainty as to
the presence or absence of even the smallest of growths
is obtainable by digital exploration. In spite of the comparison plausibly unfavourable to digital examination of the
bladder, drawn by Mr. Hurry Fenwick, in his advocacy of
the cystoscope (*Brit. Med. Journ.*, May 4th, 1889), there
can be no doubt of the certainty afforded by the perinæal
exploration in all but exceptional cases of enlarged prostate.

The finger of the experienced surgeon can inform him
as surely as can his eye, and indeed more surely, unless the
cystoscope is used when the bladder is quite free of blood.

The value of the cystoscope in diagnosing tumours of
the bladder is that it may reveal their presence without
the necessity of making an operation of an exploratory
nature ; but in the case of the female it is an absolutely
needless adjunct in diagnosis, for with the finger passed
through the dilated urethra we can at once learn all we want
to know ; and that, too, without submitting the patient to any
more risk or unpleasantness than with the endoscope. Even
in the male, the functional symptoms and physical signs give
such clear indications that the exploratory incision is made
in most cases with the confident assurance that we shall find
a growth to be the cause of these symptoms, and at the same
time be able to extract it, if removal is possible.

The chief question and difficulty, in most instances, is
to ascertain whether the hæmaturia is of renal, or of vesical
origin. This will be decided if we find, on the one hand, a

swelling in the renal region, or on the other, an abnormal condition of the bladder, by the mechanical means just related. It is quite an exceptional thing—though such may, of course, happen—that there exist in the same individual at the same time an enlarged kidney, and a source of vesical hæmaturia. Difficulty occurs, too, if the examination of both renal and vesical regions afford negative information. We must then have recourse to distension of the bladder, which, if it provokes hæmorrhage, affords proof of vesical trouble. The examination of the shape of the clots (if any) by floating them out in water will often tell us much, especially if the clots are elongated and "worm-like," and have been preceded by renal colic. I have known patients to preserve and bring to the surgeon for examination partly discoloured elongated clots, casts of the ureter, with the conviction that they were dead worms, "like earth-worms" twisted or curled up, as we see worms on the ground.

The cystoscope is certainly a valuable aid in doubtful cases, and by it blood or pus may occasionally be seen trickling from one or other ureter. From the hæmorrhage attending acute and chronic cystitis, tubercular disease of the bladder, calculus, and chronic enlargement of the prostate, the diagnosis will be readily made by a careful attention to the history of the case, and to the cardinal symptoms of the respective diseases.

There are cases of hæmaturia in which it is impossible to be sure of the source of the bleeding; in some of them, possibly, it is due to congestion or varicosity of the vessels of the bladder, and in these it is justifiable to make either the hypogastric or the perinæal exploration of the bladder, as the operation is very likely to prove curative as well as explorative in these cases. As between malignant and benign tumours, it is sufficient to repeat what has already been stated, viz. that the presence of infiltration, nodulation, or thickening of the vesical walls, as felt per rectum or per vaginam, or with the sound in the bladder, indicates malignancy, whereas the absence of any such condition is indicative of the benign growths, and such as are capable of being removed.

Prognosis.—This is always serious. The malignant are unfavourable for removal as they infiltrate the vesical walls, and quickly recur. The benign tumours are often easily removable; but some, especially the villous polypi, are prone to grow again. Then there is the danger from hæmorrhage, which alone may kill; or from cystitis running on to pyelo-nephritis, and from intermittent hydro-nephrosis. (*See* paper by author in the Med.-Chir. Trans., vol. lix.) Both of these causes of death arise from the innocent as well as from the malignant growths. If hæmorrhage does not rapidly kill the patient, it may so reduce the strength and vital powers as to quite unfit him to bear a radical operation. This is apt to be the case with persons who either dread an operation too much to submit to it, or who obstinately argue time after time that, as they have "got over" previous attacks of hæmaturia or cystitis, so will they manage to do again.

It is said that tumours have retrogressed and even spontaneously become detached and expelled. We see this occasionally in uterine myoma; and it may occur in pedunculated tumours of the bladder, but it cannot, of course, be reckoned upon as a probable termination.

As to the duration of life, Féré gives for malignant tumours eighteen months to two years, Barling three years; whereas Guyon has operated upon patients for epithelioma in cases in which the first symptoms of bladder tumour dated back ten years previously. Such cases indicate either that cancer progresses much more slowly in the bladder than elsewhere, or that tumours benign at first can subsequently become malignant; as we know to be the case in uterine myoma, and in other tumours in other parts of the body.

Vesical malignant growths only slowly, and by no means invariably, end by causing secondary infection of other parts or organs.

The benign growths may exist for years, causing only occasional hæmorrhage at longer or shorter intervals, and of greater or less severity. I have known cases go on for ten years and more, and when at last an operation has been absolutely necessary, a mass of villous polypi enough to fill a breakfast cup, has been removed.

Tumours of the bladder, if left alone, almost always cause death, though their progress, especially in the benign cases, may be very slow. It is mostly by hæmorrhage that the fatal result is brought about; in other cases it is by pyelo-nephritis, the sequel of cystitis. We have to bear these facts in mind when considering the treatment.

Treatment.—This may be either palliative or curative. I do not propose to dwell upon the treatment by astringent drugs, because they are of only temporary use. When a patient declines any surgical treatment they must be employed, and as further safeguards against hæmorrhage the diet must be unstimulating and bland, the bladder should never be allowed to become distended, and violent and prolonged exercise, and straining at stool should be avoided. To relieve pain nothing is so beneficial as morphia, or morphia combined with belladonna in suppositories.

The best palliative means are incision and drainage of the bladder; the excision of the tumour is, of course, the only method of cure.

It will be well to consider, first of all, the indications and contra-indications for the active treatment of vesical tumours. As hæmorrhage is, in these cases, generally, a very grave symptom, the sooner it is checked the better; and, therefore, when once the diagnosis has been made, and the probabilities are in favour of the tumour being of small size or of benign nature, an operation ought not to be delayed.

And, in cases where the hæmorrhage is not so considerable, but in which the pain and frequency of micturition caused by supervening cystitis are very severe, an operation should be undertaken with the double object of relieving these symptoms, and of possibly removing the cause.

When the bladder wall is not largely involved, and if the condition of the kidneys does not forbid, the curative treatment should be carried out where possible, but when, after opening the bladder, the disease is found to be too extensive for removal, the surgeon has to fall back upon the palliative means at his disposal.

When a growth is felt, per rectum or per vaginam, or with the sound, to be involving a large surface of the bladder wall, to be infiltrating its coats, especially in the neighbourhood of the ureters and neck of the bladder, no operation whatever should be proposed unless the hæmorrhage is copious or the symptoms of cystitis severe, and then an incision for palliative purposes only should be made. This should be the vesico-vaginal boutonnière in the female, the perinæal boutonnière in the male, unless the prostate is very large, and then hypogastric cystotomy affords the best drainage. By these means we place the bladder at rest; and thus, by drainage, we remove the septic urine from an inflamed bladder, and by preventing the alternation of distension and contraction of the bladder, which is the chief cause of the bleeding, we check the hæmaturia. When the disorganised state of the kidneys is unfavourable to any prolonged operation, drainage is still indicated to check hæmorrhage, or for the relief of the sufferings caused by cystitis. These operations are slight and quickly performed; they do not tax the resources of the patient in their performance, whereas they afford much comfort when accomplished.

Palliative treatment.—This has for its object the relief of hæmorrhage, pain, and frequency in micturition, by incision into and drainage of the bladder. The French surgeons, and perhaps most of the English and American, now prefer the hypogastric operation in men, considering it affords excellent drainage, and gives the opportunity of inspecting the interior of the bladder and of converting, if possible, what was commenced as a palliative, into a curative operation. Sir Henry Thompson, who was the great exponent of the perinæal incision, has more recently had great success with the supra-pubic operation, and for the last ten years or thereabouts has never done a lithotomy, or a tumour removal, by any other method. Mr. Harrison, who thinks highly of the perinæal operation for many purposes, considers that in operating for vesical tumour, whether with the object of cure or relief, supra-pubic cystotomy is on all grounds to be recommended. When the patient is very stout, or his perinæum is very deep, or his prostate gland is much enlarged, the hypogastric route is certainly, I think, to be preferred. When the growth is in the more usual position, the tube, if passed through the perinæum, is apt to chafe the diseased part, and thus provoke hæmorrhage. In certain cases, on the other hand, of malignant infiltration of the front of the bladder, drainage through the hypogastrium is impossible without going through the diseased tissues. In one case of this sort

I had to abandon this route and employ the perinæal opening.

In the female, the best incision for palliative purposes is through the vesico-vaginal septum ; sutures should unite the vesical with the vaginal mucous membrane over the edges of the incision so as to secure a permanent opening.

Curative Treatment.—The object of this is the extirpation of the tumour. In men this has been accomplished in three ways—(1) through the urethra ; (2) by median urethrotomy ; (3) by supra-pubic cystotomy. Von Antal has removed small tumours through the urethra by means of the lithotrite, after careful observation of their exact position and size by the cystoscope. This is on the same footing as the removal of small foreign bodies, after carefully observing their position and direction with the electric light.

But it will not often be of any avail ; and owing to the difficulty of inspecting the whole of a large tumour with this instrument, as at present formed, there is the probability of removing only a tuft or portion of a large growth instead of a small entire tumour.

The perinæal incision is objected to because—(1) it does not permit of inspection of the bladder ; (2) it affords only a " narrow straight " through which to operate ; (3) in a fat deep perinæum, or where there is an enlarged prostate, it is diffi-cult even to reach the cavity of the bladder, still more to thoroughly examine the growth with the finger before com-mencing to extract it ; and (4) another objection arises out of the foregoing objections—this is the great probability of mul-tiple small growths remaining, some or all, undetected. There is much truth in these objections in many cases, and probably almost unanimous preference is to-day given to the hypogastric cystotomy. It is probable, however, that surgeons will return to the perinæal operation for tumours situated at the neck or base of the bladder, should resection of part of the bladder wall with the tumour ever come to be practised.

The hypogastric cystotomy has lately been much extended in severity in certain cases by Helferich, Koch, and Tuffier : the first two advocate resection of the pubes, and the latter symphyseotomy where the growth occupies the front part and region of the neck of the bladder, and a large field for

operation is required.   Tuffier has twice performed the supra-
pubic operation with satisfactory results when the growths
were on the anterior wall of the bladder.

In women, urethral dilatation enables many tumours to be
removed easily and thoroughly through the canal, and as the
urethra can be dilated so as to admit easily the forefinger
without fear of after ill consequences, this route is the most
satisfactory for the majority of cases suitable for curative treatment.   Where the growth is too large to be removed through
the female urethra, the hypogastric cystotomy should be done
as in men.   Should resection of part of the neck or base of
the bladder, together with the tumour, come to be practised
in females, the vesico-vaginal route will probably prove to
be the best.   At present, these operations have not found
favour, or been much attempted by surgeons, for this, amongst
other reasons, that the results of the few cases in which they
have been performed, have been very discouraging.

It is not my intention to describe the details of the various
methods of removing the growths after the cavity of the
bladder has been reached.   It must suffice here to say that
these methods are by—(1) tearing them away, (2) crushing
them off with forceps or ecraseur, (3) curetting, (4) torsion,
(5) excision with the bistoury and closing the wound in the
mucous membrane by sutures, or searing the surface with the
cautery, (6) cauterisation alone.   The method will vary with
the tumour, partly as to whether it is pedunculated or not,
partly as to its size, and partly as to its malignant or benign
nature.   Undoubtedly, the removal by dissecting out the base
of the growth and closing the wound on the inner surface
of the bladder with fine sutures, is theoretically the best,
and will, perhaps, in future be more frequently adopted.
For this treatment supra-pubic cystotomy is required.

Extirpation of the growth with portion of the bladder wall
is advocated, on the grounds that malignant disease of the
bladder so comparatively seldom invades the lymphatic system
or distant organs; but the usual situation of these growths about
the orifices of the ureters forbids this radical procedure, and,
except in the practice of Pawlick (*Congrès Internat. de
Berlin*, 1890), it has not so far given satisfactory results.

When any operation is undertaken for the purpose of

cure, the ideal plan would be to close, by sutures, the wound in the bladder. No doubt, as the operations become perfected, this will be the practice, and the bladder will be drained for a day or two subsequently by a catheter passed through the urethra; possibly even the catheter, in some cases, may be dispensed with.

Tuffier has collected the results of different operations in 180 cases. The mortality was 42—*i.e.* 23·3 per cent.; 23 of these deaths were undoubtedly the result of the operation. In man, the supra-pubic operation was performed in 51 cases with a mortality of 29·4 per cent.; the perinæal operation in 60 cases, with a mortality of 28·3 per cent. In women, 43 operations were performed through the urethra without a death, and 5 supra-pubic operations all successful. As regards late results of the operations, Tuffier's figures show 35 operations for cancer with 16 cures, 13 recurrences within a year, and the rest not followed long enough to make a return; 55 operations for papillomata show 41 cures and four others cured after recurrence.

CHAPTER XII.

VESICAL FISTULÆ. URACHAL FISTULÆ. URACHAL CYSTS.

VESICAL FISTULÆ.

URINARY fistulæ are of many varieties, and might be classified (1) as to the part of the urinary organs with which they communicate; (2) as to the part of the surface at which they establish an opening; (3) as to their causes; and (4) as to their characters—namely, as to whether they are simple, or callous, or attended by loss of tissue. Many of the forms of urinary fistula which arise, for example, from stricture or abscess of the perinæum, I have already described (Chapter X. Part II., p. 257). I shall here refer especially to those connected with the bladder which open on some part of the surface of the abdomen; and shall merely enumerate others which consist in a communication between the urinary bladder and the viscera within the cavities of the abdomen and pelvis.

1. **Vesico-Abdominal Fistulæ.** — Wounds, gunshot and otherwise; sub-parietal rupture of the bladder; ulceration of the coats of the bladder from disease of its walls, or from the presence of a foreign body within the organ; and inflammation beginning in the peritoneum, pelvic cellular tissue, or ovary, or other pelvic organ—are all causes of vesico-abdominal fistula, that is, of fistula opening externally upon some part of the abdominal wall, and communicating with the bladder.

(*a*) Dr. Otis gives records of a number of very satisfactory recoveries after shot-wounds of the bladder. In several of them the missile traversed the distended bladder obliquely, passing in at the left or right side of the hypogastrium, and out at the opposite buttock; in some instances the ball entered above the pubis; in one, it passed in at the iliac fossa, and perforated the fundus of the bladder on its way out at the opposite buttock. In some of these cases the wounds healed very rapidly, urine escaping from one or both orifices, but generally from the supra-pubic, for a short time, and then the wound closed without ultimate derangement of the function of the bladder. In others, a troublesome urinary fistula remained for two or three years, and then permanently closed. In some cases the patients recovered, but with persistent urinary fistulæ, the persistence of which was in several instances due to the presence of dead bone, though in others there was neither dead bone nor any other foreign body acting as a source of irritation. Patients are reported as recovering from recto-vesical fistulæ from gun-shot wounds with similar uncertainty, *i.e.* early in some cases, but in others the fistula remained pervious for a long period. The surgical historian of the War of the Rebellion remarks, " It is rare to find the functions of the bladder perfectly restored after shot injury."

(*b*) Stricture of the urethra may lead to ulceration of the parietes of the bladder, and this to an external fistula. Experience shows that, in cases of old and neglected stricture, abscesses may form above the pubis, owing to vesical ulceration, and the surgeon may be deceived into fancying that the supra-pubic tumour is a distended bladder. Such an abscess is likely to lead to a vesico-abdominal fistula.

(*c*) An abdominal fistula may form after rupture of the bladder. Sir P. Hewett reported the case of a man aged fifty-three who suffered rupture of the bladder behind the pubis, and by the twelfth day afterwards three distinct tumours had formed in the lower part of the front of the belly. ·An incision was made into one in the left iliac region, and about three pints of fetid pus with large sloughs were let out. Urine afterwards passed through this opening. The man died on the twenty-third day.

(*d*) A foreign body may find its way from the bladder by ulceration, and lead to a fistula in the groin. An interesting case is mentioned by Sir Hans Sloane in his reply to the Marquis of Caumont, who had sent Sir Hans " a very remarkable stone taken out of a man's bladder after death." Sir

Hans writes :—"I have likewise a common pin, which, by some means or other, had got into the bladder of a young woman, and was there coated all over by a calculous matter; but having occasioned a fistulous ulcer in her groin, it was discharged thence with the matter of the fistula."

(*e*) In other cases, a foreign body may ulcerate into the bladder, and likewise through the abdominal parietes, and thus give rise to a vesical urinary fistula. A very remarkable case was related by M. Hippolyte Larrey, before the Académie de Médecine, of a dermoid cyst of the ovary, complicated by a urinary fistula in the median line of the abdomen, half-way between the pubis and the umbilicus. It occurred in a previously quite healthy woman, aged thirty-three, who had borne three children, and had had rapid recoveries after her confinements. Some days after the third, however, she felt a severe pain, with heat and swelling, in the left iliac region, and pus was passed with the urine. For five years all symptoms subsided; then the tumour increased, and spontaneously opened below the umbilicus, and a quantity of hair and pus was discharged. Afterwards, urine in large quantities passed by this abdominal opening. Some of the hair from the cyst likewise escaped into the bladder, through a fistulous communication, and there, phosphatic matter being deposited in the hair, so considerable a calculus was formed as to entirely prevent any urine flowing off by the urethra, so that at length the whole of it passed through the fistula. The patient was cured by a single operation, which consisted in introducing a bistoury at the abdominal fistula, and laying open the cyst by cutting the abdominal parietes downwards along the median line; then, with a sound in the bladder and the finger in the lower part of the cyst, the fistulous communication between the cyst and the bladder was found and enlarged, and the calculus was removed through the incisions thus made.

(*f*) Inflammation of the peritoneum, or of some one of the pelvic viscera, may lead to adhesion with and ulceration of the bladder, and then to a circumscribed abscess, which, bursting through the abdominal wall, results in a urinary fistula indirectly communicating with the bladder.

(*g*) Similarly, inflammation of the sub-peritoneal cellular tissue may lead to suppuration around and ulceration into the bladder; and, by the burrowing of pus, an external opening may be formed on the abdomen, above the pubes, at the groins, by the side of the anus, or in the adjacent parts of the nates, or over one of the large foramina of the pelvis, a complete urinary fistula being thereby established.

2. **Vesico-visceral Fistulæ.**—Urinary fistulæ are not unfrequently established between the bladder and rectum, bladder and vagina, or bladder and small intestine, as the result of inflammatory adhesions and ulceration between those parts. Vesico-rectal fistulæ are sometimes caused by penetrating bodies passing through the anus and rectum into the bladder. (*See* page 350.) They may follow punctured wounds of the rectum, which do not penetrate the vesical wall, in consequence either of suppuration or sloughing. A case of this sort is recorded in the *Medical Press* (Dec. 6, 1893) by Mr. T. Myles: it was that of a young man who fell on the broken leg of an upturned chair, which passed through the wall of the rectum without wounding the peritoneum or bladder or injuring the anus. A fistula followed, and was cured by continuous drainage by means of a catheter *en demeure*.

When the small intestine becomes matted together, and adherent to a sloughing or ulcerating bladder, a firm tumour may be formed in the hypogastrium and be mistaken for a distended bladder. I have elsewhere reported a case somewhat in point (*Med. Times and Gazette*, July 28, 1883, p. 92).

Simple chronic inflammation, tubercle, cancer of the bowel, uterus, or vagina, and cystic and other diseases of the ovary are common causes of these forms of urinary fistula. Stricture of the urethra, calculus, or, indeed, any cause within the bladder which excites adhesion to parts around and ulceration of the bladder-walls, will conduce to them. In the female sloughing followed by fistula sometimes results from prolonged pressure of the head of the fœtus and other complications of parturition.

Treatment.—In the treatment of vesico-abdominal and vesico-visceral fistulæ each case will require special consideration and management; but the following general rules may be stated:—

1. Any cause of urethral obstruction should be removed, and a free and direct channel should be obtained for the discharge of the urine.

2. If this cannot be done by way of the natural passage, an operation will be required for the purpose of establishing direct temporary drainage of the bladder.

3. Any foreign body in or near the bladder, or any other cause of inflammation of the bladder or neighbouring parts, should be removed if possible.

4. Any abscess, suppurating tumour, or cyst, and diffused suppuration in the cellular tissue of the pelvis, or in connection with the pelvic or abdominal organs, must be treated on the general principles of surgery applicable to these cases.

5. Callous fistulous tracks should be laid open, erased or excised, or treated by strong escharotics or the cautery, so as to stimulate them to granulate healthily, and cicatrise.

6. Where the fistulæ persist, in spite of all effort to close them, the skin must be protected, as far as possible, from continual contact with the pus and urine; eczematous excoriations must be treated with antiseptic lotions or emollients; and the garments of the patient must be kept clean and sweet if possible by his wearing a suitable and well-adjusted urinal. When the fistula opens by a wide and single orifice, and it has a direct track to the bladder, the adjustment of an urinal is often easily accomplished.

Foreign bodies sometimes pass into the bladder from the peritoneal cavity without leaving even a temporary fistula. In a well-known case a pair of torsi-pressure forceps which were left in the peritoneal cavity at an ovariotomy, ulcerated through the bladder wall, and were subsequently extracted from the bladder. I have also known the silk ligature of an ovarian pedicle ulcerate into the bladder and set up cystitis. The ligature became coated with phosphates and was then mistaken for a calculus. A lithotrite was passed, and after crushing the supposed calculus the instrument could not be disengaged. Some considerable traction was used and at last the lithotrite became free and was withdrawn, having entangled in its blades the loop of silk ligature. The patient immediately afterwards recovered.

URACHAL FISTULA.

Most writers on the development of the bladder have referred to the occasional patency of the urachus at the time of and after birth, and to the discharge of urine from its umbilical extremity, which, under these circumstances, is likely to take place. Very frequently, perhaps generally, the urachus at birth is tubular for a short distance above the bladder, and in after-life it becomes a mere fibro-muscular cord. The urachus retains the tubular character of the allantois till about the thirtieth week of fœtal life, but the exact time at which the metamorphosis of the allantois is complete varies in different animals, and in different instances in the human subject.

At birth, according to some observers, the urachus very frequently does not extend as far as the navel, but at about five or six centimetres from the bladder passes into a number of tendinous threads, which unite with the right and left lateral ligaments of that organ. Luschka, who holds this view, says, however, that in many cases a tubular elongation of the mucous membrane of the bladder may be found, the commencement of which is indicated by a minute opening passing from the cavity of the bladder; but that generally, in place of this opening, only a depression is to be seen, and even this is often absent and thus all trace of tubular communication is lost.

Rokitansky says, "The urachus may remain patent to a certain distance from the bladder, or throughout its entire extent."

Cruveilhier, following Boyer, states that in urachal fistula the urethra is always obliterated; and Boyer goes on to remark that the fistula ceases to exist as soon as the obstruction at the neck of the bladder is removed, so that the urine can flow by the urethra. That these distinguished anatomists were wrong in this opinion some of the cases on record conclusively prove: thus Lannelongue (*Sem. Med.*, Aug. 21, 1895) reports the post-mortem of a child three months old, who died of broncho-pneumonia. The infant micturated at the umbilicus through a slit-like opening on a hernial protrusion of the urachus which resembled a penis; and at the same time through the penis, which was quite natural. It was found that the bladder was continuous with a patent urachus right up to the umbilicus by a channel as large as the fore-finger.

Boyer was further of opinion that many of the cases supposed to be urachal fistulæ were really herniary protrusions of the mucous membrane of the bladder through the rest of its coats, near the point of connection of the urachal ligament, and caused by some urethral obstruction; and that this herniary protrusion extended as far as the umbilicus, and subsequently ruptured. He, however, records no case in favour of his hypothesis, though the perusal of Mr. Thomas Paget's description inclines me to think that there may be instances which support it. In Mr. Paget's patient the umbilical orifice of the fistula measured three inches by two inches; through it a hernial protrusion, the size of a goose's egg, had occurred, and along this the surgeon's fingers could be passed right into the bladder. Though the man had no difficulty in voiding urine, and though a catheter could easily be passed when he was under Mr. Paget's care, it is quite possible that some obstruction had existed in early life before the fistula had formed. I have made a dissection in one case, and reported another, in which there was extreme saccular dilatation of the kidneys, ureters, and bladder, in a fœtus; and where the only cause of obstruction found was a thin membranous septum, easily broken down with a small catheter, in the membranous part of the urethra. A less complete septum might, perhaps, give rise to the umbilicovesical hernia described by Boyer, and, from the ease with which it yields to an instrument passed along the urethra, such a septum might altogether escape detection. Agnew has briefly mentioned a case seen by him, which, in the absence of proof to the contrary, is capable of being explained on Boyer's theory. It was that of a child, who had no fistulous opening at the umbilicus; but when urine was allowed to accumulate in the bladder, the navel became distended.

The *character of the orifice* is not the same in all urachal fistulæ:—

1. In some, a peculiar button-like papillary or columnar projection at the umbilicus, having an orifice at its summit, has been described. Mr. Bryant mentions a case in which the

projecting mass was about the size of, and not unlike, the glans penis. The orifice was constantly moist, but especially so when the bladder was distended. The boy was eight years old, and the condition was congenital. It was regarded as a case of open urachus. Mr. T. Smith gives a brief note of a case very similar to Mr. Bryant's. The boy was two years old, and had a button-like protrusion at the umbilicus which was constantly moist, and the discharge, though slight, had the odour of urine.

2. The urine may escape at several points on the surface of a hernial protrusion, as in the case described in the *Medicinische Zeitung*, No. 19, 1837. An infant, aged four weeks, had a urachal fistula discharging urine copiously through several points on the excoriated surface of a hernial swelling, which projected three-quarters of an inch. The excoriated area was one-quarter of an inch long and one line broad. The urine was normally discharged by the urethra.

3. The orifice may be a mere deficiency—circular, oval, or irregular—in the linea alba. In the adult male patient under the care of Mr. Paget. of Leicester, it was circular, with a thick margin of cartilaginous hardness.

4. It may be situated in the cup-like depression of the navel, or hidden from view by the falling together of the skin of the umbilicus. In a second case described by Mr. Paget, that of a female child aged four months, the orifice was thus hidden, but on drawing aside the folds of skin, urine always escaped; the lining membrane of the tube was cuticular for a short distance, and then became mucous membrane; the orifice was large enough to receive an ordinary cedar pencil.

5. There may be, as already mentioned, a hernial protrusion at the umbilicus; the external covering of such a hernia, instead of being skin, is mucous membrane, which, however, becomes pale and dry after prolonged exposure. In these cases the fistulous orifice is at the side, or on the summit, of the hernia. In some cases the hernial protrusion acts like a plug to prevent the continual escape of urine, but is withdrawn during the act of micturition by the pull of the vesical muscular fibres, and thereupon urine is ejected at the fistula, as well as along the urethra. This was the condition in Mr. Paget's adult patient; the first contraction of the bladder

had no other effect than to draw into the abdomen the whole of the protruding parts, and until this was accomplished no urine passed by the urethra. The jet of urine from the umbilicus which then followed was sudden, and quickly ceased, not to be renewed except by a violent accelerating action of the expulsor muscles. The bladder would retain a pint of urine without any escaping; and it seems to me that this case sheds light on the capacity for retaining urine, and for passing it naturally, which has been possessed by several patients after rupture of the bladder.

6. The fistula may be indirect. It will probably be so when an abscess precedes it, as in the case reported by the late Sir William (then Mr.) Savory. This patient was a male child aged thirteen months, in whom an abscess, which had been forming for eight weeks, pointed, and was opened at the umbilicus. The symptoms were pains in the lower part of the abdomen and frequent desire to micturate. Vesical calculus was suspected. Subsequently there was a discharge of pus, and of nearly all the urine through the umbilical fistula. The child died nine days after the abscess was opened. At the autopsy it was discovered that a polypus of the bladder had led to obstruction at the orifice of the urethra, and this to dilatation and suppuration of the ureters and kidneys. A small papilla on the upper part of the vesical wall represented the unobliterated urachus, but a probe could not be passed from the urachus into the bladder. Sir Wm. Savory surmised that a valvular communication with the bladder had existed, and that the urine, having been propelled into the urachus, had set up suppuration around, so that by degrees the urachus had been destroyed, and an abscess cavity formed between the peritoneum and the rest of the abdominal parietes. The abscess extended in the course of the urachus from the bladder to the umbilicus. Though no opening could be detected after death between the bladder and abscess, or urachus and abscess, there is the fact that during life, for some days, nearly all the urine passed through the umbilical fistula, and the fair inference is that the urachus had communicated with the abscess cavity.

Urachal fistulæ may be either **congenital** or **non-congenital**.

Congenital Urachal Fistula may commence as soon as

the umbilical cord separates; it may or may not be associated with dilatation of the ureters and kidneys, or with urethral obstruction and hypertrophy of the bladder; and the urachus may subsequently be shut off from the bladder, and then a urinary may be converted into a pus-secreting, fistulous tract, as in the case of the infant referred to and illustrated on pages 162 and 163. In this instance the urachus remained very large and patulous, and, as soon as the umbilical cord sloughed away, urine alone, then urine mixed with pus, and subsequently pus alone, escaped at the umbilical extremity of the urachus. In this case the penis was bent laterally and twisted half a turn round its own axis, and it was, no doubt, due to the obstruction thus caused that the bladder was hypertrophied and contracted, and the urachus, ureters, and kidneys were dilated and sacculated. The child lived from November 30th to March 2nd, and nephrotomy was performed in each loin twenty-two hours after birth. It was thought that no urine had been passed by the urethra prior to the operation, but afterwards, on a few occasions, two or three ounces were voided at a time *per vias naturales.* The bulk of the urine was discharged through the fistulæ established in the loins, but for many days a good deal of urine escaped along the urachus and through its umbilical opening; this subsequently ceased, and at the post-mortem the urachus was abruptly shut off from the cavity of the bladder and was full of creamy pus.

Non-Congenital Fistula.—When an abscess precedes the fistula, as in Sir Wm. Savory's case, and in some cases where there has not been an abscess, the fistula is not congenital, though in all instances the defect which makes it a possibility, and which indeed predisposes to it—namely, the non-obliteration of the urachal tube—is, of course, congenital. Dr. Francis Cadell has reported the case of a girl aged eight, who from earliest infancy had had difficulty in micturition, with frequent desire to pass water. From four years of age the symptoms of cystitis had increased, and when she was eight years old, after a few days of great pain, with swelling and hardness of the belly, urine was observed to come in a small stream from the navel. A No. 6 catheter could be passed through the fistula into the bladder. The child died four months afterwards from cystitis, with sacculated and suppurating ureters and kidneys. At the autopsy the umbilicus was found to be natural, save for the fistulous opening, which presented neither fungating granulations nor induration about its margins. The bladder was contracted and thickened, and the little finger could be passed from it into the unobliterated urachus, which gradually narrowed towards the navel. In this case the urachus must have been in part patent from birth, and having become gradually dilated, subsequently gave way altogether, and an urinary fistula was thus established.

Mode of Origin of Non-congenital Fistula.—When the lower end of the urachus remains open, some of the urine is forced into it at each act of micturition, and especially at the commencement of the act, as was shown by Paget's case. If the bladder becomes after a time the seat of inflammation, the difficulty and straining in micturition will increase the dilatation of the urachus, as it does that of the ureters and pelves of the kidneys. Again, if, as Luschka seems to indicate, the vesical orifice of the urachus becomes very minute, or even closes, we see how the tube of the urachus may be converted into a shut sac; and then if any urine or mucus is enclosed within it, inflammation and abscess will be caused, and the abscess may either burst spontaneously, or be opened by the surgeon, at the umbilicus, where it will point. In either of these ways a non-congenital fistula may be formed, quite independently, as it would seem, of any mechanical obstruction at the neck of the bladder or in the urethra.

In Dr. Cadell's case the fistula was direct, complete, and unassociated with any abscess, but it was non-congenital and urinary. When an abscess occurs after the obliteration of the vesical end of the urachus, and opens at the umbilicus, the resulting fistula is non-congenital, and will or will not discharge urine, according as it does or does not subsequently communicate again with the bladder.

Complications of Urachal Fistula.—Some of the complications are causes, others are results, and others again merely coincidences. Of the first set, there are polypus of the bladder, urethral calculus, phimosis, congenital stricture, and everything which prevents the free discharge of urine along the natural passage. That these act only partially as causes is clear, as there must be also a patent state of the urachus to admit of a true urachal fistula. When this patency does not exist, the bladder, ureters, and kidneys may all become sacculated, without any alteration of the urachus. This is proved by cases of congenital hydronephrosis.

A remarkable complication or result of fistula was witnessed in Paget's adult patient: a ring calculus was formed by the deposit of uric acid on a small hair from the pubes which had found its way into the bladder through the umbilical opening. Cruveilhier also met with a calculous concretion within the urachus, and he goes on to remark that Huller and Harder have made similar observations. Boyer says that in 1787 he dissected the bladder of a man aged twenty-six, whose urachus formed a canal an inch and a half long, and contained twelve urinary calculi as large as millet seeds, one being larger and resembling a grain of barley. Though a fistula did not exist in this case, the calculi were a very sufficient exciting cause of abscess or ulceration, either of which might easily have resulted in a fistula. Luschka has suggested that the cells of the lining mucous membrane of the urachus may occasionally be developed into cysts and need surgical interference; he does not, however, record any case of the sort.

Prognosis.—When the fistula is congenital and caused by some obstruction to the outflow of the urine, the prognosis is . unfavourable, as death from renal disease is likely to result, unless the cause of the obstruction can be removed, like phimosis or a urethral calculus. When the fistula is non-congenital, and follows cystitis or abscess, the health of the patient will have been greatly destroyed, in all probability, before the fistula is established, and death will occur subsequently from exhaustion, cystitis, or pyelo-nephritis. In cases of simple patency of the urachus without urethral obstruction, there is no reason why life should be interfered with, though the comfort of the individual necessarily is so.

Treatment.—There are two clear indications—namely: (1) to remove any source of obstruction to the natural discharge of urine, and (2) to close the fistula when there is nothing (like suppuration or obstruction) to require it to be kept open. When phimosis exists circumcision should be performed, as in a case recorded by Dr. J. J. Charles, of Belfast. When a calculus is present it must be, of course, removed. If cystitis is a complication, irrigation of the bladder or drainage by means of dilatation of the urethra in the female, and median external urethrotomy in the male, may effect a cure of the fistula.

With a view to closing the umbilical orifice of the fistula, different methods have been tried, and each may succeed, though all may fail. If the opening is a vent for pus, or for urine which cannot, or can only with difficulty, pass through the urethra, no attempt at closure ought to be made. When the opening is upon a papillary outgrowth, it is sometimes sufficient to apply a ligature around the base of the papilla which in a few days will then dry up and fall off, and the fistula be permanently closed. In some cases the application of nitric acid, or of the actual, or galvanic, or Pacquelin's cautery to the edges of the fistula has been followed by healthy granulations and cicatrisation. In other cases, again, the plan of dissecting off the skin around the opening, and bringing the raw surfaces together with hare-lip pins, as was so successfully done by Mr. Paget in his two cases, should certainly be tried. In Mr. Paget's first case, the operation was performed when the patient was fifty-five years of age.

CYSTS OF THE URACHUS.

Besides the permanently tubular condition of the vesical end of the urachus, to which attention has been drawn above under the heading of urachal fistula, pouches or cyst-like dilatations of the urachus are sometimes found in the abdominal wall, or at the umbilicus. These cysts are the results of the imperfection of the embryonic changes which should entirely obliterate the tube of the urachus. They are situated in the cellular tissue immediately outside the parietal peritoneum, and though often small, they may attain such a size as to simulate ovarian cystic disease. Their contents vary, being either mucus or mucus and epithelium, or urine, or pus; their growth is slow and painless; and they may be either single or multiple. The cyst wall is composed of a mixture of fibrous and non-striated muscle tissue, covered with cells like those lining the interior of the bladder and the allantois.

In certain cases the urachus remains patent throughout its length between the urinary bladder and the umbilical cyst, which is thus subject to intermittent enlargement by propulsion of urine into it when the bladder contracts in micturition. One instance at least has been reported in which there were three immense cystic dilatations. When situated at the umbilicus they may be mistaken for umbilical hernia; but the soft, elastic, and perhaps fluctuating feel—possibly the translucency—and certainly the history and irreducibility of the swelling, will assist to a right diagnosis.

Small cysts of the urachus, either single or in a string of three or four, are occasionally met with when dividing the abdominal wall in laparotomy; and Mr. Lawson Tait has related twelve cases of large extra-peritoneal cysts which he believes to have been urachal, and which in some respects closely resembled in their clinical characters ovarian or parovarian tumours. These large cysts were situated between the transversalis fascia and the thickened peritoneum; a large quantity of thick brown, purulent fluid, mixed with large masses of fibrinous deposit, was contained within them. In one case the cyst had been tapped, and ten pints of this fluid had been drawn off; subsequently thirty pints were withdrawn from it, and the cyst was removed in its entirety. The intestines and pelvic organs were non-adherent and apparently healthy, and could be felt through the exposed but unopened peritoneal membrane. The inner surface of the cyst was formed by broken-down mucoid epithelium, infiltrated everywhere with pus, and lying upon a basement-membrane of muscular fibre. The tumour, though entirely extra-peritoneal, dipped into the pelvis on the right of the median line. In a second case the cyst was gangrenous. Both patients succumbed to the operation. It is a remarkable thing, if the theory of their urachal origin is correct, that these cysts remained so many years in abeyance, and then suddenly developed to such an enormous size.

Treatment.—The fatal results point out the risk there is in excising large extra-peritoneal tumours from the abdominal parietes. The vitality of the exposed and disturbed peritoneum is likely to be destroyed, and therefore incision and drainage would seem the better practice and certainly has been the most successful. If excision is resorted to, it would be best to remove a large portion of the denuded peritoneum and bring the edges together with buried sutures, or to fill the gap with a plug of omentum.

INDEX TO AUTHORS.

E E

INDEX.

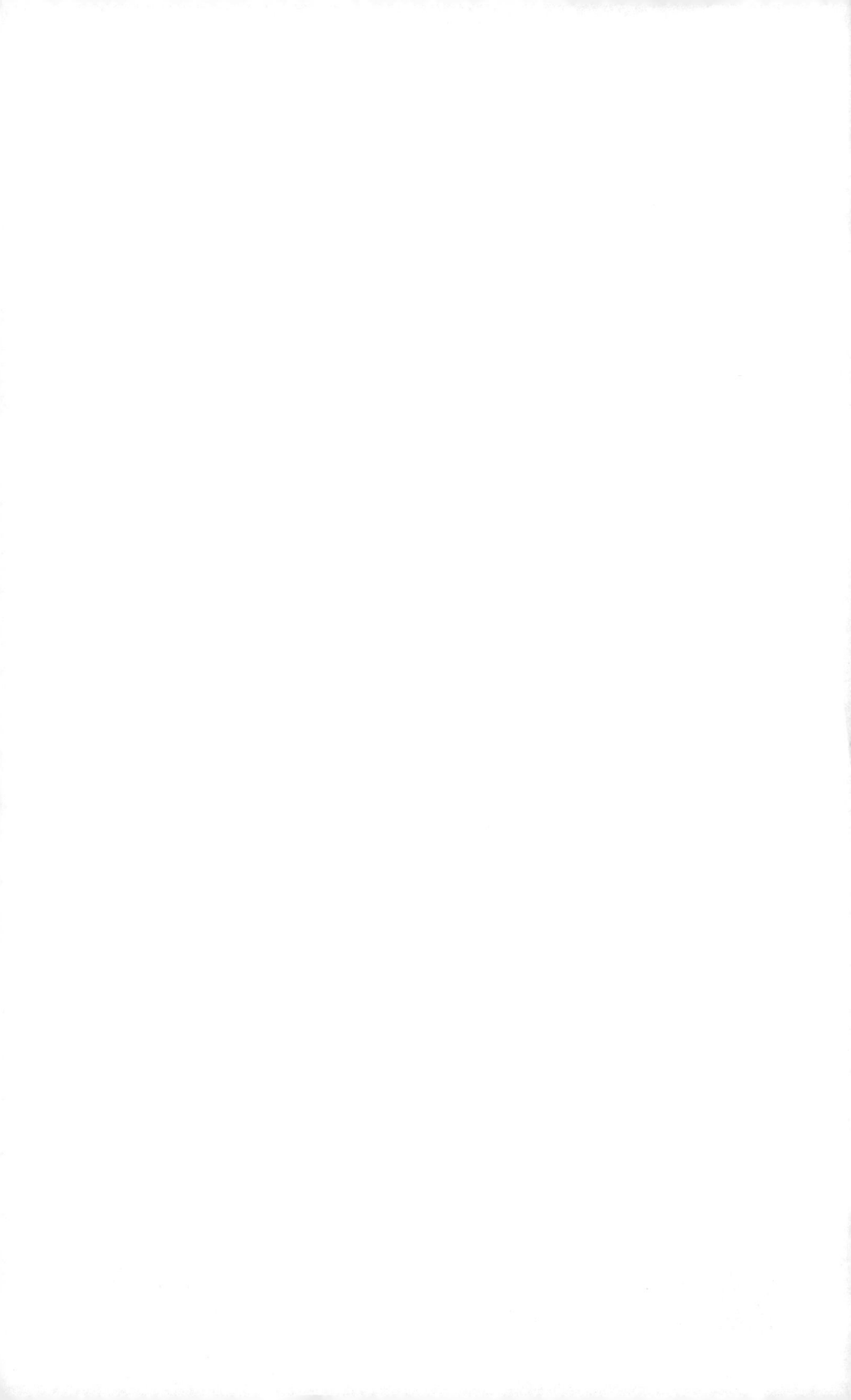

Lightning Source UK Ltd.
Milton Keynes UK
UKHW020159260219
337978UK00012B/1351/P